critical social work

critical social work

theories and practices for a socially just world
second edition

edited by
june allan
linda briskman
bob pease

Routledge
Taylor & Francis Group
LONDON AND NEW YORK

First published 2009 by Allen & Unwin

Published 2020 by Routledge
2 Park Square, Milton Park, Abingdon, Oxon OX14 4RN
605 Third Avenue, New York, NY 10017

Routledge is an imprint of the Taylor & Francis Group, an informa business

Cataloguing-in-Publication details are available
from the National Library of Australia
www.librariesaustralia.nla.gov.au

Index by Jo Rudd

Set in 11/14 pt Minion by Midland Typesetters, Australia

ISBN-13: 9781742370927 (pbk)

contents

preface

Six years after we edited the f rst edition of the book, the purposes of a second edition remain substantially unchanged. At the time of compiling the f rst edition, all three editors were employed at RMIT University. Linda Briskman and Bob Pease are now based at Curtin and Deakin Universities respectively, while June Allan remains at RMIT. The impetus for the f rst edition of the book arose from ongoing efforts by social work staff at RMIT to develop a critical curriculum in social work education at that university. The origins of those endeavours dated back to the early 1980s when the then School of Social Work at Phillip Institute of Technology adopted structural (Moreau 1979), developmental (Benn 1981) and feminist approaches to social work practice. Although there were changes to the educational philosophy of RMIT's social work curriculum over the years, the core value commitments remained in place and the f rst book aff rmed the basic premise that a central goal of social work practice is social change in order to redress social inequalities and injustice.

Staff in social work courses at other Australian universities increasingly articulate critical social work approaches in their curriculum and research priorities. Furthermore, other Australian and international writers have produced critical texts in social work over the last six years that have inf uenced curriculum content in social work courses. In acknowledging the increasing scholarship in critical social work, this new edition incorporates new writings and approaches, particularly in the light of an increasingly complex socio-political context that besets social work.

Several of the chapters in this new edition have been updated by contributors to the f rst edition of the book. In addition, we have invited a number of new writers, including early career researchers and doctoral students, who are at the cutting edge of critical social work scholarship.

Our dear friend and colleague Wendy Weeks, who wrote a chapter in the f rst edition of this book on feminist practice in women's services, died in 2004. We take the opportunity here to acknowledge and honour the deep and lasting contribution that Wendy made to critical social work through her feminist-inspired scholarship and activism.

The development of critical social work courses in Australian universities is an ongoing process and remains a struggle in the light of conf icting interpretations about the purposes of social work, the diversity of social work theories and competing pressures on the curriculum. This book is offered as a constructive approach to address the prospects and limitations of critical theories and practices in social work.

We hope that the book will resonate with the many social work educators who struggle with the various tensions and contradictions that we analyse. The f rst edition of the book was intended as an introduction to critical social work for students and human services practitioners. While this second edition does not require previous knowledge of critical social work, we have endeavoured to move the debates forward and to avoid the sometimes polarised discussions about structure versus agency that have plagued social work's transformative project. We hope that those inspired by the critical tradition in social work will f nd much in this book to sustain their critical hope and to inform their progressive practice.

contributors

June Allan holds a PhD from La Trobe University, Melbourne, and is Senior Lecturer in Social Work at RMIT University, Melbourne, where she teaches in the MSW and BSW programs. Her current teaching and research interests include group work, loss trauma and grief, cross-cultural work and critical social work perspectives. Over the last several years June has complemented her teaching at RMIT through working in the bereavement sector and as a counsellor/advocate with refugees and asylum seekers. She holds a Specialist Graduate Certif cate in Bereavement Counselling Practice and is on the Committee of Management of the Australian Centre for Grief and Bereavement. She was a member of the International Scientif c Committee for the Eighth International Conference on Grief and Bereavement in Contemporary Society held in 2008. June co-edited the f rst edition of *Critical Social Work: An introduction to theories and practices* (Allen & Unwin 2003).

Uschi Bay is a lecturer in Social Work at Deakin University, Geelong. Prior to working at Deakin University, Uschi was a member of an academic team that set up undergraduate and Master's programs at the Coffs Harbour campus of Southern Cross University. Recently, Uschi was part of a Desert Knowledge Cooperative Research Centre team using a community-based research approach to research the sustainability of desert settlements. She holds a PhD from RMIT University on the politics of empowerment in critical social work. Her social work practice experience includes direct client work as well as equity policy development and implementation. Currently, her teaching is in the areas of community development, anti-oppressive and empowerment social work practice and a critical social work unit that introduces students to critical ref exivity using contemporary social and political theories.

Barbara Black has a wealth of experience working with older people in many different capacities. She worked as a carer in residential aged care while completing her social work degree and conducted her honours research into the area of retired people who volunteer. After graduation, Barbara worked as an aged care advocate for a number of years before deciding to return to study. Her PhD research examined the human rights experiences of people in residential aged care. Barbara has recently been working as the Executive Off cer of the Alliance for the Prevention of Elder Abuse: Western Australia, developing policy and research in the area of elder abuse.

Jacques Boulet has lived, studied and worked in f ve continents, obtaining a social work undergraduate degree in 1965 in Leuven, Belgium. He worked for three years in a major community development project in Africa, did a postgraduate diploma in community development and social planning at the Institute for Social Studies in Holland and subsequently was a curriculum developer in social work education programs in Germany throughout the seventies. He completed his MSW and PhD (in social work and in sociology) between 1980 and 1985 at the University of Michigan, USA. He became Senior Lecturer and Associate Professor at Melbourne University and RMIT between 1985 and 1996, leaving academia in 1997 to become involved in the Borderlands Cooperative, a community learning and action centre in Hawthorn, Melbourne. He is Head of School of *oases*, an accredited program in integrative and transformative studies.

Linda Briskman holds the Dr Haruhisa Handa Chair in Human Rights Education at Curtin University, Perth. Her social work practice, policy and research interests are in the areas of Indigenous rights and asylum seeker rights and she has published extensively in both areas. Recent publications include *Social Work with Indigenous Peoples* (Federation Press 2007) and *Human Rights Overboard: Seeking asylum in Australia* with Susie Latham and Chris Goddard (Scribe 2008), which received the 2008 Australian Human Rights Commission award for literature (non-f ction). Linda was a co-editor the f rst edition of *Critical Social Work: An introduction to theories and practices* (Allen & Unwin 2003).

Susan Costello is a social work practitioner who has worked with families from diverse backgrounds in child protection, family support, disability, psychiatry, family therapy, health and institutional settings. As program coordinator of family resource and community support programs, her roles included direct practice, group work facilitator, staff development and supervision. She is a Clinical Member of the Victorian Association of Family Therapists. She now teaches the core practice courses in the

RMIT University's undergraduate and postgraduate social work degrees. She has a PhD from RMIT. Susan's publication and research interests include critiques of behaviour change groups for men who use violence against women, Indigenous homelessness, practitioner supervision and consultation, cross-cultural education and international social work in Thailand and Burma. Susan maintains a small private practice.

Christine Craik has spent the last two decades as a social worker supporting women and children who are affected by violence and abuse. She has done this in many roles, including counselling and support of victims of violence, advocacy, group work with survivors of sexual abuse, community work and leadership of programs. She is now a Lecturer in Social Work at RMIT University, where she has developed a very successful subject called 'Working with Violence and Abuse'. Christine's research has focused mainly on gender-related issues, such as access to university for girls from government schools, and the body image of young women, particularly in relation to plastic surgery and the normalisation of sexual standards. Christine is active in wildlife rescue, social justice campaigns and the community life of her local village.

Heather D'Cruz is Senior Lecturer in Social Work, Deakin University, Victoria. Her research interests include child and family policy and practice; child protection; identity, diversity, inclusivity/exclusivity; and critical discourse analysis. She has a PhD from Lancaster University, UK. She is the author of *Constructing Meanings and Identities in Child Protection Practice* (Tertiary Press 2004), and (with Martyn Jones) *Social Work Research: Ethical and political contexts* (Sage 2004). She is an International Diversity Community Online Conversations Facilitator and a member of the International Advisory Board, for Common Ground Publishers. Her current research projects include Reconstructing Child Welfare through Participatory and Child-Centred Professional Practice (with Karen Stagnitti), and Silenced Voices: Perspectives of Parents and Children involved in Child Protection Services (with Philip Gillingham). She was an Invited Visiting Leverhulme Fellow at the University of Salford, UK, from November 2007 to July 2008.

Christine Fejo-King is an Aboriginal woman from the Northern Territory. Her mother is a Warumungu woman from the Tennant Creek area and her father was a Larrakia man from the Darwin area. Her social work practice spans a wide variety of experiences. Christine is currently employed by Reconciliation Australia, an agency working with Reconciliation Action Plans for all government, schools, peak bodies and State and Territory Reconciliation Councils. She is Chairperson of the National Coalition of Aboriginal and Torres Strait Islander Social Workers Association. Christine was heavily involved in the background work for the recent Apology to the Stolen Generations as the then Indigenous Chairperson. She is currently in the process of completing a PhD through the Australian Catholic University on the topic of 'The Aboriginal Kinship System: Informing Social work theory and practice in Australia'.

Heather Fraser is Senior Lecturer in Social Work at RMIT University, Melbourne. Heather is interested in all forms of inequality, disadvantage and oppression, especially those related to gender, class, sexuality and race. Identifying as a feminist, she has longstanding aff liations with women's services in Melbourne, especially those related to sexual assault and domestic violence and has recently published a book called *In the Name of Love: Women's narratives of love and abuse* (Women's Press 2008).

Nick Halfpenny has experience working in remote Aboriginal health, education, research and practice and service development. For the past four years, Nick has worked as Coordinator of Practice Development with MacKillop Family Services, a child and family welfare organisation in Victoria. Nick is undertaking a PhD at Curtin University exploring how to interpret what motivates or informs the practice of human service workers to examine how to understand practice and the inf uences that can lead to change.

Kelley Johnson is currently Professor of Disability: Policy and Practice and Director of the Norah Fry Research Centre, University of Bristol, UK. She has been a researcher and advocate with disabled people for the past f fteen years in Australia and overseas. This research has included a focus on deinstitutionalisation, inclusion of disabled people in community life, women's life issues and inclusive research.

Selma Macfarlane is a lecturer in social work at Deakin University, Geelong. Her interests include diversity and inequality, mental health, and the development of critical social work practice. Her PhD thesis was entitled 'Support and Recovery in a Therapeutic Community'.

Catherine McDonald is Professor of Social Work in the School of Global Studies, Social Science and Planning at RMIT University, Melbourne. Her research interests and publication areas are the non-prof t sector and the mixed economy of welfare, the functioning of service delivery systems, welfare to workfare, the impact of social policy on vulnerable and disadvantaged people, the role of social theory in social policy and the future of social work. Her current research projects are on the functioning of the Job Network, urban inequality, gender and care work in the community services. She has a practice background in social policy, and has a longstanding involvement in policy activism.

Philip Mendes is Senior Lecturer in the Department of Social Work, Faculty of Medicine, Monash University. He teaches the three social policy and community development subjects, and is also coordinator for the on-campus undergraduate Bachelor of Social Work. He has published widely in peer-reviewed academic journals (over 80 publications in total), and is the author or co-author of six books, including *Harm Minimisation, Zero Tolerance and Beyond: The politics of illicit drugs in Australia* (Pearson 2004), *Inside the Welfare Lobby: A history of the Australian Council of Social Service (ACOSS)* (Sussex Academic Press 2006), and *Australia's Welfare Wars Revisited* (UNSW Press 2008). He completed his PhD on the peak community welfare lobby body, the Australian Council of Social Service.

Christine Morley currently works as Senior Lecturer in Social Work, University of the Sunshine Coast, Queensland. She has been a social work practitioner and academic for the past ten years. Her practice experience has predominantly been in the f elds of grief and loss, and sexual assault. Her main teaching and research passions include critical social work, anti-oppressive theory and practice, and critical ref ection, and she has published widely in these areas.

Sharlene Nipperess has worked as a social work practitioner and educator in Queensland, Western Australia and, most recently, Victoria. As a practitioner she has considerable experience working with refugees and asylum seekers, people who experience mental health issues and Indigenous Australians. She is also interested in rural, regional and remote social work and environmental issues. As an educator she has taught a wide range of subjects but her particular interests lie in social work theory, specif cally human rights and critical social work and its relationship with practice. Sharlene is currently completing her PhD through the Centre for Human Rights Education at Curtin University, Western Australia, which brings together her experiences as a social work practitioner and educator and her interest in and commitment to human rights more broadly.

Bob Pease is Chair of Social Work at Deakin University, Geelong. He has research interests in men's violence against women, cross-cultural and global perspectives on men and masculinities and profeminist approaches to working with men in the human services. His publications include *Recreating Men: Postmodern masculinity politics* (Sage 2000), *Working with Men in the Human Services* (co-editor: Allen & Unwin 2001), *A Man's World? Changing men's practices in a globalized world* (co-editor: Zed Books 2001), *Men and Gender Relations* (Tertiary Press 2002), *Critical Social Work: An introduction to theories and practices*, 1st edition (co-editor: Allen & Unwin 2003) and *International Encyclopedia of Men and Masculinities* (co-editor: Routledge 2007). He is currently co-editing a book titled *Migrant Men: Critical studies of masculinities and the migration experience* (Routledge, forthcoming) and writing a book titled *Undoing Privilege* (Zed Books, forthcoming).

Marjorie Quinn is a Senior Lecturer in Social Work at RMIT University, Melbourne. Her current teaching and research interests are in the areas of community development in the contemporary context, anti-racist and cross-cultural social work, community development in cross-cultural and international contexts and in the complexities and challenges for critical theory approaches to social and community work. She coordinates the RMIT study tour to Bangladesh. Marjorie has extensive practice experience as social worker, community worker and manager, especially in Broadmeadows (City of Hume) and most recently in Zambia. She is co-editor of *Issues Facing Australian Families*, 3rd edition (Pearson Education 2000).

PART I

introduction

1

introducing critical theories for social work in a neo-liberal context

Linda Briskman, Bob Pease and June Allan

When we were in the process of writing the f rst edition of this book and discussing the project with academic colleagues and practitioners, we were sometimes asked: Is there still a need to articulate a 'critical' social work? Is not all social work 'critical' in the sense of being committed to social as well as individual transformation? Some contemporary social work writers at the time believed that to be so. Ife (1997), for example, argued that 'social work is, by its very nature radical' (1997: 178) and he stressed the importance of bringing radical social work in from the margins of the profession. He argued that the task was to 'conceptualise social work in such a way that its inherent radicalism is recognised and incorporated into "mainstream" understandings of social work practice' (1997: 178). Alston and McKinnon (2001) have argued similarly that professional social work is concerned with human rights, social justice and support for marginalised people. We still believe, however, that the notion of a social work as a 'radical profession' is as elusive now as it was when Rein (1970) wrote about this possibility almost 40 years ago. This issue is even more crucial six years on from the f rst edition, as critical social work has, regrettably, not made a signif cant impact on mainstream social work and there is still reticence by many organisations in which social workers are employed to engage with critical and emancipatory frameworks.

Given the context in which social work is practised, this elusiveness is not surprising, for Australia is aligned with global trends—particularly in Western nations, which focus on valuing the individual over the collective and pursuing economic gain at the expense of community and social development. Alongside this prevails a fear of 'difference' that contributes to the failure of reform in areas of fundamental importance to social work—f elds as diverse as immigration, disability and criminal justice. Such factors, which may contravene social work's core values, should ideally point to a social work of resistance and challenge. However, the contextual and political trends can serve to limit social work's critical engagement and in this book we hope to encourage social workers to contemplate that their own practice might be strengthened by critical social work frameworks.

For these reasons, and for others that will become apparent throughout this book, we continue to stress that it is still important to name and promote critical perspectives in social work. Most of these perspectives are informed by some form of critical theory, including Ife's (1997) 'critical practice', Pease and Fook's (1999b) 'postmodern critical perspectives', Thompson's (2006) 'anti-discriminatory practice', Baines' (2007a) 'anti-oppressive practice', Mullaly's (2007) 'structural social work' and Ferguson's (2008) radical social work. Feminist, anti-racist, postcolonial and human rights perspectives in social work are also informed by revised versions of critical theory. Thus, it is important to set the scene by examining some of the key debates within critical theory and by exploring some of the criticisms that have been levelled at it.

Critical theory as a foundation for critical social work practice

It should be stated at the outset that the term 'critical theory' does not designate a unif ed theoretical perspective. It is a term that embraces a variety of different theoretical positions (Alway 1995; Cheek et al. 1996). On a narrow level, it is a school of Western Marxism known as the 'Frankfurt School', encompassing the writings of Herbert Marcuse, Jürgen Habermas, Theodor Adorno, Erich Fromm and Max Horkheimer. These writers attempted to integrate elements of Marxism with an understanding of subjectivity. At a broader level, critical theory has involved a variety of analyses which have endeavoured to link the concern with subjectivity, with the structural focus on the social and political context of people's lives (Thompson 2000). From the point of view of critical theorists, contemporary Marxists neglected the impact of dominant ideologies upon people's consciousness. Unlike structuralist Marxists, who spoke about the inevitability of the structural contradictions of capitalism in bringing about transformation, critical theorists stressed the importance of people's agency—that is, their capacity to be actively involved in the process of social change (Alway 1995).

Most critical theorists are concerned with emancipatory education that enables people to see the links between their experiences and the material conditions and dominant ideologies in society. In this regard, over twenty years ago Fay (1987) emphasised the capacity of critical theories to explain the sources of oppression in society in such a way as to encourage those affected by oppression to take action to transform it. In the words of Alvesson and Willmott (1996: 13): 'The intent of critical theory is to challenge the legitimacy and counter the development of oppressive institutions and practices.' Critical theory thus places a signif cant emphasis on ref ecting upon how dominant ideologies or ways of thinking, as well as societal institutions, impact on people's lives. Critical theory also questions the place of existing institutions, such as the family, educational establishments and governance, with a view to constructing a more just society.

Critical theory has not been without its critics. Some have argued that critical theory in general, and the Frankfurt School in particular, failed in its attempt to link individual and social consciousness with institutional analysis and political economy (Held 1980). Others suggest that critical theory 'exaggerates the importance of consciousness in the processes of radical social change' (Alvesson & Willmott 1996: 86). Feminist writers also note that critical theory has not adequately engaged with feminist theory and subsequently has been unable to appreciate the signif cance of gender analysis (Cheek et al. 1996; Alvesson & Willmott 1996).[1] Further, Alway (1995: 73) argues that, rather than imposing a particular claim or interpretation, emancipatory politics should be 'expanding the opportunity for groups to determine and live according to their own claims and interpretations'. This development is consistent with some forms of postmodern thinking.

Influences of postmodernism on critical theory

A number of writers have commented that postmodernism shares many of the concerns of critical theory (Cheek et al. 1996). Just as the origins of critical theory came out of a project to reappraise and reconstruct Marxist theory in light of changed historical conditions, so critical theory itself may now need to be reappraised for the same reasons. The vision of emancipatory politics in critical theory has thus been rethought by many critical theorists in light of postmodernism (Yeatman 1994; Nicholson & Seidman 1995). A more detailed analysis of the rise of postmodernity is provided in our 2003 edition, but for the purposes of the current text we provide a brief overview of the contest that postmodernism poses to enlightenment thinking and some of the key tenets of postmodernism, as these ideas are implicitly and explicitly woven into the chapters that follow.

Just as modernity implies a departure from earlier ways of thinking about the world that incorporated superstition, paganism and traditional forms of authority associated with religion and feudalism, postmodernity has emerged as a break from modernity. The notion of modernity is usually associated with the Enlightenment project, which has sought to replace fear and superstition with consent and truth, and the establishment of a social order based on reason and natural law (Macey 2000). Distinguishing features of the age of modernity are the understanding of history as having a def nite and progressive direction; the idea that reason can provide a basis for all activities; the attempt to develop universal categories of experience; and the creation of order, boundaries, classif cations and certainties through formal reason, laws, typologies, uniformity and universality. Importance is placed on the objectivity of knowledge, the universality of values and the progress of science and society, and truth is centred in human reason (Seidman 1994; Parton & O'Byrne 2000a). Modernity's 'grand narrative' (the form of knowledge seen as legitimate) is emancipation of all people and production of a universal knowledge that speaks for all.

This fundamental belief in the value of scientif c knowledge in the human sciences as a means of public enlightenment and social progress of modernity has been debated and challenged by thinkers as diverse as Jürgen Habermas and Michel Foucault. Scepticism has emerged about the Enlightenment's promise that humanity will be or can be emancipated by rational knowledge. Such scepticism is 'one of the hallmarks of the age of postmodernity' (Macey 2000: 111).

For the purpose of the current book, we understand postmodernism to refer to a cultural phenomenon in contemporary society characterised by fragmentation brought about by an explosion of information and new technologies, consumer capitalism with its proliferation of products and images, political shifts and upheavals, and new experiences of space and time (Best & Kellner 1991; Bordo 1993). Key elements of this social transformation include the growing signif cance of difference, plurality and the developing awareness of the social construction of 'reality'.

Postmodernism emphasises attention to difference rather than sameness, awareness of the importance of language and the part played by discourses in the construction of social reality, as well as recognition that power is operating in many ways, creating opportunities for the individual to resist and to be other than a victim of 'an oppressive and monolithic social order' (Leonard 1984: 5).

Along with O'Brien and Penna (1998a: 53), we reject the view that 'one true theory will overturn the system of false ideas and lead to the elimination of exploitation, oppression, and domination'. If, as Pozzuto (2000) suggests, no singular answer to the question of what is critical social work is necessary or even possible, it may be more appropriate to follow Hekman's (1999: 22) exhortation to develop 'an epistemology of truths rather than the Truth. This will enable us to avoid both a new form of universalism and 'an "anything goes" relativism.' Leonard (1997) refers to these multiple critical views as 'radical pluralism'. Such perspectives would draw upon Marxism, critical theory—modernist and postmodern—along with feminism, postcolonialism and anti-racism among others. We encourage linkages between these perspectives without attempting to develop an integrated theoretical framework.

As we are opposed to the idea of a single model of critical social work, we encourage the reading of this book alongside other recent attempts to construct a critical social work practice (Fook 2002; Davies & Leonard 2004; Healy 2005a; Hick et al. 2005; McDonald 2006; Thompson 2006; Baines 2007a; Mullaly 2007; Ferguson 2008; Ife 2008a). We call upon readers to extend their understanding of the contribution that each has to make to the development of critical practices in social work, and in so doing offer this book as a contribution to ongoing dialogue.

The changing socio-political context of social work

The current edition of this book is substantially informed by the social and political context in which social work is practised, and this is raised by many of the contributors. Theory on its own is inadequate unless it guides forms of practice that embrace criticality, are ref ective, grapple with questions of universalism and relativism, adopt diverse knowledges and do not see alternatives to Western norms as deviant. This necessitates the critical social worker engaging in some of the wider debates that have an impact on practice and being attentive to policies that may be antithetical in nature to social work values.

To do so may require social workers to move from their comfort zones and to consider how the new world order requires them to engage with the most pressing concerns facing the world today, as well as to understand their interconnectedness with local practice contexts. Social workers need to understand and question the pervasiveness of the ideologies in relation to the market economy and minimalist government intervention when these are among the tenets that fail to redress inequality. There remains a lack of concerted attention to world poverty, even though there is some global agreement through the setting of the United Nations millennium goals which aim to substantially reduce world poverty and achieve other human rights goals such as tackling child mortality and reducing the incidence of HIV in many parts of the world. Closer to home, social workers need to be cognisant of the impact of international conf ict on groups within our own society. In taking this stand, we argue that the critical social worker must be vigilant and be aware that the prevailing economics-driven policies can have detrimental impacts on the most vulnerable members of society: those groups and individuals who are the key concerns of the social justice mission of social work. In this way, critical social work and politics converge in adopting an ethic of a responsibility for humankind, and not just those with access to economic and social resources.

The dominance of economic paradigms reveals itself to social workers in a number of ways, including the increased corporatisation of the human services sector, including contractual arrangements which see services delivered less and less by government itself. Social workers are both perpetrators and victims in this process. On the one hand, social work operates within a policy subset that is governed by dominant ideologies; on the other hand, these policies are determined by those with little connection to the world of everyday social work practice. For example, dominant discourses may suggest that economic development is the key answer for Indigenous Australians. Resulting from this is a set of policy constructs that ignores historical, colonial and experiential viewpoints. Hence social workers and their organisations seemingly have little choice other than to engage with the funded programs and the policy directives. Similarly, in child welfare the increasing resourcing of the 'hard edge' of policy, child protection, may mean that many social workers are limited in their endeavours towards prevention and family support. In such situations, a critical framework, including structural and feminist analyses, is pushed from prominence. To resist the dominance of the prevailing paradigms means to engage in political practice, something for which social workers are either not equipped in their training or are inhibited from doing by the organisational context.

Social work is a profession laden with contradictions, for despite an increasingly conservative practice environment, there are directives and principles enshrined in social work ethics which call on social workers to aff rm human rights and to challenge unjust principles. As we will see in Chapter 5, both the International Statement of Principles on Ethics in Social Work and the Australian Association of Social Workers Codes of Ethics proclaim that the principles of human rights and social justice are fundamental to social work (IFSW & IASSW 2004; AASW 1999). The New Zealand Code (1996) goes further by including such headings as Liberation Through Solidarity; Non-Discrimination; Democracy and Human Rights; and Dismissal of Brutality. To exercise moral courage in order to bring together practice imperatives with political undertakings is an immense but surmountable task for critical social workers.

The rich knowledge base of social workers provides much of the answer. The knowledge base is predominantly derived from practice wisdom, which means that we can position ourselves as critical ethnographers, participant observers in our work where we are witness to the impact of subjugation, oppression, racism and structural disadvantage. Critical theories, including postcolonialist, anti-oppressive and anti-racist ideals, can assist us in working towards emancipation and liberation (Mullaly 2007). Through our connections and observations, there is the prospect to challenge the taken-for-granted ways of doing things, which for practitioners may equate with complacency or unquestioning compliance. This means that social workers need to move to the centre stage of activism in order to position themselves as key actors in the policy realm. At the practice level, this book contains many examples of how social workers can apply a critical approach in diverse practice arenas, and the exemplars contained in the chapters provide leads for how this can occur.

Overview of the book

The remainder of the book is divided into three parts. Part II provides an introduction to the historical and contemporary debates about critical social work theories and practices. Part III surveys the implications of critical theories for developing critical practices in relation to different sites of domination and oppression. Part IV outlines the challenges facing critical social work in shifting contexts of practice.

Part II begins with a chapter by Philip Mendes tracing the history of critical social work in Australia, the United States and the United Kingdom. He draws attention to the historical split between individual and structural approaches in the 1970s, and traces the emergence of feminist social work theory and the later development of postmodern critical theory in the 1990s. The strengths and limitations of these historical developments are critically analysed with reference to their inf uence on mainstream social work theory and practice.

In Chapter 3, June Allan reviews contemporary approaches to social work theory. She notes that while the transformation of social structures and institutions is at the core of these various approaches, they place different emphases on the various systems of oppression and highlight a range of ways for achieving change. She shows that structural approaches emphasise addressing the material conditions of the vulnerable and marginalised through politicisation and collectivisation of social problems. In contrast, postmodern approaches focus on aff rming diversity and emphasise the multiple identities of people in their particular historical, socio-political and cultural contexts. This revised chapter examines some of the more recent debates in the literature concerning social work practised from a critical perspective, which highlight the continuing tensions within critical social work and its evolution as a transformative practice.

In Chapter 4, Bob Pease examines the tension between critical social work theories that are concerned with human rights and social justice and the development of models of evidence-based practice that are focused on quantif cation of outcomes and experimental ways of knowing. He observes that, while evidence-based practice in social work has been subjected to numerous criticisms from a critical theory perspective, no alternative epistemological base for critical social work practice has been proposed. In this chapter, he articulates an alternative knowledge base for critical social work that encompasses critical social theory, quantitative and qualitative research, tacit knowledge, critical ref ective practice, social justice values and consumer-based knowledge. In his view, it is only when we value knowledge from diverse sources that our commitment to social transformation can be fulf lled.

Chapter 5, by Sharlene Nipperess and Linda Briskman, advocates a human rights perspective on critical social work. They demonstrate that the relationship between a human rights discourse and critical social work has remained largely unexplored. In this chapter, they argue that human rights frameworks meld with a range of theoretical perspectives within the critical genre, including anti-oppressive and anti-colonial constructs. Drawing upon key examples of relevance to contemporary social work, they explicate the connections and the prospects in a context where core social work values are increasingly eroded by the state and its institutions. The chapter demonstrates how the melding of human rights and critical theories can be signif cant in the emancipatory project that underpins critical social work.

In the f nal chapter in Part II, June Allan considers the implications of critical social work perspectives for practice in social work, discussing issues and processes central to these perspectives. She highlights the importance of the consideration of power and the use of ref ective practices in this work. The updated chapter explores recent developments in ways of opening up choices and options for service users through practices which enable individuals to develop new understanding, awareness and conf dence, and which foster social change through resistance to oppressive social relations and conditions.

In the f rst chapter in Part III, Marjorie Quinn outlines the principles for anti-racist and culturally aff rming practices in social work. She observes that, in our contemporary world, differences of culture and race are often centrally involved in injustice, oppression and violence. Therefore, the pursuit of justice requires effective capacity to work in and across these differences. Using the concepts of culture and race and drawing upon critical theory perspectives, she examines the diversity of cultural meanings and practices, and looks at the implications they have for critical social work practice. The chapter is updated on the basis of new literature and the changing demands on us as citizens of the contemporary world.

Continuing the theme of race and culture in Chapter 8, Christine Fejo-King and Linda Briskman examine the complex relationship between social work and Indigenous peoples in Australia. They observe that in recent years social work has begun to retheorise its practice to engage more effectively with Indigenous peoples, to incorporate Indigenous knowledge and to adopt a more political approach for change. At the same time, however, they also note that while the profession is moving forward in partnership, policy imposition that acts against Indigenous interests is increasing. In this chapter, they examine the impact of the policy domain on Indigenous communities and consider how social workers can adopt critical anti-colonialist frameworks that can inf uence social change in the spheres of direct practice, advocacy, research and policy.

In Chapter 9, Susie Costello focuses on working with families from a critical theoretical perspective. She observes that the prevailing concept of the traditional family has oppressive implications for the lived experience of diverse family lives. In this revised chapter, Costello offers a critique of theories, practices and policies that have currency in work with vulnerable families with children, and she reviews the shift in government policies that have increasingly devolved responsibility from the state to community organisations. Against this background, she considers the critical social worker's use of power, critically reappraising psychological theories and exploring ways of working with vulnerable families that are progressive, empowering and respectful of cultural diversity.

The chapter by Heather D'Cruz examines the identity of the child and the meaning of childhood in critical social work practice. In the chapter, she critically engages with taken-for-granted ideas about the child by drawing on social theories that explore questions of identity, ref ected in personal assumptions about the identity of the child, and the legal, social and cultural contexts in which the identity of the child is constructed. The chapter also considers how the identity of the child is related to complementary identities of parent and adult. She argues that such ref ective critiques are central to critical social work practice with children to be able to attend to the different needs and rights of individuals identif ed as children and parents, and the power dynamics between such identities within a grouping called the family.

In Chapter 11, Christine Morley demonstrates the use of critical ref ection to improve and enhance feminist practices in social work. She notes that while feminist practitioners have used modernist emancipatory ideals to guide practice, the changing practice context has led some commentators to argue that feminist ideals have lost their contemporary relevance. In this chapter, she highlights the continued importance of feminist analyses to critical social work and explores how feminist practitioners have responded to changing, more complex and uncertain practice contexts, through engaging with some of the newer theoretical developments such as critical postmodernism.

Again on the theme of gender, Chapter 12 by Bob Pease explores the challenges and directions for profeminist practice with men in social work. He argues that we must locate our understanding of men's lives in the context of patriarchy and the divisions of class, race, sexuality and other forms of social inequality, while at the same time exploring ways in which patriarchal belief systems become embedded in men's psyches. He identif es six main arenas of men's practices where patriarchy is either reproduced or resisted: sexuality; intimacy and emotional expressiveness; health and wellbeing; family and care of others; paid work; and violence against women. He concludes by outlining the practice implications of a profeminist approach to men, as individuals, in men's groups and in working for structural change at the community and societal levels. This revised chapter also explores the dilemmas and tensions of men working with women as allies in movements against men's violence and for gender equality.

In Chapter 13, Barbara Black outlines empowering and rights-based approaches to working with older people. Drawing upon critical theories and their practice applications, she examines social work with older people in the areas of aged care and elder abuse. She analyses how age discrimination, combined with poverty, disability, and cultural and linguistic diversity, places some older people at risk of marginalisation and unequal access to resources and entitlements. Theoretical perspectives such as human rights, advocacy and empowerment are examined as a foundation for constructing a critical social work practice with older people to address these issues.

In Chapter 14, Kelley Johnson explores the ways in which theories and their resulting practices in relation to people with disabilities have impacted on their lives. She draws upon original research to analyse how different discourses have shaped 'professional practice' in relation to people with disabilities. Adopting a discursive approach to disability, Johnson explores the key discourses to which disabled people are subject. She concludes that for social workers to work effectively with disabled people they need to critically appraise the knowledge they receive and the ways in which they exercise this knowledge in practice.

The chapter by Selma Macfarlane explores a range of critical perspectives in relation to the construction of mental health and illness, and the practices engendered by these diverse belief systems. Macfarlane problematises the dominant medical model constructions and discusses counter-discourses, such as those posed by consumer and recovery movements, critical psychiatry and anti-oppressive practice proponents. She examines the ways in which race, class, gender and other structural factors intersect to create complex experiences of mental distress or wellbeing. Drawing upon postmodern thinking about power, discourse and subjectivity, she concludes by examining the role of critical ref ection in opening spaces for alternative understandings and more emancipatory practices.

June Allan in Chapter 16 illustrates ways of understanding and responding to the losses and the resultant grief experienced by individuals and communities, from critical social work perspectives. She views loss and grief as social experiences and argues that working with people to live constructively with their grief can only be understood through the knowledge that the personal, political and cultural are intimately bound together. Allan discusses themes and contradictions in our understanding of grief and ref ects on theories and practices for responding to grief in f exible ways.

In the f nal chapter in this section, Heather Fraser and Christine Craik explore how the many forms of violence and abuse adversely affect societies, groups, families and individuals. While recognising institutional violence, as well as child abuse, intimate violence, queer and elder abuse, they demonstrate that violence and abuse are gendered and sexualised crimes steeped in history, religion and political ideology. They also show how susceptibility to violence and abuse is connected to social status and access to resources, and illustrate why special attention needs to be given to women oppressed by class, race, ethnicity, sexuality, age, ability and/or geographical location. They emphasise the importance of working towards social, not just personal, change and advocate the promotion of egalitarian and democratic social processes at the local, national and international levels.

In the f rst chapter in Part IV, Catherine McDonald examines the changing socioeconomic and political context of critical practice in social work. Using a post-Fordist-informed political economy approach, she discusses the broader factors which have destabilised the 'professional project' of social work, encompassed by the erosion of welfare states and the rise of workfare. McDonald mounts an argument for why social work needs to renew itself in the light of contemporary conditions, particularly by reference to the importance of reviving the ethical impulse embedded in and propelled by the original vision of what social work could and should achieve.

In Chapter 19, Nick Halfpenny examines the degree to which social work has developed and evolved as an institutional activity, and how its location within and outside the bureaucracy has shaped social work practice. He explores how social workers practise in a context where public services are increasingly accompanied by a range of regimes to monitor and prescribe practice. Using social work practice in child and family services in Victoria as the context, he concludes with a consideration of how social workers can critically engage with the increasing prevalence of techniques of surveillance and control in their practice.

Often overlooked, rural and remote communities are the focus of Uschi Bay's work in Chapter 20. Bay observes how Australian rural and remote communities are facing increasingly challenging interactions between their geographical locations, place-based policy, livelihood strategies and various forms of inequality. She argues that framing critical social work practice with these communities requires an engagement with these socio-political and discursive changes. In this context, she critically examines how notions of 'social capital' have made local rural communities responsible for addressing structural issues that they may have no control over. In contrast, she explores how a critical theory-informed approach that emphasises dialogical and participatory processes, with sensitivity towards power differences within and across community groups, can generate an effective response to recent socio-political policies impacting upon rural and remote communities.

In the f nal chapter, Jacques Boulet critically examines the relevance of the emerging global and international context within which social work theory, practice and education are enmeshed. He inserts social work practice into the context of development, globalisation, human rights and social justice discourses alongside neo-colonial inequalities and exploitations, and the violence of massive military interventions and occupations. The revised chapter deepens the critique of the development/growth discourse in the context of the reality of global warming, deteriorating life systems and the growing recognition of the uncertainty of the survival of our own species. He concludes by examining the transformations of which critical social workers should be cognisant of and in which they should be involved, against a background of demands of adaptation to an increasingly turbulent socio-ecological environment.

In the second expanded edition of this book, we have been able to address some of the omissions of which we were acutely conscious when we published the f rst edition: disability, childhood, later life, rural poverty, and violence and abuse. There were many other sites of domination and oppression on our wish list, however, that we were not able to include. We hope that the book continues to inspire critical theory-informed frameworks for practice which address domination and oppressions wherever they arise, and that it provides impetus for others to address the new questions that arise as critical social work theories and practices evolve.

PART II

developing conceptual frameworks for critical social work

2

tracing the origins of critical social work practice

Philip Mendes

From its very beginning as a profession, social work has been divided between those who would emphasise the treatment and cure of individual problems and def ciencies, and those who prefer to emphasise structural inequities and the importance of social reform. As noted by Drakeford (2002: 294), there are 'those who see their primary task as changing the individual to meet the needs of society and those who see themselves as changing society to meet the needs of the individual'.

This individual/structural dichotomy was typif ed by the philosophical clash in the early twentieth century between Mary Richmond and Jane Addams in the United States. Mary Richmond's highly inf uential 1917 text *Social Diagnosis* argued for a case-by-case analysis of individual problems. She rejected any involvement in broader social change campaigns. Richmond worked in Philadelphia and later in New York for the inf uential Charity Organization Society movement, which emphasised the moral and character def cits of those who were poor. In contrast, Jane Addams and her Settlement House colleagues in Chicago identif ed the social and economic causes of problems, and campaigned for social reforms such as minimum wage laws, widows' pensions, factory safety regulations, the outlawing of child labour and tenement reform (Woodroofe 1968; Ehrenreich 1985; Reisch & Andrews 2002; Alston & McKinnon 2005b).

Some authors argue that these different approaches have increasingly converged, and that social work has assumed responsibility for both individual and structural (social change) interventions. Reference is often made to what is called the 'person in their social environment' focus (Trainor 1996). To be sure, numerous social work bodies and publications assert the need for social workers collectively to be involved in broader political action, and also def ne advocacy based on promoting systemic and social change for service users at both individual and societal levels as a core professional requirement (Schneider & Lester 2001). As a result, some social workers in Australia and elsewhere have been involved in social and political activism. However, many (perhaps most) social workers do not participate in social action, and many appear to believe that any activism that goes beyond individual advocacy is incompatible with professional practice (Haynes & Mickelson 2003).

The Canadian social work academic Bob Mullaly argues that there exists a continuing division between what he calls the conventional view of social work and the progressive or critical view. The former view, which is arguably dominant in the profession, recognises that social problems exist, but constructs social work practice around the specif c needs of the individual. It is assumed that social work interventions can empower service users without requiring any fundamental change to existing social structures. In contrast, the minority critical view holds that services users can only be empowered by eliminating oppression and inequality. A successful intervention will require fundamental social change and transformation (Mullaly 2007). The remainder of this chapter explores the historical tension between conventional and critical views.

Historical beginnings: a class emphasis

The emphasis of Jane Addams and other social reformers on the social environment, rather than psychological inadequacy as the basis of social problems, had a signif cant inf uence on American social work in the decade leading up to the First World War. But subsequently US social work was largely dominated by the views of Freudian psychiatry, which prioritised therapeutic work with individuals rather than addressing the broader social context and social change. This 'psychiatric deluge' ref ected the conservative social and political climate of the postwar years. In contrast, the United Kingdom continued to be inf uenced by sociological explanations of poverty and disadvantage, and psychoanalysis was less inf uential than in the United States (Woodroofe 1968).

Critical views seem to have had a renewed impact in the 1930s, when a group of radical and progressive workers in the United States responded to the hardship of the Depression by forming a Rank and File Movement. The movement urged the social work profession to build alliances with the labour movement, and to take a stronger stand in favour of social and economic justice. Some of the key leaders of this movement, such as Bertha Reynolds, were connected with the Communist Party, and later blacklisted by an anti-communist backlash (Fisher 1980; Powell 2001; Reisch & Andrews 2002).

These radical views had no inf uence on the small and f edgling social work profession in Australia, which was mainly directed by the psychoanalytic tradition emanating from Britain and the United States. There was a strong emphasis on casework at the expense of alternative methods such as social and community development (Lawrence 1965; Weeks 2000). Some critical views emerged in Australian social work education in the late 1950s and early 1960s involving the identif cation of structural causes of social problems, and the use of sociological techniques in research. For example, Melbourne University academic Geoff Sharp examined the impact of a mother's employment on her children, and used the insights of labelling theory to explore the relationship between a medical diagnosis of epilepsy and institutionalisation. But these ideas were quickly suppressed by the *Bulletin* magazine's attack on alleged communist inf uence in the Melbourne University Social Studies Department. The attack also discouraged social work involvement in broader social reform activities (Bryson 1997; Mendes 2001; Anderson 2005).

A renewed critique of conventional social work emerged from left-wing radicals in the early to mid-1970s. Key authors included Galper (1975) in the United States, Bailey and Brake (1975) and Corrigan and Leonard (1978) in the United Kindom, Moreau (1979) in Canada and Throssell (1975, 1976) in Australia. There were also organised radical groups such as Case Con, a revolutionary organisation for social workers in the United Kingdom, Catalyst, a group of radical social workers in the United States, and Inside Welfare, a socialist group of welfare workers in Australia (Langan 2002; Reisch & Andrews 2002). The radicals were strongly inf uenced by Marxism and associated intellectual movements such as anti-psychiatry, the sociology of deviance and sociological critiques of welfare approaches to poverty (Fook 1993). They argued that social work was a form of social control and coercion utilised by the ruling class to 'cool out' socially marginal groups and under-classes in society, and encourage conformity with prevailing conservative values.

According to an oft-quoted study by Pemberton and Locke (1971: 101), 'the social worker is a double-agent; while claiming to be working on behalf of the client, he is really an agent of socio-political control, bolstering the existing social order by reinforcing and interpreting moral, social and political rules'. Similarly, Skenridge and Lennie (1978: 47–8) argued that: 'Social work, by operating in and by ideology, has as its effect the reproduction and maintenance of the relations of domination and subordination which characterize the capitalist social formation, while at the same time repressing consciousness of this effect.' Their view was that the structure of capitalist society precluded any form of progressive social work practice.

Further, they contended that the emphasis of social work (particularly casework) on individual problems and solutions led to a 'blaming of the victim', rather than a broader critique of society. Individuals were discouraged from identifying the structural causes of their problems, or engaging in collective actions to change the existing socio-economic environment. Casework was held to preserve the class structure of an oppressive and unequal capitalist society (Pemberton & Locke 1971; Throssell 1975; 1976; Tomlinson 1975, 1977). They also maintained that social work's emphasis on professional discourse such as competencies, standards, accreditation, continuing professional education and ethics undermined the politicisation of social workers, and the potential for alliances with oppressed communities and service users (Withorn 1984; Reisch & Andrews 2002). In place of social work's allegedly consensus-based or ordered view of society, radicals offered a conf ict perspective. They called on social workers to develop a radical practice that would identify the linkages between individual problems and socio-economic causes, and critique existing inequitable social, political and economic arrangements (Mullaly 2007).

Many of the key social work radicals in Australia were associated with Inside Welfare (IW), a socialist group of welfare workers formed in Brisbane in January 1975. Groups were also formed later in Sydney, Melbourne, Perth and Adelaide. They consisted mostly of academics and practitioners, and don't seem to have included any welfare consumers. IW strongly rejected the professional discourse underpinning conventional social work, arguing that 'professionalism dissociates social work from its links with political action . . . Striving for professional status separates welfare workers from those dependent on their service and it encourages the introduction of business-like career structures where correct and professional behaviour is rewarded with advancement' (Hennig 1975: 5–6).

Inside Welfare was involved in a number of social welfare policy campaigns, produced a booklet of working papers, published an annotated bibliography of Marxist welfare literature, and hosted a national conference in April 1976 to provide a Marxist critique of the Henderson Poverty Commission Report (Inside Welfare 1975; 1976, 1979; Lennie 1976; Hayes 1992). A further priority was to promote the unionisation of welfare workers within the newly formed Australian Social Welfare Union. The organisation was active in the political campaign against Queensland premier Joh Bjelke-Petersen's street-march ban in 1977–78, but seems to have dissolved in the late 1970s. In the ensuing years, the radical critique contributed to changing some of the often apolitical and oppressive practices of social work. In particular, radical social work practice assumed an end to overtones of moral or personal failure, and the value of collective action to tackle structural problems. These ideas began to inf uence conventional social work education and practice (Langan & Lee 1989; Mullaly 2007).

The f rst and perhaps most successful attempt in Australia to translate macro-structural ideas into micro-practice and intervention strategies was the Brotherhood of St Laurence's (BSL) Family Centre Project of the early to mid-1970s (Benn 1981). The BSL experimental project provided a small group of 60 poor families who had been long-term welfare clients with a guaranteed weekly income supplement, the purpose of which was to overcome material poverty so that other pressing social and personal issues could be addressed. The structural basis of the project was a multidisciplinary staff team rather than a conventional social work service with an emphasis on developmental work rather than traditional casework. There was also a commitment to the deprofessionalisation of service provision with management of the program being transferred from social workers to service users. The BSL's aim was to demonstrate that changes in economic and social conditions and opportunities were a precondition for change in family and societal relationships, and that it was at such changes (redistribution of resources and power) that social work intervention should be directed.

The project f ndings suggested that the social disadvantage of participants ref ected a complex interaction between structural or material deprivation, and individual lives and experiences. An effective model of practice needed to address both social change via a self-help and welfare rights perspective, and the development of greater personal skills and self-conf dence (Liffman 1978; Benn 1981; Martin 2003). Unfortunately, the small-scale nature of the project meant that the wider application of its outcomes and knowledge base was limited. In addition, the project was criticised for failing to acknowledge the class basis of poverty, and for not developing a more critical analysis of the political implications of an alliance between professional social workers and relatively powerless and often apolitical service users (Wiseman 1978).

As suggested by the f ndings of the BSL project, the radical critique of conventional social work contained some obvious weaknesses or limitations. While radical social work may help some clients, it assumes client competence and is not likely to help all clients. Clarke (1976: 504) notes that some clients are 'fundamentally helpless, crushed and damaged by the experience of institutionalization, unemployment, poverty and oppression'. Furthermore, not all problems involve material deprivation.

Many social work clients suffer from emotional or psychological aff ictions such as grief, sudden illness, job loss, disability, exile, and so on, which require immediate counselling or therapy rather than material assistance. Yet arguably the radical social work movement failed to develop a psychology of personal troubles (Langan & Lee 1989; Payne 1997), although to be sure some authors acknowledged the need to address personal concerns as well as promoting consciousness-raising (Moreau 1979; Leonard 1984).

Radical approaches may also be viewed as recommending a utilitarian approach—that is, using people as a means to an end, rather than respecting the needs and wants of individuals. As Fook (1993: 145) notes, clients have a 'right not to be politicized at the expense of being helped'. In addition, radicals failed to address oppression based on gender and race as well as class. Fook (2002: 8) would later comment that radical theories actually seemed to reinforce a 'status differential between men and women', whereby men were elevated as macro-theorists and women devalued as micro-practitioners. Radicals also made the assumption that all statutory social work—whether corrections, juvenile justice, child protection or psychiatric assessment—is solely about coercion to maintain the existing social order (Galper 1980). Yet when social workers act to protect a young baby from severe physical assault, or to prevent a severely psychotic person injuring themselves or others, it seems obtuse to argue that their sole purpose is one of social control (Simpkin 1979).

As with the broader radical critique of the welfare state, the specif c critique of social work contained a number of contradictory tendencies. On the one hand, radicals claimed the welfare state acts to repress and control the working class, and to reinforce the institutions and values of capitalist society. On the other hand, they viewed the welfare state as the result of protracted struggle by the working class to attain their political demands, and so acknowledged that welfare programs do improve the lives of the poor and disadvantaged. These political and ideological contradictions were also present in the radical approach to social work practice which included differences between evolutionary Marxists, who viewed social work as a potential path to socialism, and revolutionary Marxists, who dismissed social work as inherently connected to the capitalist state. Overall, radicals seemed to recognise that the role of social workers was potentially both to control clients, and to meet their needs and interests (Galper 1975; Watts 1979; Mullaly 2007).

Finally, most radical critiques arguably failed to provide any effective guide for practice. At best, they suggested various forms of collective action such as community work, social and political action, and trade union activity. There were also some attempts to develop Freire's ideas about consciousness-raising in order to mobilise client groups. Yet little or no attempt was made to relate the radical perspective to an actual social work practice model with specif c strategies for engagement with, assessment of and intervention with individual clients (Fook 1993). However, some veterans of the radical social work movement (e.g. Langan 2002) dispute the validity of this conclusion.

The influence of feminist ideas

The emergence of feminist ideas targeting gender inequality as well as class-based oppression, and linking personal experiences and the political, served to address some of the def cits of earlier critical social work approaches. Feminist social work has been def ned by Dominelli (2002a: 7) as 'practice that starts from an analysis of women's experience of the world and focuses on the links between women's position in society and their individual predicaments to create egalitarian client–worker relationships and address structural inequalities'. Martin (2003) summarises a number of the key strategies of feminist social work. They include: def ning personal problems as political and requiring social change campaigns to allocate greater resources to gender-specif c programs around domestic violence, rape and incest; creating collectivist organisational structures to manage the funding and resourcing of these programs; focusing counselling and therapy on legitimising female emotions and developing the skills and conf dence of individual women; focusing social work in statutory settings on addressing issues of gender and social injustice; and challenging examples of gender inequality and discrimination in the workplace.

A number of women, including Norma Parker and Lyra Taylor, played prominent roles in establishing the social work profession in Australia. Yet feminist ideas took some time to impact on social work practice. Lawrence's (1965) history of Australian social work argued contentiously that the numerical dominance of women was problematic, and that a greater male presence was required to lift the recognition and prof le of the profession. Lawrence's history (which arguably ref ected the values and attitudes of his time) has been criticised on a number of grounds including his sexist-based denigration of female social workers, and his failure to acknowledge their role in wider social activism (Mendes 2005).

It was not until 1973 that a Radical Women's Group (RWG) was formed by Australian social workers in the state of Victoria to examine the status of women in social work, and to discuss discrimination against women social workers and women clients (AASW 1973–74). An associated article by a Victorian social worker involved in the RWG, Jane Nichols (1973), lamented that men were represented disproportionately in senior social work positions, and that there appeared to be ongoing discrimination and bias against female social workers. A later article by Nichols (1977) complained that the Women's Liberation Movement had left Australian social work untouched, and that sexist bias had continued in areas such as staff ng, student selection and course content in social work courses.

However, a growing feminist consciousness developed among Australian women social workers in the 1980s concerning their own career opportunities, and broader patriarchal inf uences on social welfare policies and social work practice (Martin 1990, 1992). This consciousness resulted in the formation of a national caucus of the Australian Association for Social Work and Welfare Education, called Women in Welfare Education, which addressed issues of specif c concern to women (Weeks 2000). There were also a number of key publications, such as a special issue of *Australian Social Work* in 1985 devoted to the theme 'Women in Social Work', and a study by Marchant (1985) of the early development of the social work profession in New South Wales. She argued that control of social work training and education had passed from social activists who were women to the male-dominated medical profession, and suggested that contemporary social workers needed to address this connection between professional development and patriarchy.

In addition, Marchant and Wearing (1986b) edited a volume of papers titled *Gender Reclaimed*. The two editors explored three particular concepts linking feminism and social work practice: the wider social factors inf uencing women as clients or as workers in the social work profession; the practices by some males within the profession which had reinforced gender inequality despite the numerical domination of women; and the identif cation of broader strategies for overcoming gender-based disadvantage. By the mid-1980s, most social work courses offered at least one feminist subject—even if most of the mainstream literature ignored gender issues—and some attention was also paid to the development of profeminist men's studies. Structural feminist ideas also had a signif cant impact on particular f elds of practice, such as centres against sexual assault (Weeks 2000).

Towards a critical social work practice approach

Over time, social workers inf uenced by socialist and feminist assumptions developed a number of practice-based approaches to critical social work theory and practice. The critical perspective was characterised by two major themes: the structural basis of personal and social problems, and an awareness that many social problems are not amenable to individual, family or subcultural solutions; and the need to work at both the personal (through individual consciousness-raising that connects private troubles with structural sources) and political levels to challenge oppressive and inequitable structures (Thorpe & Petruchenia 1990; Healy 1993; Mullaly 1993).

One of the most comprehensive critical practice approaches for individual casework was developed by the Australian scholar Jan Fook in the late 1980s and early 1990s. Fook (1990: 27) def nes radical social casework as 'individually orientated help which focuses on problems caused by the interaction of individual person and socio-economic structure'. According to Fook, structural factors may cause personal problems in a number of direct and indirect ways. First, social structures may complicate or exacerbate individual problems such as psychiatric illness. Second, the role assumptions imposed by socio-economic structures such as marriage and lack of equal pay in the workforce may create personal problems by inf uencing and limiting people's choices about their lives. And third, structural factors may directly cause personal problems by determining the unsatisfactory material conditions under which people live. For example, young single mothers may become depressed due to living in rundown housing, or disabled people may become socially isolated due to a lack of accessible public transport.

In order to demonstrate the difference between radical and traditional casework, Fook (1993) provided six case examples in which both approaches were used. The emphasis in the radical approach tended to be on empowering the client by linking them with broader support networks, and tackling oppressive social or economic structures that were contributing to the presenting problem. In contrast, the traditional approach concentrated on addressing the individual inadequacies or deviancy of the client, and helping them to conform to mainstream values and expectations.

Fook's distinction between radical and non-radical practice was criticised on two grounds: that what she described as radical practice was in fact practice commensurate with conventional social work values and ethics (Ife 1997); and that her description of non-radical practice as based on individual blaming and indifference to socio-economic inf uences misrepresented the nature and ideology of conventional social work (Trainor 1996). However, it would be naïve to believe that all social workers adhere to a structural framework, or that conventional and critical beliefs have converged. Many social workers almost certainly adhere to small 'l' liberal or conservative ideologies which emphasise individualistic rather than structural analysis. In this sense, Fook's distinction between radical and non-radical assumptions remained valid. Nevertheless, the key question that remained unanswered was the extent to which (if at all) there could be demonstrated a qualitative difference in outcome between critical and conventional social work interventions (Webb 1981; Fook 1993).

Potential research which could have resolved this question might, for example, have focused on the interventions of critical and conventional social workers in child protection. Case scenarios could have been devised linking structural factors such as poverty and unemployment with alleged child abuse or neglect, in order to assess whether social workers were more likely to offer structural supports to families, or alternatively to take out protection applications and place children in care. The project could then examine whether the critical interventions were actually more successful than the conventional interventions in providing fairer and more socially just outcomes for the families involved.

Similarly for Centrelink social workers, a case scenario could have been devised involving gender discrimination by pension off cers against female recipients of the Parenting Payment to assess whether social workers were more likely to use individual bureaucratic or broader collective/advocacy approaches to addressing the problem. Again, the project could have examined whether the critical rather than conventional approaches were more effective in promoting a socially just outcome for the service users involved. In the absence of such research, it is diff cult—as Fook (1993) acknowledged—to prove or disprove the effectiveness and uniqueness of radical casework approaches.

The diversity of contemporary critical social work practice

Over the last decade or so, critical social work approaches have integrated older modernist forms of structural analysis and newer postmodern ideas which emphasise more diverse sources of power and emancipation. There is a broad range of approaches including anti-racist and culturally aff rming social work practice, anti-oppressive and anti-discriminatory social work, anti-colonial social work, feminist social work and structural social work. These perspectives recognise inequities of class, gender, race, ethnicity, age, ability and sexuality, and target social change at both the individual and societal levels (Pease & Fook 1999a; Dominelli 2002b; Healy 2005a; Ife 2005a; Mullaly 2007).

For example, anti-oppressive and anti-discriminatory approaches emerged in the United Kingdom in the 1980s and 1990s as a response to new social movements representing oppressed groups such as women, new immigrants, black people[1] and those with disabilities. These approaches recognise a wider range of structural inequities and oppression than earlier economic or class-based radical approaches, and particularly target the failure of individualistic theories of social work to recognise the impact of discrimination against minority groups in society. They also suggest a more active alignment between social work practitioners and oppressed groups in developing an understanding of the needs to be addressed, and designing empowering solutions (Payne 2005).

Australian authors appear to have made a signif cant contribution to recent critical social work ideas and practice (Payne 2005; Baines 2007d). One inf uential theorist is Healy (2000), who argues that critical approaches offer three specif c criticisms of conventional social work: it focuses on individuals rather than structures; it fails to recognise the power and authority of the social worker compared with that of the client; and it validates a professional ideology which grants the social worker control over the client. In contrast, critical social work practice emphasises the prioritisation of the social structure in the analysis of problems; a shift from a focus on individual pathology to a concentration on individual or group oppression; the development of more egalitarian practice relations; the adoption of practice strategies such as consciousness-raising that recognise and challenge the structures of oppression; and the involvement of the worker in social-change activities.

A signif cant practice approach is provided by Fook (2002). Her approach is based on a number of key assumptions of critical social theory: domination is created structurally but experienced personally; false consciousness means that people accept rather than challenge structural inequities; but fatalism should be rejected because even those who seem powerless have the capacity to facilitate personal and social change. A number of core actions are necessary to achieve change, including the deconstruction of dominant sources of power and knowledge, resistance to and questioning of the dominant discourse, challenge via labelling prevailing or hidden discourses, and a reconstruction of new knowledge and structures.

Nevertheless, Payne (2005) argues that critical social work still contains some of the weaknesses of earlier radical or Marxist approaches, such as the emphasis on collective action that may lead to a neglect of the immediate personal needs of clients, the highlighting of material and structural issues at the possible expense of emotional and personal problems, and a Western-oriented bias that fails to recognise and tackle the fundamental abuse of civil and human rights that occurs in many non-Western countries. However, critical social work theory, unlike earlier radical theory, does provide some practical strategies for engaging with clients, and ensuring that marginalised voices—particularly of those suffering from sexism and racism—are heard.

The extent of the impact of critical approaches on Australian social work practice is uncertain. Some authors have used critical ideas to dissect the conventional ideological perspective underpinning the current AASW Code of Ethics, and to develop a critical alternative (Noble & Briskman 2000; Fraser & Briskman 2005). In addition, research reports document the teaching of critical social work skills to students (Fraser & Strong 2000), the application of critical ref ection in the training of practitioners (Morley 2004) and the use of critical perspectives to inform the development of a peer support and advocacy group for young mothers who had experienced violence (Healy 2000). However, most of these reports don't seem to include any ongoing evaluation processes that would provide evidence of actual impact on and/or changes in practice. There also appear to be few case examples of critical practice interventions implemented with individuals and families. But this does not mean that a narrow evidence-based approach should be used in isolation to judge the merits of critical social work.

Regardless, there is some limited evidence from practitioners that critical ideas are useful to and incorporated in practice strategies. For example, one Australian social worker (Goldsworthy 2002, also cited in Mendes 2008) has identif ed critical ideas as central to effective practice with either individuals or communities. Other research has conf rmed the use of critical ideas by some social workers in a number of practice contexts (Mason 2005; Osmond & O'Connor 2006). There is clearly a need for further research into the application of critical social work practice, although Healy (2000) warns that such research may be politically risky. She recommends that the research be conducted by social workers themselves rather than by external evaluators who may wish to censor or exclude activist social workers.

On balance, it appears that the majority of social workers in Western countries favour conventional rather than critical approaches to social work practice (Gilligan 2007; Mullaly 2007). A number of Australian authors (Ife 1997; Alston & McKinnon 2005b; McDonald 2006) acknowledge that critical social work appears to sit at the margins of Australian social work practice. Further development of critical practice might arguably be assisted by the establishment of critical social work networks similar to the Social Welfare Action Alliance in the United States and the radical social work group Case Con in the United Kingdom (Reisch & Andrews 2002; Shearing 2005) as a means of mentoring practitioners, particularly including new graduates. It has also been suggested that critical practice based on linking the personal and the political be prioritised in the planning and implementation of student f eldwork placements (Ife 1997).

Conclusion

The early Australian critical social work approaches provided a useful critique of potentially oppressive forms of social work practice, but generally failed to provide detailed intervention strategies for linking individual powerlessness with broader political action. However, the emerging inf uence of feminist theory and later theories inf uenced by postmodern thought assisted the development of more sophisticated approaches which addressed many of these earlier def cits. Critical social workers now have a range of approaches which they can use to promote both individual and social change with a diverse range of oppressed groups. International research conf rms that Australian authors have made a signif cant contribution to the history and development of critical social work theory and practice (Payne 2005; Gilligan 2007; Mullaly 2007).

The specif c contribution of critical social work approaches to Australian social work practice is less evident. To be sure, conventional social work theories appear to have incorporated some ideas from critical practice, such as the key role of the social context in shaping individual behaviour, and the importance of linking social work practice to the promotion of social justice values. But we still need more case studies that document the implementation of critical approaches in the casework and case management positions that are held by most social workers, and particularly in those f elds of practice that involve statutory power (Healy 2005b). We also require further research to assess whether critical approaches actually promote different (and more socially just) outcomes than conventional social work practice approaches.

3

theorising new developments in critical social work

June Allan

Social work scholars and practitioners continue to grapple with the development of approaches to practice that recognise the power imbalances in society, endeavouring to bring about social change while simultaneously providing a humane and respectful response to people in their everyday struggles with social problems. In this chapter, I explore the development of critical social work theories. While the desire for social change is at the core of these theories, they highlight a range of ways for achieving change. On the one hand, there is an emphasis, inf uenced by modernist ideas, on addressing the material conditions of the vulnerable and marginalised through challenging structures and politicisation and collectivisation of social problems. On the other hand, the chapter's focus is inf uenced by postmodern thinking—on aff rming diversity, on the multiple identities of people in their particular historical, socio-political and cultural contexts, and on challenges to disabling discourses. After reviewing these approaches, I will consider some of the more recent developments and debates concerning critical social work. These developments highlight the continuing tensions within critical social work and its evolution as a transformative practice.

Various terms fall within the rubric of 'critical social work', each with its own particular interpretation of what transformative social work means. They include radical social work (discussed in Chapter 2), structural social work (Moreau 1979; Mullaly 2007), anti-discriminatory and anti-oppressive practice (Dalrymple & Burke 1995; Dominelli 1998; Thompson 2006; Baines 2007a), human rights-based practice

(Ife 2008a), postmodern critical social work (Pease & Fook 1999b), progressive social work (Reisch & Andrews 2001) and critical best practice (Jones et al. 2008). A number of these are referred to in this chapter, illustrating the varied and different ways in which critical social work is constructed.

Structural approaches within a modernist tradition

Structural approaches to social work practice emerged in the 1970s. Inf uenced by the modernist tradition and arising out of the radical social work movement, practice frameworks developed that focused primarily on the materialist dimension of people's lives, although there was some beginning recognition of the diversity of people's experiences. Among these scholars were a number from North America, including Moreau (1977, 1979; Moreau & Leonard 1989; Moreau et al. 1993), Carniol (1990), Mullaly (1993, 1997, 2007) and Lundy (2003). The approach can be termed 'structural' for its focus on structural oppression (particularly class) and a concern for social change. Middleman and Goldberg (1974) from the United States f rst coined the term 'structural social work' in 1974, but their framework was based on a conservative view of the social environment as the location of social problems that left the fabric or structures of society unchallenged and unchanged.[1]

Conceptualisations of a structural approach that followed Middleman and Goldberg were based on socialist ideology and grounded in critical theory. They emerged out of disenchantment with the inequities and social injustices perpetuated by the capitalist system and an emphasis within mainstream social work at the time on a casework approach that individualised social problems and typically saw them as being the 'fault' of the individuals experiencing them. Emphasising solidarity among oppressed peoples and collective action, these conceptualisations of a structural approach linked the 'personal with the political', making it possible for people to consider their personal experience of oppression within a broader political understanding (Moreau 1979; Mullaly 1993, 1997, 2007).

Focusing on oppression as the root cause of social problems, the approach aimed to develop people's awareness of how capitalist society shapes, limits and dominates their experiences, thus alienating them from society, each other and themselves. Social workers were challenged to change the oppressive conditions of institutionalised structures (political, economic and social) rather than the individual, the family or the subculture adversely affected by social problems. According to this perspective, there were two goals. The f rst involved alleviating the effects on people of exploitative and alienating practices; the second was concerned with bringing about change in the conditions and social structures that cause these negative effects (Mullaly 1993, 1997, 2007). Thus the change process involves immediate relief or tension-reduction for the individual/s experiencing the problems, along with longer-term institutional and structural change (Moreau 1979). There was recognition of the need for both 'radical counselling' and collective action through social networks and social-change movements, to increase pressure on established institutions to make changes (Carniol 1990).

There was acknowledgement that the structural approach incorporated tasks that social workers had always undertaken as part of their professional commitment and responsibility. What was new was the way in which social problems were conceptualised and objectives formulated. The new approach was political in nature and moved from dichotomising person and situation, directing 'attention to the transactions between people and specif c social, political and economic situations' (Moreau 1979: 78). In that regard, the structural approach was seen as a generalist model of practice focusing not only on social institutions but also requiring knowledge and skills for working with individuals, groups, families and communities (Mullaly 1997, 2007). An assumption in the approach is that the prevailing ideology, policies, practices and procedures of most social organisations maintain the power of workers and reduce the power of the users of their services (Moreau & Leonard 1989). Intervention, therefore, required social workers to work towards a more equal power relationship between themselves and their clients to overcome the usual sanctioning in professional relationships between workers and clients of emotional, physical and social distancing.

Structural approaches dominated the critical social work literature from the late 1970s through to the 1990s and were valuable for challenging the status quo through highlighting the impact of structural oppression on people's lives and for raising awareness of the need to address the root causes of oppression, especially through solidarity and collective action. However, they paid limited attention to the human, communicative, relationship face of social problems as they are often presented, and did not develop ways of engaging effectively with the multiple realities of people's lives. Because structural approaches relied on an analysis at a general and abstract level, based on universal discourses of structural oppression that transcend different cultures, they also did not adequately allow for the consideration of difference within and across cultures (Fook 2000a; Ife 1997). This denied the experience of many groups in society.

The growing inf uence of postmodern ideas was seen as a way forward by many social work theorists from within a critical tradition. A growing body of practice literature questioned the truth status of modernist critical social work perspectives, their top-down notion of power that left disempowering practices continuing at the interpersonal level, and the usefulness of a structural approach in ever-changing and diverse local policy and practice contexts (Fook 2000b; Healy 2001).

The influences of postmodern ideas

There has been acknowledgement of the complexities of trying to capture the meanings of such a complex and varied body of thought as postmodernism (see, for example, McDonald 2006). My concern here is not to review the postmodern literature itself but rather to consider critical social work approaches that have drawn on postmodern ideas. The approaches to critical social work inf uenced by what Healy refers to as 'post' theories—postmodern, poststructural and postcolonial (2005a: 197)[2]—have appeared in the literature over the last decade (e.g. Pease & Fook 1999b; Fawcett et al. 2000; Fook 2000a, 2000b, 2002; Healy 2000, 2001, 2005a; Leonard 2001). They are concerned with social change and freedom from oppression, but in ways different from modernist approaches, which are inf uenced primarily by a concern for the impact of social structures on people's life opportunities and experiences. Although critical social work approaches inf uenced by postmodern thinking do not discard outright the notion of the inf uence of these structures, they question the modernist notion of one universal truth or reality. Instead, they engage with diversity in society by viewing individuals as having multiple and diverse social identities or realities; they rethink power relations in society in terms of how these are maintained through language and discourse and how they play themselves out at local levels, not simply at macro levels such as government emphasised by the modernist approaches. Such understandings allow for dominant understandings and structures to be disrupted and changed so that they can be more inclusive of different interest groups (Fook 2002: 18). These features of postmodern thought in critical social work will now be explored in greater detail.

Critical social work inf uenced by postmodern ideas challenges the grand narratives of modernism, proposing instead that there are multiple truths or realities, all of which are valued equally and are understood through language and discourses (Healy 2005a; Baines 2007a). Discourse can be referred to as 'the ways in which we make meaning of and construct our world through the language we use (verbal and non-verbal) to communicate about it' (Fook 2002: 63). Language as a medium for communication is not neutral as in the process of channelling communications and their meanings; it includes some ideas and omits others (Fook 2005). Discourses as sets of meanings therefore actively construct how we understand different phenomena or experiences (for example, refugees, or who is 'allowed' to grieve in a given culture). In society, particular discourses become dominant and are sustained according to 'the kinds of knowledge that are valued and whose knowledge is valued' by the discourses (Healy 2005a: 200).

Associated with the notion of discourses is the concept of deconstruction. Discourses need to be unpacked or critiqued to uncover hidden and marginalised meanings and assumptions, and unsettle taken-for-granted power differences (Fook 2002). Often represented in discourses as polar or binary opposites (for example, powerful/powerless, working class/middle class, male/female, able-bodied/disabled), these binaries establish hierarchies between the two terms and hide differences within and between them (Healy 2005a). As Healy notes, one person can move from the 'working class' to the 'middle class' during their lifetime, and even within the one category there are many variations. Thus deconstruction can be thought of as 'ongoing interrogation of that which is excluded in the processes of representing anything' (Healy 2005a: 205).

Critical social work within a postmodern tradition challenges assumptions about power, which in modernist terms is seen as something that is possessed, repressive and operating in top-down ways 'as a force imposed by one set of subjects on others' (Healy 2005a: 202). Influenced particularly by the ideas of Foucault (e.g. 1977, 1980), the power people have available to them is seen as arising out of their historical and contextual location in society, not just their material location. The dominant negative view of power is rethought and regarded as being both coercive and productive, something that 'people use and create rather than simply possess' (Fook 2005: 52). For example, social workers use their professional power and authority to gain needed resources for oppressed and marginalised people, and to provide people with necessary knowledge and information. Invisible networks of power in the relations between social workers and their institutions are also seen to influence the social worker and get translated into practice as power is played out in everyday actions like interpreting evidence and in the 'walk and talk' of the office, where there is flexibility despite narrowing frames of policy and accountability (McBeath & Webb 2005).

The notions of identity and subjectivity have been scrutinised by critical social work theorists influenced by postmodern thinking. Modernist categorisations of people based on the binary opposites referred to earlier overlook the changing identities that individuals typically experience throughout their lives, deny their ability to change and reinvent themselves in changing contexts, and potentially disempower those with marginal identities through being placed in a fixed category. Postmodern perspectives recognise that, through their life experiences in different contexts, individuals' identities or 'subjectivities' may change and be multiple and contradictory (Fook 2002). The challenge, as Fook notes, is to create meaningful categories to order our world without denying or stigmatising the experiences of marginalised groups (Fook 2002: 82).

Postmodern ideas have led critical social work theorists to question the modernist claim that people can change the way they live simply through rational thought and action. Instead, approaches to social change that are f exible, pragmatic and sensitive to the person's context are advocated (Pease & Fook 1999b; Fawcett et al. 2000; Fook 2000a; Healy 2001). Multiple systems of oppression, each of equal signif cance, are identif ed and many different ways of knowing are recognised (Healy 2000). Individuals are also recognised as being irrational, embodied and inf uenced by tradition. Rather than follow a grand vision of transformation and change, the aim is to move towards the creation of conditions for ongoing dialogue and contestation in relation to change so that multiple views and realities are represented. From this perspective, workers additionally need to be critically ref ective and self-ref exive, ref ecting on their practice but also on their own values, feelings and actions and the way these inf uence their work. Critical social work informed by postmodern understandings thus values both the lived experience of service users and the knowledge of the professional, through ongoing scrutiny of the knowledge that both bring to the relationship (Fook 1999, 2005; Healy 2000; de Montigny 2005; Fook & Morley 2005).

Through the inf uence of postmodern thinking and its emphasis on language and discourse, the idea of narrative therapy has attracted particular interest (see, for example, White & Epston 1990; White 2000; Parton & O'Byrne 2000a; 2000b; Pozzuto et al. 2005). Narratives can be thought of as the stories that people construct to make meaning of their lives through language by 'arranging their experiences of events in sequences across time in such a way as to arrive at a coherent account of themselves and the world around them' (Freedman & Combs 1996: 30). But as there are multiple realities, people give power to some stories over others (often their problem stories) so that alternative (more positive) stories remain buried and unheard. Narratives play a central role 'in organizing and maintaining and circulating knowledge of ourselves and our worlds' (Freedman & Combs 1996: 30) and exist at many levels—individual, family, organisational, national and cultural, such as Western beliefs about 'Orientalism' (Freedman & Combs 1996; Fook 2002).

Through its capacity to examine the 'taken-for-granted', narrative therapy can open up possibilities because it locates problems in the relationship between the individual and social structures, which mutually inf uence each other. As the individual changes, so do social processes and hence 'the stuff' of social contexts. Narrative therapy thus has the potential to alter the continued reproduction of social relations (Pozzuto et al. 2005). The client–worker relationship becomes the space for seeking or creating alternatives through questioning and destabilising the 'taken-for-granted', opening up possibilities and choice. Pozzuto et al. (2005) acknowledge that this process is not easy in the face of support of the taken-for-granted by existing dominant power relations and knowledge systems, but regard it as not impossible.

Although not claiming to draw on critical theory but noting the inf uence of postmodern thought on the development of their ideas, Parton and O'Byrne (2000a, 2000b) developed the concept of 'constructive social work' as a way of acknowledging the importance of language and narrative. Like Ferguson (2008) more recently, Parton and O'Byrne (2000a) were responding to the developments in social work in the United Kingdom of the mechanistic process of assessing needs and determining categories of risk and vulnerability in functional, proceduralised and bureaucratic ways. Their social constructionist approach to practice prioritises dialogue, and listening to and talking with the other. Also adopting a critical stance to taken-for-granted ways of understanding the world and ourselves, the approach is centrally concerned with the social processes that bring this about and that can be changed, and the negotiated understandings and different kinds of actions that result from these processes. The approach revalues the daily interactions between people, and provides some valuable ways of understanding and theorising practice in a fragmented world that demands attention to uncertainty and diversity. Despite a professed commitment to social justice and empowerment, Parton and O'Byrne's emphasis is entirely on personal agency and personal empowerment to the neglect of social transformation and collective empowerment (e.g., see 2000a: 59–60).

There has been continuing debate and ambivalence about the place of postmodern perspectives in critical social work theory from many quarters (e.g. Rees 1991; Dixon 1993; McDonald 2006; Ferguson 2008). Postmodern perspectives are treated sceptically because they are regarded as retreating from such universal notions as social justice, the realities of the effects of neo-liberalism and global power, and the redistribution of resources at a time when structures such as class, gender and race remain such virulent social divisions (Walby 1992; Taylor-Gooby, in Jamrozik 2001; Mullaly 2007; Ferguson 2008). Postmodern perspectives are seriously questioned for adopting a politics that privileges difference and locality and that draws attention away from the power of the state (Fook 2000a; Healy 2000; Mullaly 2007), and are perceived as offering little in the way of alternatives to address social injustices at the macro level (Leonard 1995, cited in Healy 2001; Ferguson 2008). Questions are raised about how a social work practice informed by postmodern perspectives can challenge oppression and inequality because of its individualism and moral relativism—even though some challenge this by arguing that they make even more explicit the moral choices and responsibilities central to social work practice (see Parton & O'Byrne 2000a). In contrast to Parton and O'Byrne's postmodern approach, there has been a growing interest in approaches within a critical tradition that explicitly acknowledge the signif cance of structures in people's everyday lives but at the same time incorporate ideas from within a postmodern tradition. It is to this shift in emphasis that I now turn.

Shifting emphases

Over the last few years, we have seen the development of approaches within a critical tradition that are explicitly inf uenced by both modernist and postmodern ideas. These approaches purport to recognise the limitations of both sets of ideas and endeavour to draw on the strengths of both to inform a social justice-oriented approach that takes account of the diversity amongst those who are oppressed and marginalised. This section explores some of these approaches and their efforts to address the central challenge of creating unity between people while acknowledging their differences.

Writing out of a concern for the impact on social work practice in Australia of the growth in neo-liberalism, Ife (1997) adopts a human rights framework that combines a structural analysis and an understanding of oppression that can lead to action and change with an interpretive understanding that allows for multiple and diverse realities. He acknowledges the tension in the position he takes, through its competing narratives of unity and difference.

Ife attempts to deal with this tension by negating the dichotomy between structural and post-structural,[3] arguing that radical practice must incorporate both. He argues that although universalist accounts such as humanism can readily incorporate a vision of social justice, they can reinforce marginalisation by ignoring the voices of difference. On the other hand, by rejecting the dominance of a single explanation, relativist discourses such as postmodernism run the risk of removing themselves from a universal commitment to social justice. Ife warns that, without a structural analysis, humanism can merely reinforce existing relationships of power and oppression. A structural analysis is necessary in order to identify the causes of people's oppression or disadvantage within a wider context, since the felt needs of people may result from forces of which they have no understanding or knowledge. The structural analysis provides an overall perspective within which individuals construct meanings and take action. Thus, for Ife, a critical approach incorporates both structures and discourses. His approach is built on the belief that power is def ned within changing discourses and is also present in structures of domination such as class, race and gender.

How Ife takes account of the interplay between structures and discourses in practice is not entirely clear. Recognising that policies can reinforce structural disadvantage unless relevant structural issues are addressed, Ife calls for practices such as consciousness-raising, education and community action. But he does not pay detailed attention to how power actually becomes entrenched in structures, nor to how this power in turn impacts on the thoughts and actions of individuals. Issues of identity and subjectivity are not addressed.

More recent approaches that draw explicitly on modernist and postmodern ideas can be found in the Canadian work of Donna Baines' (2007a) 'anti-oppressive practices' (AOP) and Bob Mullaly's (2007) 'new structural social work'. Recognising the extreme diff culties social workers face because of the complex, uncertain and sometimes hostile environments in which they work, both Baines and Mullaly provide optimism about practising social work in ways that challenge and resist social injustices at micro and macro levels and heed the diversity amongst those who are marginalised. Baines' edited collection in particular provides many examples of the approach in practice and refreshingly illustrates the energy and inspiration that can accompany such work.

In his 'new structural social work' approach, a revision of his earlier work (1997), Mullaly (2007) weighs up the pros and cons of both modernist and postmodern positions. He concludes that postmodernism is a positive inf uence which acts as a corrective to important differences that modernism glosses over, such as its lack of attention to complexity and the diversity of people, cultures and interests. Mullaly, like Ife, recognises the tension between solidarity, or unity, and difference. He argues that to overcome oppressive inclusions/exclusions from coalitions or groups, differences within these groups need to be acknowledged. The silencing of the voices of marginalised groups through the power of dominant discourses must be acknowledged and ways found for marginalised voices to be heard and to come together in solidarity.

Continuing a tradition of anti-oppressive practice discussed by others before her (for example, Dalrymple & Burke 1995; Dominelli 1998; Thompson 1998) and informed by a social justice-oriented framework, Baines' AOP approach is shaped by theories or beliefs that 'bring together multiple theories and perspectives that challenge orthodoxy and fundamentalism' (2007a: 22) and emphasise the importance of everyday experience. For Baines, an approach that draws unashamedly on a variety of critical approaches offers the greatest potential for social justice-oriented practice. Baines sees the debates about the blending of postmodern with critical theories as a necessary part of theorising contemporary social work through social workers helping clients, communities and themselves to understand why they are oppressed and how to f ght for change. At the heart of her approach is the dual aspect of supporting individuals 'while simultaneously politicising all aspects of everyday life and engaging in efforts to transform society on many levels' (2007a: 192). Part of this involves social workers developing alliances with other groups such as social movements and activist organisations to work towards large-scale socio-political changes and engaging in self-ref exive practice (Baines 2007a).

Drawing on the experiences of the chapter authors in her edited collection, all of whom have extensive backgrounds in social justice and frontline practice, Baines (2007a) concludes that successful anti-oppressive practice results from engaging in resistance and f ghting for change, and from advocacy or community-based work mixed with specif c practices designed to relieve people's emotional pain and shift resources and power to service users. Baines argues that anti-oppressive practice is possible in most practice settings but acknowledges that it is diff cult in the current socio-political climate, and concedes that in some settings that are 'narrow, conservative and limiting' only some beginning AOP may be possible (2007a: 29).

While anti-oppressive practice is valued for its attention to the cultural, political and social contexts of people's lives, it has been critiqued—especially for the lack of critical ref exive thinking about its own position and practices and for its taken-for-granted assumptions about what is true and correct (Healy 2005a; McDonald 2006). Like the approach taken in the United Kingdom, Baines' approach adheres to a universalist anti-oppressive framework but appears to allow for greater ref exivity as it is not a single unif ed approach but rather a set of practices that evolve to address changing social conditions and challenges. Other concerns have been raised about AOP. These include the oppositional stance embedded in AOP which may create obstacles to work in situations that require careful negotiation and compromise for workable outcomes to be reached on behalf of service users (Healy 2005a). The principle of minimal intervention promoted in the UK approach (Dalrymple & Burke 1995; Healy 2005a) in response to the perceived oppressive effects of social work intervention can also be problematic as it does not provide for a way of prioritising the needs of service users when these are in conf ict (see for example, Healy 2005a: 189–90).

Yet again, other recent writers from within a critical tradition have deplored the shift away from attention to structural issues and consider new ways of collectivising people's problems. For example, Trevor Spratt (2005), drawing on his experiences in the child welfare system in the United Kingdom, endeavours to link common experiences of oppression with their sources through methods derived from radical drama. Spratt uses forum theatre with schoolchildren to raise their collective awareness of oppression and to develop solutions.

Thoroughly disillusioned with the developments of the Third Way under Tony Blair and New Labour in Britain, and sceptical about the direction of intellectual ideas and their implications for social work, Iain Ferguson (2008) also suggests a re-emphasis on collective strategies, especially at the global level. Ferguson f rmly rejects postmodernism as a plausible theoretical basis for the struggle against oppression and injustice. In contrast to Mullaly and Baines, he voices concern that the inf uence of postmodern ideas in social work and social policy actually leads to a neglect of issues of inequality and oppression. Drawing from the successful social movements of recent times—in particular, the anti-capitalist or global justice movement and the mental health service users' movement in the United Kingdom—Ferguson sees the value of 'unity in diversity' and proposes, amongst other things, that social workers should develop the use of community work, group work and social networking approaches to draw together very disparate groups of people in the name of a common cause. He also urges social workers to reclaim a structural understanding of society, eroded in recent years due to a lessened emphasis on the part played by the structural determinants of service users' lives, and to reclaim the political through 'analysis of social work's role within the State and society' (Ferguson 2008: 132–6). Ferguson does not dismiss the therapeutic encounter, and indeed encourages reclaiming the signif cance of the worker–service user relationship, but his real interest is in building a social movement in which social workers and service users alike can be involved.

Implications for critical social work theories

Although challenged by postmodernism's questioning of grand narratives, critical social work's concern for addressing issues of social justice and equality continues to be pertinent in a world in which personal and social oppression persists unabated. While the foregoing discussion reveals different ways of understanding critical social work, several core principles that are common to these different positions have emerged:

- a commitment to work towards greater social justice and equality for those who are oppressed and marginalised within society
- a commitment to working alongside oppressed and marginalised populations
- an analysis of power relations which serve to marginalise and oppress particular populations in society

- a commitment to question taken-for-granted and dominant assumptions and beliefs
- an orientation towards emancipatory personal and social change.

As we have seen, although the differing approaches seek the transformation of social structures and institutions with attention to power relations in society, they place different emphases on the various systems of oppression and underline different ways for achieving change, ref ecting the complexities of contemporary social work practice.

So where does this leave us? Structural approaches informed by modernist ideas provide a lens for challenging social injustice and inequality through social transformation. They emphasise the need to consider injustice and inequality, and provide ways for analysing and strategising responses to disadvantage, particularly at the broad collective level. However, because of their universalist assumptions, they provide little guidance on understanding and dealing with difference within and between oppressed groups. For example, what does Ferguson's (2008) analysis of the mental health service user movement in the United Kingdom have to offer an analysis of such a movement in Australia?

Critical approaches informed by postmodern thinking, on the other hand, run the risk of overlooking or obscuring the material realities of disadvantage and injustice but raise questions about the 'truth' of a modernist approach, highlighting multiple oppressions, difference and the multiple sources and sites of power within a particular historical moment and cultural context. But as we have seen, some critical social work theorists are calling for reclaiming the structural, fearing that structural disadvantage and oppression are overlooked in the desire to acknowledge diversity and the operation of power at local levels. Other theorists have sought to abandon the dichotomy in the interests of drawing on the strengths of the different approaches. As Fook (2005: 237) has argued, it may be more constructive to focus on ways in which the different theoretical positions might be used to throw light on the problem at hand rather than continue to focus on the differences.

The issue here is how to hold together the different approaches and so practise in ways that pay attention to inequitable material arrangements and their impact on individuals and communities, at the same time heeding difference and diversity while maintaining an open, ref exive and self-critical stance. This means maintaining the tensions between the different positions and working with the contradictions, debates and uncertainties that emerge. In noting the various critical perspectives in social work, each of which offers its own solutions to the quest for empowering the oppressed and vulnerable, Pozzuto (2000) concludes that perhaps no singular answer is necessary or even possible. To have a f xed answer risks perpetuating the present into the future rather than supporting many alternative futures.

There are a number of challenges for critical social workers, which are addressed in a general sense in the principles outlined at the beginning of this section. More specif cally, a central concern—and one that has been a recurrent theme throughout this chapter—is that of how to achieve unity or solidarity amongst oppressed groups while recognising differences within and between them. How readily can solidarity in groups or movements be achieved to advocate for social change in Western societies where individualism is so dominant? Is resistance in small ways at local levels of any value? In the pursuit of social justice and equality, individuals who are disadvantaged and oppressed should at the very least be provided with opportunities to understand oppression within a socio-political framework and to benef t from that understanding. Does the provision of such opportunities at individual and local levels detract from or contribute to possibilities of unity on a much larger scale in social movements that perhaps have the greatest chance of achieving social change? The sorts of approaches (such as narrative work and forum theatre) that engage individuals and groups in addressing individual oppression and question 'taken-for-granted' knowledge can open up opportunities for awareness and action through the rejection of any determined nature of the world or people. In this regard, opportunities for these small-scale and local resistances are important, if individuals and groups are willing to participate, so that oppression at a local level is not perpetuated; such small-scale resistance may even contribute to building resistance more broadly. The mental health users' movement in Britain, for example, led by people with experience of mental ill-health and the psychiatric system and supported by professionals, grew from the development of mental health user groups. Collectively, these groups have contributed to, among other things, a growing recognition of the need for different service responses and to the involvement of service users in the development of new Scottish legislation (Ferguson 2008).

Another challenge that requires ongoing consideration is how to realistically promote social change in a neo-liberal context with its stringent managerial controls and accountabilities. A critical social worker understands that political struggle occurs everywhere and that exploring opportunities for advocacy, organisation and resistance is central. Drawing on her own experience and research undertaken with a small group of female Canadian frontline workers, Kristin Smith (2007) discovered various ways in which frontline workers in mainstream practice settings found spaces and gaps for the potential to resist in the face of heavy workloads, restricted resources and limited opportunities for advocacy and activism. Resistant practices able to be used in the interests of higher quality practices for clients included 'stealth social work practices' such as continuing to use policies and practices no longer off cially sanctioned in an organisation; practices that divert attention from resistance, such as silence and avoidance; and 'hidden and transitory coalitions' that involve building supports and networks within unwelcoming environments. Such strategies were found to provide some possibilities for democratic opposition in work arenas that are sites of signif cant struggle (Smith 2007). Baines (2007a) also notes that, to increase possibilities for social justice, managerial and supervisory positions need to be taken up by critical social workers, and students and practitioners should be better prepared for management positions. Drawing on the work of Yeatman (1998a), Healy (2001: 9–10) reminds us that we should not overlook the sometimes invisible effective forms of activist work that can be found among government bureaucrats.

Similar to the critique of anti-oppressive practice referred to earlier, critical ref exivity must be practised and caution is urged against any tendency for critical social workers to impose truths on others (Healy 2005b; McDonald 2006). Healy (2005b), for example, urges care to be taken against the 'will of truth' couched within a critical social worker's desire to emancipate others. In a similar vein, Baines (2007a) warns against concepts such as social location and identity being used in authoritarian ways in education and practice. When individuals identify themselves in particular ways, they can be demobilised by feeling that their fate has been predetermined, rather than using these ways as tools for understanding and learning how to use the privileges they might have to challenge everyday oppression.

Another challenge is to include the 'missing voices' in theorising critical social work. Much work is still to be done to incorporate the voices of clients and practitioners in this theorising. Such a development, Healy (2005b: 226) asserts, would enrich the theories and recognise differences between academics, clients and practitioners.

Conclusion

There are many challenges facing critical social work, a set of approaches that cannot be singularly def ned. Yet the passion for social justice and equality underpinning critical social work is what attracts many social workers concerned about injustice and oppression. It is out of the differences within critical social work and the challenges it faces that it will continue to evolve as a set of approaches aimed at moving towards a society which is more inclusive and supportive of the various groups within it. For critical social work to continue to be relevant in the challenging contemporary contexts, practitioners will do well to practise self-ref exively, to constantly ref ect on the interplay between their own knowledge and values and the situations that they encounter, as well as the economic, social and political contexts of which they and the marginalised people with whom they work are part. Pozzuto (2000) suggests that questions and possible solutions are not static. His words remain as pertinent as they ever did: 'the task of critical social work is to lift the veil of the present to see the possibilities of the future' (2000: 2).

4

from evidence-based practice to critical knowledge in post-positivist social work

Bob Pease

While critical social work theories have articulated the socially constructed nature of knowledge and moved away from positivism, science and experimental ways of knowing, social policy, public management and some forms of social work practice have moved in the opposite direction to embrace scientif c and evidence-based practice (Trinder 2000). Evidence-based practice in social work has been subjected to various criticisms from a critical theory perspective. However, few writers have explored the implications of these critiques for developing alternative epistemological foundations for critical social work practice. In this chapter, I consider the limitations of attempts to incorporate elements of evidence-based practice into critical social work. I argue that we need to develop an alternative knowledge base for critical social work, if it is to fulf l its emancipatory objectives.

Interrogating the evidence-based research and practice tradition in social work

Evidence-based practice 'encourages social workers to use empirically-tested methods of helping to formulate their reasoning and to evaluate their own work rigorously' (Munro 1998: 23). In this view, social work interventions should be based on the best evidence available (McDonald 2006). At f rst glance, it is hard to argue against the idea that social work should be based on evidence. However, the questions are: what constitutes evidence and who chooses it? Is the best evidence produced within a positivist social science paradigm? The reality is that there are competing claims as to what counts as evidence (Webb 2006). What must be remembered is that evidence-based practice is a construct. As a theoretical entity, it has to be operationalised (Westen & Bradley 2005). For critical social workers, it is a question of whether it contributes to social justice outcomes or not.

The dominant view of evidence-based practice originating in North America emphasises the importance of 'empirically supported' interventions that are able to be validated by research evidence through randomised controlled trials (RCTs). Randomised controlled trials have become accepted in medicine as providing the best evidence for medical interventions. They are at the top of the hierarchy of levels of evidence. There is thus an evidence-based pyramid with randomised controlled trials, cohort and case studies at the top of the pyramid and ideas and opinions at the bottom (Webb 2001).

So this form of evidence-based practice in the social work and counselling f elds is analogous to drug trials, and is thus predicated on a pharmaceutical model (Westen & Bradley 2005). Experimental methods in medicine are able to determine the effect of specif c chemical substances on the body. While it can be argued that patho-physiology and pharmacology can establish relationships between cause and effect in bodies and forms of treatment (Meagher 2002), how transferable are the principles of evidence-based medicine to the human services and social work (Marston & Watts 2003)? Feltman (2005) says that it is totally inappropriate to apply methods associated with physical medicine and drug-oriented treatment to therapy and counselling. Causality is more complex in counselling, and is less able to be isolated and experimentally controlled (Larner 2001).

Even within medicine, randomised controlled trials have their critics. Gupta (2003) argues that evidence-based medicine is not value neutral in that it takes certain values for granted. He points out that research on pharmaceuticals is expanding dramatically at the expense of other medical interventions, and that such research serves the drug companies and the health insurance providers. In the medical context, Griff ths (2005) expresses concern that interventions will be chosen because of their ability to be studied in RCTs. So vaccines as opposed to public health interventions will be favoured, for example.

Some doctors, however, are exploring the development of 'narrative-based medicine', where the individual narrative nature of illness is emphasised over and above population-derived evidence (Greenhalgh 1999; Carr et al. 2005). Greenhalgh (1999: 4) talks about the importance of subjective and intuitive aspects of clinical methods, and argues that 'genuine evidence-based practice actually presupposes an interpretative paradigm in which the patient experiences illness in a unique and contextual way'.

In the human services f eld, Witkin (1996) argues that evidence-based practice promotes individualism because interventions with individuals are easier to study in randomised controlled trials. Collective work and collective solutions are more diff cult to study in this way. How might community-development approaches that emphasise empowerment and participation be evaluated in relation to evidence where outcomes are hard to def ne? Furthermore, some critics of evidence-based practice have expressed concern about the lack of attention to consumer perspectives (Trinder 2000). Although there have recently been some moves to incorporate consumer views within the Cochrane collaboration (a research centre on evidence-based health care in the United States), consumer perspectives are not allowed to inform what is regarded as a scientif c process (Trinder 2000).

Any consideration given to the role of social and political forces on people's problems is likely to be denigrated as being unscientif c in an evidence-based framework. McDonald (2006) asks how, when working with Indigenous people, one could consider the impact of alienation or dispossession on people's lives within an evidence-based practice framework. How might the experiences of people with disabilities and others have their experiences validated by the epistemological standards of evidence-based practice? Listening to people's stories is an important source of knowledge. I have written elsewhere about how subjugated knowledge of service users can challenge the dominant discourses and resurrect subordinated knowledges (Pease 2002a).

The neo-liberal context of evidence-based practice

A number of commentators have identif ed a close connection between the rise of evidence-based practice and the development of neo-liberalism and the new managerialism (Webb 2001; McDonald 2006; Trinder 2000). McDonald (2006) argues that evidence-based practice can be understood as one particular response among others to the institutional upheaval and occupational instability of social work in the current context. She def nes neo-liberalism as a 'policy framework emphasising a shift from the traditional welfare state to a policy framework that focuses on creating the conditions for international competitiveness' (2006: 62). Neo-liberalism, with its emphasis on free-market economics, the privatisation of government services, free trade and user-pays services, has had a signif cant impact on human service provision. Welfare state provisions are cut back to allow for greater privatisation of human services with an emphasis on freedom of choice, small government, market values and individualism. One of the consequences of this is that the knowledge and professional judgement of practitioners is replaced by the authority of auditors and policy-makers (Davies 2003). Professional discretion is thus eroded by the changes in public service management.

Webb (2006: 38), writing in the UK context, says that 'neo-liberalism . . . monitors social welfare . . . to enforce public policy and systems of management on the basis of economic market rationality'. He argues that social work is being reconceptualised to f t in with neo-liberal strategies, giving the example of the impact of new public sector management on human service organisations where outcome-based targets and quality auditing of performance are emphasised. In Webb's (2006) view, evidence-based practice is used as a tool of public management to more effectively manage social workers and service users. Increasingly, the experiences of service users are reframed through classif cation systems based on scientif c management principles which purport to produce more eff cient use of resources and more effective outcomes.

There certainly are marked similarities between the goals of evidence-based practice and the new managerialism. Marston and Watts (2003) note that outcomes-based funding of non-government programs emphasises eff ciency as the primary political value over social justice. Evidence-based policy and practice are regarded as neutral concepts where policy-makers and practitioners will act on the 'hard facts'. The new managerialism assumes that social workers should specify their goals explicitly, select objective, evidence-based interventions for achieving them and measure the outcomes to see how successful they were (Davies 2003). In this view, there is a hidden managerialist agenda behind evidence-based practice that may have little to do with research f ndings, in spite of its claims to the contrary. Smith (2004), who is not a radical, acknowledges that managers could use the scientif c conception of evidence-based practice to privilege their view of what constitutes a good outcome.

McDonald (2006) suggests that one would expect evidence-based practice to f ourish in those countries where neo-liberalism is structuring the context of social work practice. The welfare state has undergone signif cant change in Australia in the context of the changing role of government, and this has shaped the ways in which social work is practised (McDonald et al. 2003). It has led to the contracting out of social services, cutbacks in services, increased government regulation of the community-based sector, a renewed focus on individualism, a loss of community and a declassif cation of social work positions.

One of the ways in which neo-liberalism works is by encouraging people to believe that they have no choices at the systemic level and that they need to make choices within the system (Davies et al. 2006). To develop a critical practice, social workers will need to engage in a systematic struggle against neo-liberalism. To begin, we need to become more aware of how our conceptions of practice are shaped by positivism.

Positivism, science and behavioural practice

Evidence-based practice must be seen in the historical context of attempts by social work theorists to formulate a scientif c foundation for social work practice in the context of the ongoing debate about whether social work is a science or an art (McDonald 2006). Thus any discussion of evidence-based practice must take place within an epistemological debate about the foundations of appropriate knowledge for social work (Gray & McDonald: 2006).

Most forms of evidence-based practice are located within a functionalist research paradigm and are based on positivist assumptions about the nature of social reality. In the positivist view, facts are independent of theory and are able to constitute knowledge on their own. Because evidence-based practice assumes that evidence is free of bias, numerous writers have identif ed a close association between evidence-based practice and behavioural social work and counselling (Witkin 1996; Webb 2001; Eisler 2002; Feltman 2005; Payne 2005; McDonald 2006). The main defenders of evidence-based practice in social work are all informed by cognitive-behavioural theories (Thyer 1989; Sheldon 2000; Gambrill 2001). Behaviourist theories of human behaviour provided the methods that could be most easily subjected to empirical validation and measurement by questionnaires. Such a methodological approach is even more dominant in psychology, where positivism and cognitive-behavioural theories underpin the model of the scientist-practitioner (Eisler 2002). It would also appear that evidence-based practice is primarily associated with DSM-IV categories of diagnosis (Feltman 2005). Other forms of counselling, such as family therapy and humanist approaches, do not lend themselves to step-by-step procedures that can easily be repeated and tested (Larner 2004).

The key question here is whether we can separate evidence from beliefs. Is it possible to have objective knowledge in the social sciences? As Gonzales et al. (2002) note, while the notion of scientif c evidence implies objectivity, it is also premised on epistemological assumptions and subjective understandings of what constitutes reality and what should be studied. Witkin (1996) challenges the view that evidence is value neutral, arguing that RCTs are located within a theoretical framework and value system that is unacknowledged by its adherents and that inf uences the reality it seeks to understand. Such an approach, for example, is based upon the premise that individuals are 'self-contained units' rather than 'products of relational forces' (Trinder 2000: 151). This view of the individual as a rational and autonomous being is consistent with individualism, whereby social work practice is def ned as a rational project with behavioural objectives and measurable outcomes. The issue is, to what extent can we apply a positivist epistemology to understand human behaviour when individuals make sense of the world through their subjective experiences?

From an interpretativist or constructionist perspective, there is no such thing as an objective world or objective knowledge. In this view, all knowledge is located within an historical, cultural and political context and is shaped by the experiences and values of those who create it (McNeill 2006). There is thus no such thing as 'the' evidence. Evidence-based practice does not recognise the competing epistemological assumptions about knowledge and the contested nature of social reality (McDonald 2003). Because positivists have such a narrow view of science, they are unable to engage with knowledge derived from constructivism, critical theory or postmodernism. Positivists do not seem able to grasp the reality that single system designs and RCTs are also partial ways of understanding the world (Gray & McDonald 2006).

In arguing against the dominant view of evidence, I am not suggesting that knowledge derived from empirical methods should be rejected. Clearly, survey data, longitudinal studies and off cial statistics can be important sources of information about oppression and discrimination (Oakley 2000). As someone who is committed to social justice, I am interested in empirical data about the experiences of oppression and marginalisation, and how they are connected to institutionalised processes of discrimination. What I am challenging here is the hegemonic status given to experimental ways of knowing above other approaches to knowledge development.

Oakley (2000) believes that quantitative and experimental ways of knowing can be reshaped to promote emancipatory purposes. Humphries (2008) also argues that concerns about experimental methods are more to do with the ways in which they are used than the methods themselves. She says that such methods can be used effectively to measure inequality and disadvantage. The problem for her is that when they are used to inform policy and practice, they tend to concentrate on individual and behavioural risk factors. However, quantitative methods are not value-free techniques. The questions asked in surveys and the assumptions underpinning randomised controlled trials are value laden and interest driven. Furthermore, not all forms of knowledge can be measured by quantitative methods. We need to be aware of other paradigms and different ways of knowing to understand why and how any research has political and ethical dimensions (D'Cruz & Jones 2004).

Social constructionism, qualitative social work and reflective practice

It is important to acknowledge that there is a distinction between narrow forms of evidence-based practice which rely solely on scientif c evidence and randomised controlled trials and others that recognise the importance of broader forms of knowledge and evidence. In recent years, we see some attempts to embrace a wider notion of knowledge that includes qualitative research and professional expertise (Eisler 2002). In what Trinder (2002) calls the 'pragmatist version of evidence-based practice', a much looser def nition of evidence is adopted and the notion of a hierarchy of evidence is challenged.

Some advocates of evidence-based practice have argued for the inclusion of qualitative research as sources of evidence. Larner (2004) says that it is not a choice between science and non-science but rather between a narrow positivist construction of science which only recognises RCTs, and a wider notion of evidence that includes qualitative evidence. Writing from within psychology, he argues that therapy is both science and art, and advocates the development of a 'systemic-practitioner model' that utilises both quantitative and qualitative research. Certainly, some researchers use the language of 'evidence-based practice' as inclusive of qualitative methods (Meagher 2002). Such approaches constitute better versions of evidence-based practice than the narrow positivist-based models.

From an interpretative perspective, social work practice and research are value-based rather than technical activities. Gray and McDonald (2006: 15) emphasise the importance of ethical reasoning in social work and argue that social work is primarily 'a practical-moral activity'. Most social workers emphasise the importance of values in interpreting the world. Many practitioners are concerned that scientif c knowledge will take attention away from the caring and emotional dimensions of social work where the importance of humanistic responses, feelings and interpersonal relationships is valued.

Taylor and White (2000) locate evidence-based practice in the context of technical rationality as the dominant form of professional knowledge. Donald Schön (1983) argued over 25 years ago that technical knowledge was unable to address the complexity of professional work and unable to access the tacit knowledge that informed practice. Drawing upon Polanyi's (1958) notion of tacit knowledge as habits and cultural ideas that individuals do not recognise in themselves, Schön demonstrated how knowledge internalised, often unconsciously through experiences, shaped professional practice.

Webb (2001) makes the point that practice involves a 'ref ective deliberating process' whereby practitioners choose courses of action from a range of alternative possibilities informed by theoretical understandings and values. Trinder (2000) refers to this as 'the art of practice', emphasising professional expertise and judgement over scientif c evidence. In this view, professional practice is a form of artistry (Taylor & White 2005).

In empirically supported versions of evidence-based practice, social workers use knowledge developed by experts by applying it to practice. In this view, social workers are not the makers of knowledge (Healy 2005a). An alternative tradition in social work for the development of practice knowledge is critical ref ection and ref ective practice. In recent years, the literature on critical ref ection has grown signif cantly in social work and human service practice (Fook 1999; Morley 2004; Yip 2006a). The professional social worker is encouraged to be critical and ref ective about the assumptions underpinning his or her practice. In particular, professionals are asked to critically ref ect upon how their values and theories are inf uenced by the social and political context of practice (Yip 2006a). In this view, importance is placed on recognising 'practitioners' lived experience or practice as a basis for making and using knowledge' (Healy 2005a). Fook (2004), for example, argues the case for narrative and ref ective methods to analyse practitioners' accounts of their practice as a contribution to knowledge development. Feltman (2005) also suggests inverting evidence-based practice by developing practice-based evidence.

Avis (2006) argues that it is important to construct an epistemology for critical ref ection that can provide an alternative to randomised controlled trials. In this view, critical ref ection is seen as a form of 'expert practice' that is able to interpret the diversity of evidence before making a decision about how to intervene. Thus we need to develop an 'an epistemology of practice' that recognises and validates ways of knowing that are embedded in professional practice (Clegg 1999). I have suggested elsewhere that this ref exivity should be extended to encompass the privileged positionings of the professional worker (Pease 2006a).

Plath (2006) believes that it is possible to blend critical ref ective approaches with evidence-based practice, arguing that practitioners utilise both sources of knowledge in their practice. However, where other forms of evidence and knowledge are recognised, randomised controlled trials are still regarded by most adherents of evidence-based practice as 'the gold standard'. Can evidence-based practice incorporate other forms of knowledge and values alongside scientif c knowledge without being devalued when references to practitioner-based knowledge and service users views are regarded as 'grey literature' (literature which has not formally been published)? (Feltman 2005). Beresford (2000) has documented the ways in which service users' knowledge and viewpoints have been marginalised and validated in the United Kingdom. In Australia, the Human Rights and Equal Opportunity Commission report on the Stolen Generations (Wilson 1997) was rejected by the federal government because it relied on oral testimony as the main form of evidence.

Moving beyond the quantitative–qualitative divide

As discussed earlier, the debate over what constitutes appropriate evidence and knowledge in social work is located in the wider divisions between positivists/objectivists and interpretivists/subjectivists about the nature of social reality. This debate between universalism and relativism has plagued the social sciences for many years. From an interpretivist perspective, positivism does not have a valid claim to objective knowledge. Social constructivists and postmodernists have emphasised the importance of seeing science and knowledge as being socially constructed (Lopez & Potter 2001). Thirty years ago, Burrell and Morgan (1979) maintained that objectivist and subjectivist paradigms were incommensurable. Those who hold to purist positivist and constructivist perspectives will certainly maintain that there is no possibility for accommodation between the epistemological paradigms.

From a critical social work perspective, if there is no objective reality, how can we develop the foundations for emancipatory projects? Parker (2001) argues that an uncritical pluralism undermines progressive social movements. It carries the danger of leading to what some writers refer to as the 'abyss of relativism' (Peile & McCouat 1997; Sheppard 1998; Taylor & White 2000). The relativist position considers all views equally valid, and does not allow us to develop standards to determine what is just or unjust. Alston and Bowles (2003) argue that critical social work research needs to be situated between purist objectivist and subjectivist approaches. In rejecting positivism's deductive scientif c method for studying experience, we should not reject a realist ontology that acknowledges an objective reality. As I argue later, realism provides an alternative paradigm to the positivist–constructivist divide. Thus, in critical social work, we need to transcend the limitations of these objective–subjective and universalist–relativist dichotomies.

As a critical social work theorist, I acknowledge the existence of an external reality. My concerns are more about the ways in which positivism and evidence-based practice have been used to maintain repressive regimes of power (Strega

2005). We should be careful to untangle a critique of positivism on political grounds from a critique of all realist post-positivist perspectives.

Realist and constructivist epistemologies can both be used for conservative and progressive political purposes. Thus, the epistemological dimensions of paradigms can support a variety of different political positions (Firestone 1990). However, I argue here that the transformative agenda of critical theory, in either its realist or constructivist guise, is incommensurable with those paradigm positions which argue for detached and disinterested research and practice. I thus argue against Padgett (1998), who believes that methodological rigour is compromised by advocacy-based research. I also disagree with Hammersley (1997), who argues that the political goal of emancipation undermines the legitimacy of research as the objective production of knowledge, as if this objectivity were possible. I rather believe that social workers should take sides and embrace the values of promoting social justice and human rights.

Critical social work, liberatory knowledge and participatory research

Critical social work is thus based on an alternative paradigm which challenges both the epistemological assumptions of positivism and the relativist underpinnings of the interpretative approach. In this context, Taylor and White (2000) distinguish between ref ectiveness and ref exivity. By ref exivity, they mean theoretically informed interrogations of practice that go beyond personal ref ection. Evidence-based practice advocates argue that the scientist-practitioner and the evidence-supportive models of practice are theory free. They argue that you can eliminate theoretical bias by technical means. Positivism has developed in such a way that facts are treated as independent of theory and capable on their own of leading to knowledge.

However, critical theorists regard research and practice as political processes and theory neutrality as a myth. As Mitchell (1999: 33) observes, 'all thinking is theoretical and value laden'. But evidence-based practice seems unable to recognise that practice is guided by theory, values and critically ref ective practice wisdom. In this view, 'evidence' on its own is unable to provide a direction for practice. How does one make sense of the competing empirical evidence? Only theory can offer explanations of the factors shaping individuals' experiences.

Theory, whether it refers to broad social theories concerned with the socio-cultural context and individuals' experiences of oppression or theories of practice that are focused on strategies for intervention, is very important for social work practice. One of the reasons that theory is important is that it enables social workers to identify aspects of a situation that may be unseen. Its usefulness is judged by its power to explain what is going on (Houston 2001).

As I have outlined, critical social theory is concerned with challenging oppression and inequality. This paradigm informs empowerment, anti-oppressive and critical ref ective approaches to social work practice. Critical social workers thus need to have knowledge of political and structural issues such as poverty, violence and discrimination (Scheyett 2006), and critical theories to understand them—what McDonald (2005) calls 'oppositional knowledge'. Critical social workers would argue also that values associated with challenging oppression are more compelling than those values traditionally associating with 'helping' (McNeill 2006). In this view, practice involves not only the application of knowledge but also the expression of values about the society that we live in.

Such an approach leads to the development of practice that is informed by consumer knowledge where consumers are full participants in the creation of knowledge. Participatory approaches to research are concerned with the involvement of consumers in formulating the research questions and in determining whether their interests are served by the research (Scheyett 2006). Such participatory research is essential if social work is to promote equality and social justice (Meagher 2002).

Critical realism as an epistemological foundation for critical social work practice

What would be the epistemological foundations for such knowledge? In recent years, a number of writers have argued that critical realism provides an alternative to these divisions (Sheppard 1998; Lopez & Potter 2001; Wright 2002). Critical realism acknowledges that knowledge is socially and culturally situated, but at the same time asserts that an objective reality exists. This theoretical approach was f rst developed by Bhaskar (1978) in the 1970s to challenge the assumptions underpinning both empiricism and social constructionism. In this context, others have suggested that critical realism provides the basis for an alternative to evidence-based policy and practice generally (Pawson 2002; Sanderson 2002; Clegg 2005; Wilson 2006), as well as providing a foundation for critical social work specif cally (Houston 1995, 2001; Mantysaari 2005).

Wright (2004) sums up critical realism as comprising three basic premises: that a reality exists outside of human perception; that our ability to comprehend such a reality requires subjective understanding; and that reality cannot be understood without critical and ref exive thinking that goes beyond the positivist notion of scientif c detachment. So, while there is an independent reality, research cannot accurately observe it (Parker 2001). Nor can we comprehend it, as much of it is hidden from our view. Cooling (2005) maintains that critical realism enables us to retain the possibility of human knowledge of the world while at the same time acknowledging the provisional nature of that knowledge. Because human beings produce knowledge, they can be wrong. Unexamined assumptions and ideology can distort knowledge. Thus we should be cautious and critically interrogate claims about both subjective knowledge and objective evidence.

Critical realism seems to offer a reconciliatory position between positivism and social constructionism (Houston 1995; Wilson 2006). McNeil (2006) formulates this as a 'humble realism' in that, although multiple realities are acknowledged as people endeavour to make sense of the social world, an external world does still exist even if we can only understand it in partial ways. While on the one hand we need to develop tolerance with respect to knowledge, on the other we need to take a position from which to challenge dominant and oppressive forms of knowledge (Parker 2001). In a critical realist approach, knowledge should serve the purpose of emancipatory practice (Clegg 2005; Wilson 2006). In this sense, 'evidence' outside of its narrow positivist connotations can be used for social critique and emancipatory projects (Hollway 2001; Marston & Watts 2003; Clegg 2005). As Peile and McCouat (1997) acknowledge, critical theorists do not see their analyses just sitting alongside political conservative positions. From a critical realist position, some theoretical explanations of the world are more accurate than others, and there are therefore rational grounds for preferring one theory over others (Cooling 2005). Thus critical realism does not celebrate all forms of difference and diversity, and it actively challenges anti-democratic and oppressive discourses (Connelly 2001).

Conclusion

Can evidence-based practice inform critical social work? Alternatively, are there possibilities other than the dominant form of evidence-based practice? Petr and Walter (2005) advocate a model of best practice that includes qualitative research, professional practice wisdom, consumer perspectives and a value-critical analysis of research. Brown (2006), in defence of a feminist model, also stresses the importance of drawing upon multiple forms of knowledge claims such as the above. Feltman (2005) suggests developing practice-based evidence, while Larner (2001) talks about the critical practitioner model to challenge the scientist-practitioner model.

While I accept that there are attempts to widen what counts as evidence, I am reluctant to locate my proposal for a critical knowledge base for social work within the language of evidence-based practice because it relegates non-positivist knowledge to the margins. At this historical moment, I do not believe that evidence-based practice can provide the best basis for a critical social work practice that is concerned with social justice and social change. I propose instead that critical social workers develop the foundation for 'critical knowledge-informed practice'[1] to encompass critical social theory, quantitative and qualitative research, tacit knowledge, critical ref ective practice, social justice values and consumer-based knowledge. In my view, only a valuing of knowledge from diverse sources that is driven by a commitment to social transformation will enable social work to fulf l its emancipatory objectives.

5

promoting a human rights perspective on critical social work

Sharlene Nipperess and Linda Briskman

Human rights are a contemporary global discourse. Even though ideas about human rights have been around for a long time (Wronka 1992; Ishay 1997; Freeman 2005), they have attained particular signif cance recently due to the social, cultural and economic inequality exacerbated by globalisation (Jones & Kriesler 1998; Rees & Wright 2000; Ife 2008a). The social work profession is participating in this global discourse. At an international level, the International Federation of Social Work (IFSW) has developed policy on social work and human rights, and with the International Association of Schools of Social Work (IASSW) it has agreed to a def nition of social work that specif cally states that human rights are fundamental to social work. At a national level, the Australian Association of Social Workers (AASW), in its *Code of Ethics*, makes several commitments to human rights and this is replicated by many other nations' codes of ethics.

However, despite the global discourse and the obvious importance that the social work profession has given to human rights, relatively little has been written about what social work in relation to human rights looks like, or indeed how social work academics should include human rights in the curriculum. Apart from the comprehensive work of Ife (2008a), the relationship between human rights and critical social work remains largely unexplored.

This chapter provides a human rights perspective on critical social work. It argues that the concept of human rights, though highly contested and problematic in many ways, makes an important contribution to critical social work and integrates with a range of critical theory and practice paradigms. Specif cally, the chapter explores the commitment of social work to human rights, the place of the United Nations Declaration of Human Rights, the contestation that exists in seeking common human rights principles and the synergies between critical social work and human rights.

Human rights and social work

The social work profession in Australia and internationally has a stated commitment to human rights and interest in a human rights approach for practice has intensif ed in recent times, although remaining underdeveloped.

The literature is clear about the commitment of the social work profession to the idea of human rights, and this is demonstrated in a formal sense in key policy documents and through the professional writings of some practitioners and academics. However, when the idea of human rights is raised it is often discussed cursorily and sometimes simplistically in relation to the United Nations (UN) Universal Declaration of Human Rights (UDHR). While not wishing to diminish the signif cance of the UDHR, it is also important to understand the ways in which the concept of human rights is contested. Only a handful of social workers have engaged with the critique of human rights and it is this dialogue which is vitally important to a critical social work perspective on human rights. One of the perceived barriers for social work in embracing human rights is that the concept is often seen as belonging in the legal domain, which can inhibit social work explorations of its relevance, including as discursive practice.

A stated commitment to human rights

The Australian Association of Social Workers (AASW) *Code of Ethics* (1999) makes numerous statements about the commitment of social work to human rights, and these statements are supported at the international level by the two peak social work organisations, the International Federation of Social Work (IFSW) and the International Association of Schools of Social Work (IASSW).

In Australia, the commitment to human rights is stated very clearly in the AASW *Code of Ethics* in the discussion of the Purpose of Social Work:

> The social work profession subscribes to the principles and aspirations of the *United Nations Declaration of Human Rights* and other international conventions derived from that Declaration (AASW 1999: 5).

The AASW *Code of Ethics* (1999) further explores and explicates this commitment to human rights in its discussion of the core values and principles that underpin social work in Australia. With respect to the value Human Dignity and Worth, Principle (b) states that:

> Social Workers respect the basic human rights of individuals and groups as expressed in *The United Nations Universal Declaration of Human Rights* and other international conventions derived from that Declaration (AASW 1999: 8).

Human rights are also clearly discussed in the value Social Justice where Principles (d) and (e) respectively state:

> Social Workers espouse the cause of human rights, aff rming that civil and political rights must be accompanied by economic, social and cultural rights; and
>
> Social Workers oppose and work to eliminate all violations of human rights (AASW 2002: 8).

These statements made by the AASW in the *Code of Ethics* are supported by the IFSW, which developed an International Policy on Human Rights that was approved by the IFSW General Meeting in 1996. The policy states in part:

> The social work profession accepts its share of responsibility for working to oppose and eliminate all violations of human rights. Social workers must exercise this responsibility in their practice with individuals, groups and communities, in their roles as agency or organisational representatives and as citizens of a nation and the world (IFSW 1998: 56).

Finally, in 2001, the IASSW and the IFSW reached agreement on a def nition of social work. The one-paragraph def nition ends with a specif c reference to human rights by stating that 'principles of human rights and social justice are fundamental to social work' (IASSW 2008).

Codes of ethics and policy statements by themselves are simply the 'public' declaration of the values, principles and ethics that underpin a profession, in this case social work. However, it appears that this stated commitment to social work at the Australian and international level is ref ected in the professional writings of Australian and international social workers. As it is clearly stated in one contemporary Australian social work textbook, 'the social work profession has always had a steadfast commitment to ideals of social justice and a respect for human rights' (Alston & McKinnon 2005: 5). If we use the codes as a starting point then, as Mmatli (2008: 306) tells us, it is a dereliction of our professional duty not to comply with what Mullaly (1997) calls the promotion of political will to develop a humanised society. Understanding human rights can provide greater accountability in our practice, particularly in mounting challenges to inequitable policies at organisational and government levels.

As has already been noted, there is comparatively little social work literature relating to human rights, despite the importance of the concept, and much of it is explored in a fairly cursory manner. For example, it is common to talk about being committed to human rights without fully exploring what this actually means in theory or practice. However, there is a small collection of social work academics and practitioners who have considered the topic of human rights in detail, and this literature has increased signif cantly in the last ten years.

In Australia, a number of social work academics have explored human rights in relation to a broad range of issues including people seeking asylum, Indigenous peoples, families and social work education, to name a few (Swensen 1995; George 1999; Rees & Wright 2000; Solas 2000; Yeatman 2000; Boulet 2003; Mason 2005; Briskman 2007a; 2007b; Briskman & Fiske 2008; Briskman et al. 2008). In addition, the theme of human rights runs through much of Ife's work (1997, 1999, 2002), most notably in his texts that are dedicated solely to human rights and social work practice (2001, 2008a). At an international level, one of the earliest publications on human rights and social work, *Teaching and Learning about Human Rights*, was produced by the United Nations Centre for Human Rights (1992), in cooperation with the IFSW and the IASSW. Reichert explores social work and human rights in America in a number of texts (2003, 2006, 2007a) and her most recent book (2007) brings together a collection of international social work writers on the topic, the f rst of its kind. In addition, an escalating number of authors have contributed to international journals, in particular *International Social Work*, on human rights and social work.

However, regardless of whether the literature explores human rights in detail or simply discusses human rights at a superf cial level, the literature clearly demonstrates that social workers in Australia consider human rights to be a powerful perspective for social work. As Solas notes, 'it is evident that commitment to the protection of human rights exists, and that it is particularly in evidence among those who practice activist social work . . . what remains in question and very much in contention is what it means to believe in human rights' (2000: 65, 66).

The Universal Declaration of Human Rights

According to much of the literature, 'what it means to believe in human rights' is consistent with the United Nations (UN) Universal Declaration of Human Rights (UDHR), which was proclaimed in 1948. There appears to be an uncritical acceptance of our commitment to human rights and the concomitant association of human rights with the various United Nations Declarations, Covenants and Treaties. George (1999: 15) states that 'human rights are rather like motherhood. Ask people if they support human rights they will usually say "Yes, of course!", just as we all say "motherhood is a good thing".' In the same way, most of the social work literature discusses human rights in a superf cial manner—in a way which simply presumes that there is such an entity as human rights and social workers can and should be involved in the important work of protecting and promoting these rights (Blaskett 1998; Alston 2000). When human rights are discussed, it is almost always in reference to the various UN declarations, specif cally the UDHR (United Nations Centre for Human Rights 1992; Korr et al. 1994).

It was in 1948 that the General Assembly of the UN proclaimed the UDHR. In the 30 articles of this declaration, a range of civil, political, social, cultural, economic and collective/solidarity rights are articulated. It is a powerful statement, one that is still inspiring despite the passage of 60 years, and it has been a guiding force for some social workers. It was not until the formation of the United Nations that the term 'human rights' began to be used, and after the horrors of the Second World War, the world's nations were able to surmount considerable diff culties and agreed to the UDHR, the f rst comprehensive statement of human rights. The UDHR, the International Covenant of Civil and Political Rights 1966 and the International Covenant on Economic, Social and Cultural Rights 1966 comprise the International Bill of Rights. Since the UDHR was proclaimed in 1948 there has been a plethora of human rights conventions and treaties declared by the UN, many of particular interest to social workers, including United Nations Declaration on the Elimination of All Forms of Racial Discrimination, Convention on the Elimination of All Forms of Discrimination against Women, Convention on the Rights of the Child, Convention against Torture and Other Cruel, Inhuman or Degrading Treatment or Punishment, Convention on the Rights of Persons with Disabilities and Convention Relating to the Status of Refugees.

Essentially, human rights are those entitlements that people possess simply by virtue of their humanity. The emphasis on humanity indicates that human rights are usually considered to be *universal*—that is, they belong to everyone, regardless of their gender, age, ethnicity, religion or sexual orientation, simply on the basis of being human. Human rights are also considered to be *indivisible* because they are all equally important. Finally, human rights are considered to be *inalienable* because another person, government, organisation or other entity cannot take them away (though, as Amnesty International and other human rights organisations remind us, this does not mean that human rights cannot be violated).

It is not surprising that the social work profession discusses human rights largely in relation to the UDHR and the other UN documents. Codes of Ethics provide the mandate to do this by stating that social workers are specif cally committed to these documents. However, while presented as relatively unproblematic in the literature, even the most perfunctory review of the wider human rights literature demonstrates the contested nature of the concept.

A contested understanding

The UDHR implies a search for common principles of humanity that apply to everyone regardless of class, gender, ethnicity, age, ability and religion. As Ife notes (2008a: 9), 'it is an impressive and inspirational statement, with signif cant radical implications, and it has been used in many ways since to further many important causes in the name of humanity'. But at the same time, it is important to understand that there is a signif cant critique of the UDHR specif cally and the concept of human rights more generally, in particular the claim of cultural imperialism.

The claim that human rights are culturally imperialist represents one of the main critiques of human rights. This critique of human rights essentially revolves around the argument put forth by 'universalists' and the 'cultural relativists'. A universalist position argues that human rights should be adopted by peoples and cultures all over the world. Conversely, 'cultural relativists' contend that the notion of human rights is based on Western ideas and cultures and is therefore not applicable to non-Western cultures. As Goodhart (2005) notes, 'this debate pits universalists, who hold that human rights ref ect timeless and absolute moral truths, against cultural relativists, who assert that moral truth or validity is an expression of the values and beliefs of a particular culture' (2005: 353).

Cultural relativists and others argue that human rights are a Western construct, arising out of Enlightenment/modernist thinking, which if imposed on the rest of the world results in another example of Western colonisation (Ife 2008a). It is argued that many principles underpinning this philosophical tradition, such as liberal individualism, are not part of the culture of many non-Western peoples and that the 'universality' of human rights is an ideological disguise for 'cultural imperialism' (Freeman 2002: 102).

Modern Western thinkers have clearly inf uenced much of the thinking on human rights. However, this should not mean that the idea of human rights is irrelevant to the rest of the world. Furthermore, to argue that human rights f rst emerged in modern times and in the West does two things. First, it ignores the fact that notions of human rights have been discussed for millennia, and second, it ignores the fact that cultures other than those in the West have contributed to this dialogue. The term 'human rights' is a fairly recent development but the idea of human rights has a long history, one that is not exclusively Western (Freeman 2005).

Contemporary understandings of human rights have been shaped by ideas that have been debated and discussed since antiquity in a range of cultures and religions. Notions of human rights can be found in the diverse writings of early philosophers such as Plato, Aristotle and Cicero, in the Enlightenment treatises of Thomas Hobbes, John Locke, Mary Wollstonecraft and others, and in the challenges to the liberalist ideology of the Enlightenment mounted by Industrial Age thinkers, including famously Karl Marx and Friedrich Engels (Ishay 1997). The humanist strand that informs many of the world's major religions, such as Buddhism, Christianity, Islam and Judaism, has also contributed enormously to modern ideas of human rights (Ishay 1997). Secular philosophies, such as Confucianism, also consider key moral and ethical issues relating to the meaning of humanity (Freeman 2005). Numerous legal and legislative documents also exist, such as the Magna Carta (1215), the English Bill of Rights (1689) and the United States Declaration of Independence (1776), which include some of the ideas central to the human rights discourse (Ishay 1997).

The cultural relativist position, on the other hand, has been criticised for allowing human rights violations in the name of culture. Relativists have been criticised for essentialising cultures and for assuming that cultures do not change, as well as for seeing cultures as homogeneous. The reality is that 'cultures are complex, variable, multivocal, and above all contested. Rather than being static things, "cultures" are f uid complexes of intersubjective meanings and practices' (Donnelly 2003: 86).

Ife (2007, 2008a) argues that conceptualising the debate in terms of a dichotomy is not helpful. If one views the debate in terms of polar opposites or extremes, there is no solution—a 'naïve' universalism can lead to colonialism and a 'naïve' relativism can lead to the uncritical acceptance of all practices on the basis of culture. Ife states:

> To move beyond this, the challenge is to develop an approach to the universalism of human rights that, while emphasizing our common 'humanity' and seeking to

> articulate what that humanity means, at the same time acknowledges different cultural traditions as providing different contexts within which that humanity is constructed (2007: 94).

For social workers, these debates can cause tensions in practice. As Allan (2003) explains, both social justice and human rights notions as moral concepts are problematic in their attempts to hold a universal value while valuing diversity and giving voice to oppressed and marginalised populations with which social workers engage. Globally, we are observing what Kundnani (2007), in the British context, refers to as the end of tolerance, and in Australia we have seen evidence of this in a range of policy arenas that are antithetical to human rights, including in the spheres of people movements, Indigenous rights and entrenched inequalities.

Critical social work and human rights

Is a human rights approach consistent with other critical approaches to social work? We argue that it is, and that one can inform the other. Human rights frameworks do not replace more established theorising. As well as being expressed in codes of ethics, a human rights vision builds on other emancipatory theories with particular reference to minority group rights (Cemlyn 2008). As such, other theoretical constructs and the social work value base can provide a basis for the integration of human rights perspectives, which can meld, for example, with anti-racist, feminist, structural, critical postmodern and postcolonial approaches. However, there are contradictions for social workers in implementing human rights approaches, including the complexities of balancing personal, professional and political issues, and operating within constrained environments (Cemlyn 2008) where practice ideals may be subsumed by the reality of everyday organisational practice (Lymberry & Butler 2004). Despite the rhetoric of social justice and rights, human services delivery is often framed within welfarist and needs-based paradigms (Briskman 2007b), resulting in an apparent clash of paradigms. Critical social work can be enhanced by the recognition that human rights violations can unwittingly be embedded in social work practice and policy documents that inform practice. With human rights to the forefront, practitioners can gain conf dence in advocating more robustly for groups with which they engage as they witness human rights violations and identify human rights prospects.

Many groups with which social workers come into contact have struggled with having their rights realised and use human rights frameworks to advance their humanity, which is often rejected by the mainstream. Groups may be struggling for civil and political rights (known as f rst-generation rights), economic social and economic rights (second-generation rights) or collective rights such as self-determination for colonised peoples (third-generation rights) or a combination of all. Furthermore, there is an urgency to ensure that the next generation of social workers is cognisant of human rights with intensifying concern about how the forces of neo-liberalism, unfettered capitalism and globalisation marginalise such groups as people with disabilities, Indigenous peoples and refugees (Briskman & Fiske 2008). Human rights approaches to social work hence become political practice in the challenge to dominant paradigms and policies that detract from the wellbeing of all peoples.

The f eld of disability is one area where a human rights perspective has come to the forefront. The human rights component in the disability lobby has helped raise the status of people with disabilities as well as helping to raise the consciousness of social workers (Bainbridge 1999). Rioux and Zubrow (2001) challenge the way in which people with disabilities have been constructed, and advocate moving from individual pathologising to a human rights approach. For Rioux and Zubrow, this approach sees 'treatment' from outside a bio-medical lens and through reformulation of economic, social and political policy. The adoption by the United Nations General Assembly of the Convention on the Rights of Persons with Disabilities, to which Australia is a signatory, should have a positive impact on a disability rights discourse.

In social work with Indigenous peoples, a human rights discourse is of fundamental importance. It is not possible to work with Indigenous Australians without understanding the context of their rights struggles, which are asserted in international forums and in policy advocacy within Australia. The violation of rights is apparent in a range of policy formulations applied to Indigenous peoples, where they are subject to policies and practices that are not expected of others (see Chapter 8 for examples). Adopting postcolonial theoretical approaches that shed Western dominance, combined with anti-racist practice at the institutional level, fosters an integration of human rights with other critical social work theories (Briskman 2007a).

Increasingly, social workers have contact with asylum seekers and refugees, a group that struggles for acceptance. For those men, women and children who have experienced immigration detention, there has been a denial of the most basic of civil rights and experience of loss of liberty. For those refugees and others who arrive through the humanitarian program, they frequently struggle to have their economic and social rights realised as they make their way through Australian society, where community and institutional racism are apparent. Martin (2006) proposes emancipatory practices and resistance to discourses that lead to discrimination and oppression. An understanding of these factors is a precursor to social work human rights engagement, whether at the level of direct practice, policy or advocacy. It is in the advocacy realm that social workers have taken a lead by exposing malevolent policies that breach human rights standards and are antithetical to social work values and ethics (Briskman et al. 2008).

The rights of children are of fundamental importance to social workers, as many work in the f eld of child and family services. The UN Convention on the Rights of the Child is a benchmark that can provide guidance for a human rights social worker. No person or group can feel secure in their own human rights when the rights of any children are violated (Atkinson 2008). It is in this area where a rights focus often lags as social workers become immersed in day-to-day practice complexities, particularly in child protection. In the three practice areas mentioned above, child rights need to be at the forefront. For children with disabilities, there is the question of ensuring access to the basic economic and social rights that are afforded to other children, including education and later employment. For Indigenous peoples, there remain memories of the forcible removal of their children from their families, which denied the rights of Indigenous families to raise their own children. These rights are still not totally realised, as Indigenous children remain over-represented in the child welfare system; moreover, their cultural rights are often denigrated or ignored. The incarceration of children in immigration detention centres in Australia is one practice that has been loudly condemned, and is such a severe rights violation that two social work academics describe the policies and practices as organised and ritualised abuse (Goddard & Briskman 2004).

Increasingly, violence against women is seen as a human rights violation, and an international human rights movement advances this cause, which has become the centrepiece of the women's movement and of persistent activism (Merry 2006). It is beholden on social workers to challenge this violence *per se*, by arguing for its elimination on human rights grounds that can be enshrined in legislation and policy. The direct practice experience of social workers can combine with the advocacy of feminist movements in the quest to eliminate the violence locally and internationally.

Beyond the areas of practice, a human rights approach can give social workers the tools to analyse the world about them. Some of the policies and practices of concern may, at f rst glance, seem a world apart from everyday practice. Yet they are vital in forging connections for social workers between the wider, and often global, forces and the context of practice. These may include concerns about the environment and the precedence given to the economic over the social; animal rights, in which 'development' tramples on a variety of species around the globe; and the introduction of legislation in which civil rights are increasingly eroded since the attacks on New York and Washington on September 11, 2001. Furthermore, a human rights framework creates the understanding necessary in challenging continuing world and local poverty and the disparities between rich and poor, which represent a fundamental erosion of economic rights.

As Quinn (2003) explains, if social workers are to be committed to social change, justice, inclusion, diversity and participation, they must develop theories and practices that place to the foreground the social, political and economic power relations, as well as cultural relevance. We argue that the adoption of a human rights 'culture' within social work can go far in meeting these challenges, as well as avoiding co-option into a prevailing discourse that privileges individual rights and responsibilities.

Social work education

Human rights understandings are yet to f nd their way into social work curricula across the nation. Competing paradigms of knowledge and over-stretched curricula do not always open up for new explorations. However, it is in the sphere of social work education that there is a prospect of not only introducing theoretical and practice understandings of human rights, but demonstrating the links with a range of social work theories and their application to f elds of practice. Briskman and Fiske (2008) propose a schema for human rights education that incorporates the following components:

1. *Philosophical*—understanding the evolving of ideas of human rights across the centuries.
2. *Political*—acknowledging that the causes and solutions of many human rights issues belong in the political realm.
3. *Historical*—recognising that the historical foundations of human rights are necessary to understandings, particularly those which emerged since the formation of the United Nations.
4. *Anthropological*—accepting that, while the language of rights has its roots in European thought and history, concepts of human rights can be found in every religious and cultural tradition.
5. *Legal*—appreciating basic legal concepts vested in the domestic and international human rights system.
6. *Practical*—applying the understandings to critical social work practice.

In addition, educators can work with students on how to challenge policies and practices, including through responsive practice, policy inf uence and advocacy. Through critical ref ection, confronting the tensions associated with dual loyalty—to the organisation and to the client—can assist future social workers in grappling with questions of accountability, collusion and complicity, often underpinned by power relations which are seemingly invisible to the practitioner.

Conclusion

A human rights approach does not require a total revamp of theory and practice, as there is arguably coherence with other critical social work tenets. However, social workers are not always equipped to see the connections, and hence this becomes an important role for educators. Human rights can provide social workers with a moral basis for their practice (Ife 2001) and the challenge is how to apply human rights not only in f elds of practice but in all its forms, including direct practice, policy, research and advocacy. Globally, social workers face challenges to their value base where the individual is aff rmed over the collective and where economic rationalism takes precedence over social wellbeing (Briskman 2007b). Exacerbating this trend is the fact that the social work profession is increasingly operating in managerialist organisations where the corporate planning processes have been transplanted from the private sector (Hough & Briskman 2003). In order to be a ref ective human rights social worker, it is necessary to identify how the rights of vulnerable people are increasingly displaced. International conventions can be a starting point in analysing human rights issues in relation to specif c contexts.

Rather than being at centre stage in the human rights arena, social work is a profession that is often misunderstood, ignored, practised within contradictory paradigms and sometimes lacking in self-conf dence within the hierarchy of professions. This can be overcome by adherence to core principles that recognise our common humanity. As Australian lawyer Julian Burnside (2007) tells us, we must treat people decently for the sake of their humanity. After the Second World War, the conscience of humankind resulted in a belief that what happened to one group of people affected all members of the human family (Burnside 2007). With this in mind, social workers can collaborate with others in the community 'to become a leading force for the health and welfare of all people, including the world's most vulnerable' (Reichert 2003: 226).

6

doing critical social work

June Allan

'Doing' critical social work is a contested matter, with commentators noting signif cant challenges to its practice (e.g. Harris 2003; McBeath & Webb 2005; McDonald 2007). Particularly at stake is how to engage in transformative practices at a time when the possibilities for such practices are increasingly constrained. Yet there is evidence of encouraging developments for the practice of critical social work across a range of settings, a welcome occurrence in a world where the gap between the 'haves' and the 'have-nots' is increasing.

In this chapter, I consider the implications of critical social work perspectives for practice. Based on a particular set of values in which social justice is core, I consider some of the complexities of power in social relations and their implications for working in empowering ways with service users. I explore practices and processes for assisting people who are marginalised and oppressed to develop ways of knowing and acting in order to open up their personal choices and options in life. I also consider the use of social activism and resistance to improve the access of individuals and groups to rights and resources. Underpinning these practices is the need for social workers to not only ref ect on their practice but in particular to be critically ref exive about the inf uence of their own social location, values and beliefs on their practice. Critical social work cannot be characterised by a specif c set of techniques as practice is shaped by time, place and context (Fook 2005; Hick 2005; Pozzuto et al. 2005). I argue for practice to be tailored to the particular historical, social and cultural contexts of service users' lives, and valued for its capacity to create respectful spaces, however small, from which hope can grow and change can occur.

Values, ethics and social justice

Social work is not a politically neutral activity (Weinberg 2008). A core value underpinning social work practice is respect for the worth and dignity of all people, and the rights that follow from this (AASW 2002; IFSW/IASSW 2004). A commitment to social justice, discussed in earlier chapters, is a central value underpinning critical social work practice and appears as one of the f ve core values in the AASW *Code of Ethics* (AASW 2002).

A moral concept that was once commonly regarded as having universal acceptance and applicability, 'social justice' is highly contested, neither timeless nor absolute (Camilleri 1999; Ife 1999; Hugman 2008; Solas 2008). There are inevitable tensions between the attempt to hold to a universal value such as social justice while valuing diversity and giving voice to the oppressed and marginalised populations with whom social workers engage. The debate in *Australian Social Work* (Hugman 2008; Solas 2008) between Solas and Hugman on the Australian Association of Social Workers' (AASW) understanding of social justice in its *Code of Ethics* illustrates the complexities and the need for ongoing dialogue on these matters. In addition, some commentators recognise that social work values such as social justice are being undermined by contemporary managerial priorities within an environment of tighter regulations and policies where practice is often focused on managing resources and assessing risk (for example, see Stepney 2006; McDonald in Chapter 18 of this book). Writing in the UK context about contemporary social work that is shaped by what he terms a 'quasi-business discourse', Harris (2003: 185) identif es the problems of 'f t' between the values held by many social workers and the 'quasi-capitalist rationality' of their employing organisations.

These tensions over values are clearly demonstrated in the quest for a relevant code of ethics or moral framework for practice, discussed some 30 years ago by Galper (1975) in his code of ethics for radical social workers. More recently, Briskman and Noble (1999), in their exploration of the possibilities for a progressive code of ethics, have alerted us to the complexities of universal codes that fail to represent the multiplicity of voices in pluralist societies. However, they also note that an emphasis on different voices can result in intense individualism and a lack of solidarity between people who may share similarities in their differences. They recognise that a social justice framework is necessary to provide direction for change, but acknowledge that there are different concepts of social justice. As indicated earlier, this debate continues (Hugman 2008; Solas 2008).

Similarly, others argue for the retention of a framework for social workers concerned with social justice because, by reminding us of the need to consider broad political issues, such a framework counters the relativism of poststructuralist approaches and acts as a 'moral compass', providing a direction for practitioners to take (Tew 2002; Weinberg 2008). Such emancipatory 'meta-narratives', argues Tew (2002), should not be abandoned but used cautiously without them taking on a f xed status.

Various ways of addressing these tensions in values and ethics have been suggested. In order to ref ect the interests of all groups in society, Briskman and Noble (1999) recommend a process of negotiated compromise between the different groups within society to prevent any one privileged position from emerging as dominant. Harris (2003) sees evidence of social workers holding on to values that differ from the dominant discourse, and creatively making spaces to develop practice that is more just. Centrally important to the choices available and decisions made is the context in which practitioners work (Weinberg 2008), and above all social workers are urged to embrace complexity in their work (Jones et al. 2008). In their examination of critical best practice in the United Kingdom, Jones et al. (2008) note the pattern among practitioners of moving between accepting things as they are and adopting a critical stance of ref ection on how they handle their organisations and daily interventions.

Power and empowerment

The notion of power, as we have seen from earlier chapters, is central to critical social practice, and there is now a much greater recognition of the nuances and complexities of power and its operations. Here I brief y outline the changed ways of understanding power before discussing the notion of empowerment and its practice.

Power has now come to be understood in multiple ways. Critical perspectives with a modernist structural emphasis, such as Marxist, feminist and anti-racist approaches, have identif ed patterns of domination and subordination in social relations whereby some groups in society secure privilege over others and use economic, discursive and emotional power to their advantage (Tew 2002). As Mullaly (2002) clearly describes, these traditional notions tend to view power as residing mainly in large structures, such as institutions of the state or the church, and see it as best challenged through large-scale collective action to change the power structures. Examples include the trade union and environmental movements. According to this view, individuals alone are seen as having no power and as needing to come together with others for change to be possible.

Postmodern perspectives have brought more nuanced understandings of power and its use, as power and privilege are seen as being dispersed, operating in different localities, social situations and contexts—whether that be a school, a local mothers' group or a community health centre. Power is therefore f uid and open to constant inf uence and change. It is important to ask who is exercising power in a given situation, whose interests are being served and who has def ned these interests. With this analysis comes the understanding that power is not inevitably oppressive, but can also be a positive and necessary resource that opens up social opportunities, depending on how it is used (Mullaly 2002; Pease 2002a; Tew 2002; Ferguson, H. 2008).

There are differences in power between practitioners and service users, because of the role and professional knowledge held by the practitioner. Although the relationship is not equal (e.g. Rees 1991; Healy 2005b), it is questionable that we should assume that workers always have power. A female worker who is Indigenous or disabled, for example, may have little power in particular situations (Healy 2000). But, rather than trying to dissipate or avoid the power they have, critical social workers should engage productively with the decision-making power they have in their different practice contexts, and consider how such power can be used in just and humane ways in these different contexts (Healy 2005b). They can also exercise discretion as a form of power. This issue of the power relationship between practitioners and services users is addressed again in the later discussion on dialogical or equal relationships.

A corollary of power is the commonly held notion that whenever power is exercised it is contested through resistance (Mullaly 2002). Dominelli (2004) disputes this, asserting that resistance is not an inherent part of power and 'has to be worked for, or brought into being'.

The idea that those who are oppressed need to be 'empowered' has long been popular and is a key concept in critical social work. What are the meanings of 'empowerment', a widely used term that is at risk of becoming rhetorical? And how might we 'practise' empowerment?

Empowerment

Although the notion of empowerment is seen to have many different usages and interpretations because its use is context-dependent and subject to changing theoretical perspectives (Fook & Morley 2005), a consistent theme is the idea that it is a process of change through which members of subordinate groups move from being passive to active in order to gain greater control of their lives and their social environments (Mullaly 2007). Through empowerment, people can 'access different types of power, both internal (such as personal strengths) and external (such as social networks), which they can then use to improve their lives' (Barnoff & Coleman 2007: 37).

Empowerment has three different dimensions, variously labelled: personal; interpersonal/social/cultural; and structural/political (Gutiérrez et al. 1998; Thompson 1998; Mullaly 2007). A critical perspective recognises the importance of all three. At the personal level, the emphasis is on assisting individuals to gain greater control over their lives—for example, through enhanced conf dence and self-esteem. At a social or cultural level, discriminatory assumptions, stereotypes and discourses that perpetuate the oppressive values and attitudes of dominant groups are challenged. At the structural or political level, power relations rooted in the structure of society are challenged (Thompson 1998; Mullaly 2007).

A numbers of writers believe that 'personal' empowerment is necessary if structural empowerment is to be achieved. Dalrymple and Burke (1995), for example, assert that changes at the feeling level among those who feel powerless will affect their sense of control and their ability to act. This can enable a mobilisation of resources at the level of action, which can in turn affect an individual's feelings because change has occurred. Others recognise the strong link between a sense of powerlessness related to loss of control over decisions that affect a person's life, and their mental and physical wellbeing (e.g. Lundy 2004; Ferguson, I. 2008). To avoid the traps of dualisms, critical social workers can work with people on all dimensions of empowerment—and this can be done simultaneously. For example, as Gutiérrez et al. (1998) suggest, a practitioner and an individual who have come together around issues of family violence may discuss advocacy organisations or attend a social action event together.

Empowerment practices

Empowerment is both a process and a goal, and is largely educative (Dalrymple & Burke 1995; Chenoweth & McAuliffe 2005; Mullaly 2007). However, the notion of there being such an entity as 'empowerment practices' is debated. Because empowerment is context dependent, Fook and Morley (2005) argue that its use varies widely—for example, sharing or giving of power, having choice or control in one's life or, as Hick (2005) asserts, simply having knowledge of how power is exercised. Some commentators (e.g. Pease 2002a; Dominelli 2004) maintain that the notion of empowerment has become deradicalised where it has become part of the mainstream in a discourse of 'consumer choice' to legitimate managerial policies and practices. As Harris (2003) points out with specif c reference to the United Kingdom, management has coopted the rhetoric of 'empowerment' of service users to justify services becoming 'customer-oriented' in the interests of managerialist agendas.

Fook and Morley (2005) fear that without a broader critical analysis, a single concept such as empowerment misses the bigger question of 'empowerment for what and for whom?' And like Dominelli (2004), they assert that because of factors such as lack of resources, conditions for empowering outcomes to be achieved have to be created—resistance does not just happen. So how can critical social workers empower those with whom they work, and what possibilities are there to do so in the contemporary constrained political context where, in Australia, there is a high value placed on social justice but seemingly limited access to structural change (Fook & Morley 2005)?

There are various interpretations of how empowerment can be practised, and Rossiter (2005) critiques it for being too often harnessed to a set of specif c techniques. If reduced to techniques, empowerment runs the risk of ignoring 'parity of participation' (Fraser 2001), which involves two factors needed for participation to occur—the broader distribution of resources, and freedom from discrimination within society. Strategies for empowerment practice clearly must be utilised within a framework that employs a structural and critical analysis.

Earlier interpretations of empowerment practice were seen to involve three components: feelings and beliefs associated with self-conf dence; knowledge and skills for critical thinking and action; and action strategies for the cultivation of the resources, knowledge and skills needed to inf uence both internal and external structures (Dalrymple & Burke 1995; Gutiérrez et al. 1998). These dimensions remain pertinent to the practice of empowerment, but additional elements are now emphasised. These include facilitating the voices of marginalised individuals and groups to be heard. Underpinning all of this is the development of awareness of how dominant culture oppresses subordinate groups and reinforces the entrenched power of dominant groups through dominant discourses, stereotypes and popular culture (Baines 2007a; Mullaly 2007; Ife 2008a).

The notion of an equal or 'dialogical' relationship between practitioners and those with whom they are working is an idea long promoted in critical social work. Underlying this is the assumption that each party has equivalent wisdom and expertise, born out of their respective professional and lived experiences. Sharing their expertise through a dialogue that allows for learning from each other can allow for joint action in the interests of the client and includes the authentic voices of those who are marginalised (Mullaly 2007; Ife 2008a).

Some have critiqued this notion of an equal relationship between workers and service users on the grounds that it is not appropriate to much of the work in which a social worker is engaged, or to particular organisational contexts such as juvenile justice or prison settings. Ife (2005b, 2008a) acknowledges that there will be times when a practitioner has to act against the will of a person to safeguard his or her rights, but even then such actions must be undertaken with great caution to ensure that they are not violating human rights. Even in settings where social workers represent authority in a social control role, they must strive to develop a dialogical relationship and to avoid colluding with oppressive structures and practices. If there is a genuine dialogue or exchange in which both parties can reach a shared understanding of the nature and limitations of rights and responsibilities in a given situation, then appropriate action can follow (Ife 2005b).

Almost two decades ago, a study by the Brotherhood of St Laurence in Melbourne, Australia (Taylor 1990) revealed the signif cance an equal relationship can have for those with whom social workers have contact. For the women service users in the study, an equal relationship meant being treated 'on the same level' and 'not being looked down on' (1990: 66). Someone with time to listen, who showed willingness to help, who was friendly and understanding and who acted 'human' were also important factors. More recently, a study of the views of 59 service users, carers and social workers in the United Kingdom undertaken in 2005 by Cree and Davis (2007), revealed that service users and carers wanted practitioners who would listen to them and treat them with respect. Many of the social workers, talking about their reciprocal relationships with service users and carers, described how much they learnt from service users as 'experts by experience' who taught them much about the support they needed and wanted.

Although there are concerns that empowerment practices are limited in what they can achieve, a number of recent writers maintain that empowerment practices within a critical framework can, and ethically must, be used. Harry Ferguson (2008) argues that power is a resource that can be used appropriately even in highly managerial conditions. Similarly, Baines and her colleagues (2007a) provide evidence of ways in which, despite many workplace constraints, practitioners have been able to develop strategic ways to support individuals while politicising their everyday lives and working in ways to change society at many levels. These include encouraging the voices of service users to be heard and fostering their participation in decision-making; working in collaborative ways with service users; role modelling and demonstrating possibilities; educating other service providers and service users themselves, in subtle and gentle ways; using therapeutic skills and the healing power of traditional stories, rituals and practices (see also Atkinson 2002; Bennett & Zubrzycki 2003); using advocacy and organising; and working in social movements. This work shows the place of values and hopes in working towards social justice and the importance of seizing moments and spaces to foster this.

Others assert that, although those in the human services cannot expect alone to make major structural changes, they can at least play a part in undermining inequality at the structural level. Links with local activist groups of resistance or broader social movements such as feminist or environmental groups are required (Thompson 1998; Ferguson, I. 2008).

To extend the understanding of practices relevant to critical social work beyond empowerment, I now consider factors that are especially important in opening up life choices for people through developing their ways of knowing and acting. The discussion focuses on linking the personal with the political; social-political analysis and consciousness-raising; discourse analysis; internalised oppression and internalised domination or privilege; and the reclaiming of emotions. Social activism, and ref ective practice and critical ref exivity, are then discussed.

Expanding ways of knowing and acting

Linking the personal with the political

'To politicise something or someone is to introduce the idea that . . . everything involves struggle over power, resources and aff rming identities' (Baines 2007b: 51). Traditional social work practices have separated 'intervention' into different 'levels' or methods of practice—individual or family casework and case management; group work; organisational development; community development; social policy; and social research—with practitioners tending to primarily work within one of these methods. Typically, larger socio-political issues have been left to the minority of practitioners working in community development and social policy, thus weakening the link between the personal and the political (Jessup & Rogerson 1999; Mullaly 2007). Critical social work approaches to practice do not favour one particular method over another, and instead see the need for multiple ways of working because individuals' experiences are shaped by and shape their broader world (e.g. Moreau et al. 1993; Ife 2005b, 2008a; Spratt 2005).

The following examples illustrate ways in which such links might be made. The connection can be made, for example, between the despair and exhaustion experienced by a young mother in paid work, and the type of provisions and level of support for working parents in our society as well as the dominant discourses, beliefs and practices surrounding responsibilities for domestic labour. For Ife (1997), the practitioner is expected to understand the person with whom they are working in terms of her/his community and cultural context and to work towards solutions and supports at the community level. Similarly, community workers would be expected to use interpersonal skills that are designed to build trust and rapport with those with whom they need to work. Ife suggests several ways in which links might be made between policy and practice. These include the ways in which problems are discussed with individuals, the terms used, the ways in which solutions are sought, and also linking people with others in similar circumstances. Assisting people to develop organisational skills such as advocating for themselves or making representations in meetings are other ways. Practices such as consciousness-raising and critical questioning have assisted the process of linking the personal and political, and are discussed later in this chapter.

Healy (2000) argues that the dichotomy between structural and local forms of change needs to be dismantled to allow the local concerns and goals of individuals and groups to be seen as part of a continuum of social change. Here, pragmatic and localised approaches to activism are valued, with workers engaging in social change activities through the local networks of which they are part (Healy 2000). Workers might band together with their local community, for example, to establish a drop-in centre to provide information and referral services and recreational activities, to help build social cohesion and combat isolation or fear of cultural differences. Where large-scale political action is considered, broad representation of many different political and professional interests is encouraged and ongoing negotiation of the differences between those involved is urged (Healy 2000; Ferguson, I. 2008).

Socio-political analysis and consciousness-raising

The lens through which workers analyse or 'assess' the social problems of those with whom they work is crucial to critical social work practice. The analysis of hidden oppressions and awareness of social locations is central in helping service users to view their personal experiences within a political framework (Fook 2005). The focus of structural approaches on socio-political analysis—analysing the relationship between personal problems, dominant ideology and material conditions—requires an analysis of power relationships at all levels. This involves identifying the social, political and economic barriers impinging on individuals, families, communities and organisations (Moreau & Leonard 1989). All forms of oppression and marginalisation based on sexism, racism, colonialism, imperialism, classism, ageism, disablism (physical and mental), heterosexism and others need to be considered (Mullaly 2007).

This means that practitioners need a sound understanding of political mechanisms and the workings of power. At a time when human service organisations are requiring workers to undertake 'assessments' that have become increasingly standardised and tightly scripted (Baines 2007b), social workers are urged to keep in mind the socio-political lens. Lundy (2004) recommends particular needs of individuals and families to be considered (material, social and psychological, productive, safety and self-actualisation needs), but at the same time insists on consideration of social, political and economic rights to determine the injustices people face, providing not only immediate resources but also working towards political solutions.

Consciousness-raising or 'conscientisation'—der ived from the work of Paulo Freire (1972) and popularised through feminism, among other radical traditions—is a process for undertaking socio-political analyses with service users within a dialogical relationship, as a way of assisting them to understand their personal situations in their broader socio-political context. It occurs through both ref ection and action (see critical ref ection at the end of this chapter), with an emphasis on helping groups of people gain insights into their circumstances, who holds power and how power can be used to make social change (Baines 2007b; Mullaly 2007).

The use of consciousness-raising as a process continues to be popular (e.g. Tew 2002; Mullaly 2007; Ife 2008a). But while opening up possibilities for action, consciousness-raising can be oppressive and patronising if based on the assumption that the practitioner's consciousness is superior, assuming a singular underlying truth, and if imposed on the people with whom she or he is working (Healy 2005a; Ife 2008a). This has been illustrated in efforts of workers to 'elevate' Indigenous people to state 'standards' (Grimshaw et al. 1994). By imposing their own beliefs on others about what is empowering, workers are constructing themselves as the experts, often inappropriately, with the service user expected to take on the worker's beliefs (Fook & Morley 2005).

Thus, consciousness-raising needs to be a mutual process, based on respect and a genuine desire on the part of practitioners to work together with people, whether individuals, families, groups, organisations, communities or at the national and global levels. This involves shared expertise, mutual learning in which professional knowledge and life experiences are equally valued, and joint action. An attitude of respect towards those with whom the practitioner is working, along with sound active listening skills, provides an important foundation for such practice (Ife 2008a). This means that workers need to listen for and negotiate the multiple meanings attached to dialogues, recognise the many different ways of knowing, and even take on board ways of knowing that challenge professional expertise.

Clark (2006: 1) emphasises the need for workers 'to co-create spaces for shared understanding of meanings that people use to interpret the world and their place in it' by listening for meaning in order to attend to spiritual and cultural world-views. This is not to say that service users' own analyses 'are never questioned or reconstructed'. Some reworking of ideas rather than taking them at face value may be appropriate where service users share the same oppressive beliefs as mainstream society, and so are likely to blame themselves or others in society who have little to do with the problem (Baines 2007b: 59). This process is referred to as internalised oppression and is discussed later in the chapter.

Discourse analysis

Critical social work approaches inf uenced by postmodern ideas emphasise discourses and discourse analysis, as discussed in Chapter 3. Because of the capacity of discourses as sets of meanings and language practices to generate new meanings, they can expand the possible ways of understanding different experiences and of actions available to people and are the sites of 'analysis and struggle' (Healy 1999: 118). Language cannot be regarded as producing experiences such as poverty or racism, but the experiences can only be understood through language (Healy 2000).

The term 'intervention', common in social work parlance, is one such example of how language shapes meanings. Conventional social work practices have used the term to refer to the work undertaken by social workers to bring about change to something of which they themselves are not part. The use of the term is problematic for two main reasons (Ife 2008a). First, it perpetuates an image of the social worker as an outside expert rather than a partner in an action process. Second, it reinforces a notion of disadvantaged people being the passive recipients of the expert help of the social worker who alone is responsible for affecting change. Alternatives to the language of 'intervention' can emphasise a greater degree of mutuality, such as 'work with' or 'work carried out' between practitioners and others towards achievement of goals.

As discussed in Chapter 3, the language of dominant discourses can be analysed through a process of deconstruction. Through deconstruction, cultural, community and family discourses can be f ushed out and debunked. This process can disclose ideas, beliefs and behaviours that reproduce prevailing power structures which have taught service users to succumb to their dictates, and can open up possibilities for discourses and their outcomes to be altered (Jessup & Rogerson 1999; Rossiter 2005; Goldberg Wood & Tully 2006). Goldberg Wood and Tully (2006) describe, for example, the oppressive discourse that prevents many women from reporting rape. Elements of this discourse include that once a man is sexually aroused he is powerless to control himself and that, as many authorities such as police and jury members believe this, women understand it is highly unlikely that their rapists will be convicted.

Other practices useful in discourse analysis include narrative approaches (referred to in Chapter 3) and the utilisation of critical questioning. Critical questioning, derived from the thinking of Freire (e.g. Freire & Faundez 1990) and Foucault (1979, cited in Jessup & Rogerson 1999: 165), helps individuals understand the inf uence of their stereotypical or socially conditioned assumptions in determining their life experiences (Mullaly 2007). It provides the opportunity for a person to explore their expectations and how they feel they have to act (Fook 1993). As a form of deconstruction, critical questioning acts as an invitation to another person to engage in a dialogue around reconstruction of new ideas and beliefs.

Internalised oppression and internalised domination

Internalised oppression (or 'inferiorisation'—see Mullaly 2007), as originally conceptualised by Pheterson (1986: 148), refers to 'the incorporation and acceptance by individuals within an oppressed group of the prejudices against them within the dominant society'. They thus believe and accept the prejudices against them (Mullaly 2002, 2007; Carniol 2005; Goldberg Wood & Tully 2006; Kumsa 2007). Internalised oppression includes feelings like self-hatred, fear of violence, self-doubt, isolation and powerlessness, and is the mechanism by which domination is perpetuated in oppressive situations.

In contrast, internalised domination, such as sexism in men and racism in white people, is 'the incorporation and acceptance by individuals within a dominant group of prejudices against others' (Pheterson 1986: 148). It consists of feelings such as superiority, normalcy, self-righteousness, distortion of reality, guilt, fear, and alienation from one's body and from nature, and restricts the individual's capacity to empathise, love and trust. It isolates people from one another and prevents solidarity, binding people together through their power to dominate others rather than on the basis of respect for others. Internalised domination can be countered through valuing difference, education, self-ref ection and building alliances with others, the last factor helping to counter the feelings of guilt and confusion that arise from being in social positions of dominance (Pheterson 1986). Although the term itself is no longer prominent in contemporary literature, the impact of internalised domination is a driving force behind the need for social workers to practise critical ref exivity, addressed later in this chapter.

The shift from problem-solving, therapeutic and reformative types of approaches to working with individuals and families, to educational and discursive approaches compatible with a critical discourse, has been promising in addressing the issue of how to work with people's internalised oppression or inferiorisation. Narrative approaches, for example, value the uniqueness of the individual experience and question the fundamental concepts that each individual draws on to make meaning of their world (White 1992; Pozzuto et al. 2005). Helping the individual to identify the inf uence of dominant discourses on their individual perceptions and experiences achieves this. A narrative approach provides a means of including people in challenging the dominant discourse through the exploration of alternative discourses, and is regarded as a new approach to therapy that fosters links between the individual and the social (Fook 2005). While such an approach can offer hope and optimism to people, it should not be used in isolation from a material and structural analysis of the person's situation, and the process of internalised domination should be considered as well as internalised oppression.

Reclaiming emotions

There is growing recognition in critical social work of the need to integrate an understanding of ways of knowing and transformation through the body (Cameron & McDermott 2007), emotions and spirit (Tew 2002; Wong 2004), combining the social and the psychological in new ways to attend appropriately to emotional dimensions of service users' experiences (Frost & Hoggett 2008; Stenner & Taylor 2008). In his detailed analysis of power and practice, Tew (2002) discusses a third level of social relations, emotionality (the other two levels being material and discursive). He argues that the emotions, separated from rationality in a modernist world because of their threat to the smooth running of society, are related to experiences of oppression and abuse and are a response to outcomes of power and status relations. He shows how, through modernity, emotions have been subordinated and devalued, and treated in later modernity as a commodity to be sanitised and managed within an 'emotion industry'. Tew maintains that to challenge the embedded ideologies that overlook and control emotions, two stages are necessary. First, people need to be carefully listened to in order to feel believed and understood—an experience that may be profoundly empowering. Second, emotions can mobilise energies to bring about the changes that resist oppressions and abuses, as they can bring a sense of motivation and purpose, both intra-psychically and collectively, and can forge bonds of support and alliance between people (Tew 2002).

In order to respond in an integrated yet emancipatory way to oppressed individuals and groups, rather than avoid or trivialise their emotions, critical social workers need to develop more effective ways of hearing and receiving service users' emotions stemming from discriminatory and oppressive experiences. They need to work in ways that help individuals and groups to effectively resist oppression and to channel the energy of outrage and hurt towards bringing about emancipatory change (Tew 2002).

Social activism

Activism 'involves a number of activities, such as organising, educating and mobilising people' (Baines 2007b: 54). Choices and options can be opened up for those who are oppressed and marginalised through such actions that directly challenge and resist oppressive social relations and conditions. I now consider advocacy and other collective actions, followed by some general comments on acts of resistance.

Advocacy

Advocacy involves an attempt to inf uence the behaviour of decision-makers, and is something that social workers practise on a regular basis. It aims to improve the responsiveness of social arrangements to people's needs out of a basic respect for an individual's human rights, and involves the interpretation of the powerless to the powerful (Payne 1997; O'Connor et al. 2003). Traditionally, advocacy has been divided into two types, case advocacy and class advocacy. Case advocacy involves 'the process of working with, or on behalf of, another or a small group, to obtain services to which they are entitled, or to inf uence a decision that affects them' (O'Connor et al. 2003: 190). This might occur, for example, when an individual is refused a service or benef t to which they are entitled, when an individual needs benef ts or services urgently as a result of a crisis, or when a person is denied their legal rights. Class advocacy refers to 'activity directed at changing policy, practices and laws' affecting a class of individuals (O'Connor et al. 2003), promoting social change for the benef t of social groups. This is required, for example, when groups of people are discriminated against or when organisational or government policies affect people adversely, such as the grievous effects for refugees in Australia of the former Howard government's policy on temporary protection visas.

There are three sets of strategies to inf uence decision-makers. These are normative strategies, which involve making moral arguments and generating recognition of common values; utilitarian strategies involving bargaining and negotiation, when decision-makers have a neutral view about the advocacy effort; and coercive strategies, involving the use of conf ict and complaint to force the attention of decision-makers (O'Connor et al. 2003). Skills for effective advocacy, decided between worker and individual or group, may include written and oral submissions, persuading and lobbying, f nding loopholes in bureaucratic rules, bending rules, developing familiarity with formal and informal agency rules and procedures, and skills in handling conf ict (Fook 1993; O'Connor et al. 2003; Goldberg Wood & Tully 2006).

Since the 1980s, new forms of advocacy have emerged, based on a belief in people managing their own lives, as advocacy can potentially be disempowering. For, as Ife (2008a) asserts, speaking on behalf of a person may represent profoundly conservative rather than empowering practice. Advocacy should be practised in empowering ways to develop the capacity of people from marginalised groups to act on their own behalf (Tew 2002; Ife 2008a), although Baines (2007b) questions that this applies in all instances, as will shortly be discussed. Tensions can arise where service users do not share the same social justice goals as the worker, or where actions considered empowering by a worker are experienced negatively by service users (Pease 2002a; Kumsa 2007).

Collective action, alliances and citizen participation

There is widespread agreement that for marginalised and oppressed individuals to become involved in a group process can be the most effective way for them to become politically aware of their circumstances (Mullaly 2007). Collective action and resistance through groups of people coming together provide opportunities for consciousness-raising, developing solidarity through shared views, lobbying to change opinions on oppressive rules, conditions and institutions, and developing alliances with social movements and other groups. This calls for educational, support and social change-oriented groups. Group solidarity among participants can develop as people share their individual and common experiences of frustration, anger, oppression and ideas about what might be needed to make their situations different. Full discussion on group work to help promote social change can be found in Sullivan et al. (2003), Breton (2004), McNicoll (2004), Staples (2004), Doel (2006) and Preston-Shoot (2007). Mullender and Ward's (1991) work on self-directed groups remains an invaluable source on a form of group work based specif cally on conf ict theory and empowerment practices.

Factors that act as barriers to people's participation in society need to be addressed through institutional change and reform, policy advocacy and social activism using collective resistance (Carniol 2005; Mullaly 2007; Ferguson, I. 2008; Ife 2008a) and community organising and building (Goldsworthy 2002; Staples 2004; Stepney 2006). This involves inf uencing discourses, using the law, developing alliances with other groups working for social and political change such as social justice and human rights groups and protest groups, organising public forums and social action campaigns, supporting grassroots leadership, working with the mass media to mobilise public opinion and applying political pressure against harmful institutional practices (Ife 1997; 2008a; Thompson 1998; Carniol 2005).

To return to an earlier point about power and its use, Healy (2005b) reminds us that critical social workers need to think more broadly about possible activist practice sites and processes, to make visible activism which has been invisible in conventional, bureaucratic practice settings, and to consider other possibilities for stimulating change, such as a careful analysis of specif c organisational contexts.

There are encouraging signs of the development of some highly creative collective solutions that do not locate problems within individuals, instead linking common experiences of oppression with the sources of such oppression. Spratt (2005), for example, borrowing ideas from the work of Brazilian dramatist Augusto Boal (1979), has used 'forum theatre' with a group of Irish schoolchildren on the issue of bullying as a form of oppression. The method has the capacity to raise consciousness and develop creative potential solutions that can become rehearsals for changes to be enacted in real life. Schatz et al. (2006) also discuss this creative group-oriented approach. As Sin (2007) shows through his work in a research project on gambling in the Chinese community in Montreal, participatory action research can also be used to give voice to marginalised populations and to promote social change.

Resistance within organisational, historical, social and cultural contexts

As can be seen from the preceding discussion, central to critical social work practice is resistance—those acts or actions in which people, individually or collectively, 'take a stand in opposition to a belief, an idea, an ideology, a climate, a practice, or an action that is oppressive and damaging to individual and social well-being' (Benjamin 2007). Resistance requires a strategy (a plan of action) and tactics (the specif c process for implementing the plan) as well as the use of critical analysis and critical ref ection (Benjamin 2007). Many of these practices of resistance were identif ed in the preceding section.

There is pressure for social workers to conform to organisational cultures that, despite the rhetoric around notions like social justice, are often at odds with social justice-oriented approaches to practice. Practices of resistance are therefore often limited because of the strength of oppressive everyday practices and constraints and the reluctance of social workers to take a stand. To counter these barriers, collective efforts with others are essential (Benjamin 2007). An important rider is the need to practise appropriately to the particular historical, social and cultural context and not to act on ideological clichés without critical analysis and critical ref ection.

A clear example of this is shown by Baines (2007b), who ref ects on the effectiveness of her work some years ago in a large American public hospital where class and race disparities were acute. Certain depoliticised practices rooted in white middle-class experiences did not work for the clients with whom she worked. These included individuation, encouraging women to express their anger and equalising power in the therapeutic relationship. Details of this work can be found in Baines (2007b), but some examples illustrate the point. While individuation (a process emphasising a person's separateness and autonomy) may be helpful to some individuals, especially women who might benef t from seeing themselves as separate beings from others demanding their care, it can overlook the interdependence needed, and deep meaning and support gained, from tight-knit networks that people in poverty require to survive. Similarly, the women, who were already practised at expressing their anger in order to survive their daily struggles, benef ted from assistance to develop strategies for 'using' their anger more effectively to meet their material needs rather than alienating themselves from much-needed sources of support. Finally, despite the emphasis in feminist and other justice-oriented approaches on equalising power between worker and client in the helping relationship, Baines found in her short-term crisis work with clients that they were not at all interested in understanding the therapeutic process because they needed immediate solutions and resources. Instead, Baines found that the practices which worked well with this multiracial group on low incomes were those rooted in activism: politicised practices such as critical consciousness-raising; using her privilege as a white middle-class worker in the interests of her clients; and linking with social movements and unions (Baines 2007b).

Reflective practice and critical reflexivity

Fundamental to all critical social work practice are the actions of ref ective practice. The notion of 'ref ective practice' originated with Argyris and Schon (1976) and there are now many variations of the term, often used interchangeably (D'Cruz et al. 2007)—for example, 'critical ref ection' (Fook 2002; Rossiter 2005), 'critically ref ective practice' (Tew 2002), 'critical ref exivity' (McDonald 2006) and a 'ref exive approach' (Healy 2005a).

In essence, the general concept can be understood in two main ways. The f rst concerns service users developing their knowledge and awareness for opening up their life choices through critical ref ection (see the discussion on consciousness-raising earlier in the chapter). The second focuses on social workers' critical ref ection on their own practice in relation to how knowledge about clients is generated and the operations of power in this process, but also on their ref ections on their own values, feelings and emotions and the ways these inf uence their work, a process often referred to as critical ref exivity (D'Cruz et al. 2007).

Using critical ref exivity, social workers ref ect on the inf uence of their own personality, background, social and cultural location, and perspectives on their practice (Fook 2002). Taken-for-granted assumptions are questioned and its use encourages practitioners to re-analyse situations in ways that provide for new actions and changes in power relations. The use of uncertainty is a catalyst for change, and the process of critical ref exivity draws attention to the absolute necessity for social workers to be involved in continual self-ref exive learning to work as effectively as posible for the betterment of people's lives and social relations (Fook 1999; Tew 2002; Rossiter 2005; McDonald 2006).

Conclusion

At the centre of critical social work practices is the lens through which we view social problems and their causes, involving both our emotions and our minds (Baines 2007c). Also underpinning the practices are hopes for a socially just and peaceful world that encourage us to work in respectful and ethical ways according to the values stated at the beginning of this chapter. Constraints in the workplace and in society more broadly act as signif cant barriers to working towards a more socially just world, but it is imperative that we do not lose the hope and respect. Despite these considerable barriers to the practice of critical social work in the often uncaring and alienating world of individuals and groups who are marginalised, oppressed, and largely unheard and made invisible, there are ways of working that open up alternative possibilities. A common and binding theme for 'doing' critical social work is the requirement to work in ways that link the personal with the political to ensure that people's immediate material needs are addressed and longer-term social change is acted on. We have a responsibility to continue to develop and evolve these ways.

PART III

resisting domination and oppression

7

towards anti-racist and culturally affirming practices

Marjorie Quinn

This chapter was f rst written from Zambia in central southern Africa, a long way from well-stocked libraries and conversations about critical perspectives and theories of social work, but in other ways a rich and immediate context in which to ref ect on race, culture and language—issues and concepts with which I grappled daily. Back in Australia, a little wiser from this and other experiences, I continue to grapple as citizen and social worker with these 'same but different' issues, but now from my less visible majority 'white' position. Racism is everywhere, and as Kevin Dunn writes, it is 'everywhere different' (2003: 2). Entrenched global and local processes privileging some people(s) and oppressing others on the basis of race and culture, and conf ict and violence based at least in part on these differences, mean that if we wish to strive for justice and peace, it is imperative to become more knowledgeable and self-aware about the operations of racism and about ways of combating it. This chapter explores these matters.

Critical social work theories provide a useful basis with their focus on understandings of social and personal power and their commitment to more just social, economic and political relations. They direct attention to the strength of material, ideological and discursive social structures in shaping life opportunities, including housing, education, health, food, water and decision-making, and also personal subjectivity and psychological processes. At the same time, they embrace understandings that people have some power and agency, even within oppressive structures, to shape their own lives and their own personal consciousness. Such understandings of critical theory are discussed in earlier chapters, and this chapter explores them in relation to the particular injustices and conf ict which f ow from deeply embedded racisms in Australia and across the world. First, I discuss historical and contemporary race relations in Australia and then address key concepts. Then I explore aspects of the further development of anti-racist and culturally aff rming theories and practices. As practitioners and students, we are challenged to continue a journey of self-learning in the context of race relations and culture.

Race relations in Australia: diversity and inequality

Beliefs and attitudes about race and culture have signif cantly shaped Australia's development since colonial invasion from 1788, and race relations have been the seat of tension, struggle, violence and inequality (Pettman 1992; Butler 1993; Vasta & Castles 1996; Dunn 2003). While the United Kingdom and 'white' English-speaking countries have been the major sources of immigration since that time, closer scrutiny reveals there has always been considerable diversity. Extraordinary rates of immigration and refugee movement followed the Second World War, and the distinctive waves were increasingly diverse in terms of people's countries of origin, and cultural, religious and language backgrounds. According to the 2006 census, 2.5 per cent of Australia's population identif ed as Indigenous, 22.2 per cent were born overseas and 26 per cent of people born in Australia had one or both parents born overseas. The United Kingdom, New Zealand, India, China, the Philippines, South Africa and Sudan were the top seven countries of origin (ABS 2006).

The stories of diversity are also stories of injustice, oppression and privilege. Colonial invasion and domination have left Indigenous families, communities, cultural meanings and languages fragmented and disenfranchised, and social indicators such as levels of income, employment rates, education and health status show that, overall, Aboriginal and Torres Strait Islander people remain the most oppressed and disadvantaged group. And these indicators capture only certain dimensions of the effects of colonisation; they do not portray the ways in which this history has shaped personal and collective subjectivity and suffering.

Although their experiences vary widely, great inequality also exists for immigrants and refugees. Oppression most often relates to the extent to which people differ from the dominant norms of skin colour and physical appearance, cultural meanings, religion, language and educational background, but the contributing factors are diverse, and changing within local and global contexts. Lindsay Tanner

(Finance Minister in the Rudd government) in his 2008 Redmond Barry Lecture asserted that racism in Australia is now directed mainly towards people born in Africa (*The Age*, 31 July 2008). Among the examples he cited was the announcement some months earlier by Kevin Andrews (Minister for Immigration in the Howard government) that African immigration and humanitarian intake would be reduced, ostensibly because of community concerns about crime and violence. Another face of racism in Australia can be seen in the prevailing 'fear of terror' associated with fundamentalist Islam, which extends into widespread distrust, stereotyping and abuse towards Muslim and Arabic people and communities.

At some levels, Australia claims success in meeting the challenges of building a socially just, cooperative and cohesive society across differences of race and culture. Egalitarian values are espoused, overtly racist laws and policies were abolished in the 1960s and 1970s (Vasta & Castles 1996) and many activist individuals and organisations are working towards justice and understanding. The Rudd government has made a memorable and hopeful national apology to Indigenous Australians and instigated signif cant changes to policies concerning mandatory detention of asylum seekers. Despite these important steps, the actual experience of members of minority communities, especially those who are visibly different, does not f t this picture. If we are to meet the above challenge, the intertwined knowledge and skills to combat racism and nurture emancipation, and to work across cultural and language differences, are paramount.

Race and racism

The contentious language of 'race' and 'racism' is used in this chapter, despite the controversy and strong feelings the terms engender. Language is important and Dominelli (2008) makes this point in *Anti-racist Social Work*, writing that 'Words indicate understandings of reality, shape interactions within discourses that produce them, and explore specif c conceptualisations of power relations and people's place in the world. They also inf uence action taken' (2008: 8). The language of race helps to expose the complex and particular operations of power embedded in these relations, operations which tend to be masked by alternative language such as 'ethnicity' and 'cultural diversity' (Young 2004).

By race and racism, I mean the attitudes and processes involved in categorising, stereotyping, and assigning value and power to people on the basis of their differences, including physical attributes (particularly colour), and culture and language—processes of 'racialisation' and 'politicisation' (Dominelli 2008). Stuart Hall expresses them as 'economic, political and ideological practices whereby a dominant group exercises hegemony over subordinate groups' (1980: 338). The meanings given to these terms are, however, complex, diverse and contested, shifting and changing over time and place. Race was a very powerful descriptor during the historical period of the Enlightenment and colonial expansion in the eighteenth and nineteenth centuries, when there was thought to be a scientif c basis to categorising and valuing people according to physical characteristics. Certain attributes and def cits, virtues and vices were ascribed according to physical types or 'races', and belief in the superiority of white and inferiority of black was deeply embedded. These ideas were increasingly challenged and negated during the f rst half of the twentieth century by developments in biology and genetics, the growth in social sciences and the decline of Western colonialism. As a result, the concept of race and the accompanying language such as 'pure race', 'full-blood' or 'half-caste' no longer have any scientif c support as ways of describing and valuing differences between people.

Nevertheless, despite its lack of validity in this way, race remains today as a very powerful means of categorising people and of assigning power and value. It is important 'not because it is real biologically, but because people believe it is real and therefore make it real in its consequences' (Chambers & Pettman 1986: 5). It is now recognised as a concept which is socially constructed rather than one which is inherently meaningful. However, it still has immense power to generate oppression, hatred and violence.

Racism includes not only the obvious overt acts of exploitation and oppression, but also a whole range of personal actions and institutional structures and practices in society which serve to exclude or devalue people in everyday life on the basis of factors such as appearance, culture and language. Three interrelated and interacting forms of racism can be identif ed: personal, institutional and cultural. Personal or individual racism refers to the behaviours and practices of individuals which devalue others, deny them equality or judge them prejudicially, as well as more obvious acts of violence and hatred. In the Australian context, a black African-Australian family misses out on a rental property; threats are made to an Islamic family new to a neighbourhood; and a Jewish man walking along a street is taunted then attacked.

Institutional racism refers to the ways in which the policies, practices and discourses of institutions such as governments, businesses, professions and education, health and legal systems operate to the advantage of one or some racial groups, and to the disadvantage of others. The third, and closely interconnected, element is described as cultural racism. Here, the values, beliefs, meanings and world-views from the dominant cultural group are established as not only central, but the benchmark. Other values and meanings are perceived as different and become constructed as inferior, deviant or pathological. In the Australian context, Western/white cultural meanings, values and world-views are dominant, and they are entrenched or institutionalised at the 'core' of society. Together, institutional and cultural racisms 'constitute structural racism because social resources and power are used to sustain them' (Dominelli 2008: 12). These three aspects of racism feed into and out of each other. Later in this chapter, I discuss ways in which Western/white cultural values are institutionalised in social work and human services, so legitimating individual racist practices.

White privilege

Typically, racism is thought of as an issue more for those people marginalised and oppressed by its operations than for those privileged by it. Everyone, though, has a place in the relations of race. Fine (1997) argues that to combat racism we may need to shift gears and focus not only on the unfair disadvantage accruing to people of colour, but also on the prof ts that surround being 'white'. 'White privilege' is now gaining attention and is the subject of a growing literature. 'White' is a complex and imprecise term meaning much more than the colour of skin. It is a political and cultural concept signifying status, power and identity. White privilege has been described as 'the unearned advantages and benef ts that accrue to White folks by virtue of a system normed on the experiences, values and perceptions of their group' (Sue 2003: 137). Superiority, power, privilege and identity are automatically conferred by varied processes of withholding, exclusion and denial of opportunity. 'White' is 'transparent because of its everyday occurrence' (Sue 2003: 120) and the privileges go largely unrecognised by the dominant white majority but are well recognised by people in subjugated positions.

Katz (cited in Carter 1997: 205) proposes that racism is, in fact, 'a white problem in that its development and perpetuation rests with white people'. Carter goes on to say that victims of oppression can f ght against it, protect themselves and act in spite of it, but they cannot stop something they are not creating. White people, therefore, must acknowledge, resist and challenge their position of race privilege at all levels if racism is to be addressed. I will return to this proposition later in the chapter.

Limitations of the language of 'race'

Despite the usefulness of the language of race, of 'white' and 'black', in highlighting power relations as well as difference, there are signif cant dangers and problems.

These categories quickly and easily become reif ed as f xed, separate and monolithic categories of experience and identity, rather than being understood as socially constructed, blurred, changing and intersecting with other dimensions of power. The reality is much more complex than these dualistic terms imply.

In the 2003 edition of this chapter, I wrote about my situation in Zambia to exemplify this complexity. What did it mean to be 'white' and part of the small minority constituting less than 1 per cent of the population? Contemporary race relations are very much shaped by the history of exploitation through colonisation, and the struggle for independence. Subsequently, a particular form of socialism, where consumption more than production was subsidised through the raising of an enormous overseas debt, was followed by a very diff cult decade in the 1990s where economic restructure driven by the Western world resulted in increased poverty and inequality. These stories are part of the complexity of race relations in this country. In addition, perceptions of Western culture and values are fed daily through the media, especially television. Among other things, 'white' means wealth and power, freedom, health, education, cleanliness, honesty and choices in life. It evokes resentment, together with a kind of respect at the same time. A further dimension is added to the analysis through the consideration of gender. Traditionally, women's roles and positions are culturally tied to and def ned by men in their lives—husbands, fathers, sons, employers and bosses—and women are poorly protected by law or by cultural convention from abuse, violence, exploitation, sexual assault, invisibility, exclusion and poverty. As a white woman in Zambia, I was not immune from some of this.

Within and between the categories of 'black' and 'white' there are, of course, signif cant variations which become masked by stereotypical categorisation and perceptions. For example, although many white residents and expatriates are wealthy, not all are, and despite the fact that most Zambians live in grinding poverty, there are growing numbers of wealthy and powerful black Zambians. The implications of each of these and other issues relating to social and personal power need to be teased out much further than the space here allows. Such analysis would demonstrate something of the complexity and particularity of race relations, and also their connectedness to other dimensions of oppression. This is the kind of analysis which critical theory invites. It rejects monolithic and dualistic categorisation. Many threads of my story carried with them privilege and power, others less privilege and power and even some vulnerability. While it is very important for us to identify the complex and intertwining experiences of power, privilege and oppression, we must not be blind to the fact that, overall, very real privileges accrue in our world from being white.

Ethnicity

'Ethnicity' is a term widely used in social life and is often preferred over the language of race. It, too, is a complex concept, and to some extent the two have overlapping meanings. Ethnicity refers to belonging and commonality in relation to factors such as national origin, historical experience, shared culture or physical type (Cox 1989; Hartley 1995; McFarlane 2008). It emphasises the social and historical determinants more than the physical. The term usually does not invoke the same political/power implications and judgements as the concept of race, but instead the sense of difference and belonging. It is language of difference which tends to shroud the existence of structural, material and power inequalities and oppression based on physical, cultural, national and historical differences (Frankenberg 1993; Young 2004). It operates to mask and protect race privilege and power. There are, however, differences of opinion about the use of this language within social work literature. Devore and Schlesinger (1996: 25, 28) and McFarlane (2008: 98), for example, adopt the terminology of ethnicity because (as noted earlier in this chapter) the concept of race lacks any scientif c basis and because they feel its use is often 'pejorative and divisive'.

Social work literature, theories and practices are frequently critiqued for their 'ethnocentricity'. This important concept refers to the tendency to hold 'a view of the world in which oneself or one's group is at the centre of things: a failure to take into account the perceptions of others' (Cashmore & Troyne, cited in Ely & Denny 1987: 17). The concept is similar in meaning to 'cultural racism'. Giddens (1983) argues that 'ethno-centrism is deeply entrenched in Western culture though it is also found in many (if not most) other countries as well' (1983: 23).

Culture

'Culture' is also a complex term frequently used in contemporary society, and it is currently the dominant language in Australian social policy—cultural and linguistic diversity (CALD). A range of meanings is evident, both over time and in the contemporary context. In the 2003 edition of this chapter, evolving meanings of the term were traced through time to those evident today, including the 'culture of organisations', 'popular culture' and 'high culture'. It is the anthropological tradition of def ning culture that is relevant to this chapter. This tradition evolved following colonial expansion and the development of Western social sciences. It has come to mean the distinctive ways of life and shared values, beliefs and meanings common to groups of people. With developments in anthropology and other social sciences, the emphasis is placed on processes of signif cation—on what culture does, rather than on what it is. So culture can be understood as the 'set of practices by which meanings are produced and exchanged within a group' (Bocock 1992: 233). It is often described as a complex web of meanings which underlie everyday life and behaviour, the understandings and expectations which guide actions and interactions with others. Geertz (1973) proposes that these meanings and understandings are grounded in language and other symbolic communication practices such as rites and rituals. Things and events occur, but of themselves they do not necessarily have intrinsic meaning. Meaning is given by language, through which comes the construction and exchange of understandings.

The boundaries of cultural groups, where they begin and end, are blurred and changing. They are 'constantly negotiating ambivalences or tensions' across boundaries, and within (Lee 2008: 17). They are not internally homogeneous, and intersecting differences such as class, education, gender, sexuality, rural/urban, religion, as well as personal and family factors, all contribute to diversity. Cultures are dynamic, and continually evolving and changing over time in response to all sorts of factors in the economic, political, ideological and social worlds. In addition, and for a wide range of reasons, people will be drawing on more than one set of cultural meanings. Ivey (2008) suggests we think more in terms of the 'cultural narratives that run through people's lives rather than thinking of people as identif ed in a one-to-one correspondence with a particular cultural identity' (2008: 34).

Towards theories and practices which are anti-racist and culturally affirming

Anti-racist practice calls for the development of theories and practices which privilege understandings of the complex and particular operations of race power together with relevant cultural knowledge. A range of theoretical positions can be seen in the contemporary literature, some ref ecting, as we saw earlier, an emphasis on ethnic sensitive practice and cultural diversity with little attention given to the power dimensions of racial and cultural difference. Structural and anti-oppressive approaches provide helpful frameworks for these latter considerations. However, their theoretical development has been grounded mainly in analyses of class inequality and oppression through contemporary Marxism, inf uenced signif cantly by feminism (Moreau & Leonard 1989). They therefore need to be expanded to embrace the complexities and particular operations of racism as described earlier in this chapter. These cannot simply be subsumed into narratives of other dimensions of power, oppression and privilege, or into analyses of intersecting dimensions of power (Young 2004). Anti-racist texts (such as Dominelli 2008; Constantine & Sue

2006) engage with the particular expressions of race oppression and increasingly with race privilege, as experienced historically and locally, and with intersecting dimensions such as poverty and gender relations. They emphasise the racial and cultural power embedded in professional theories and practices, social work roles, organisations and teaching institutions, and they aff rm the necessity for workers to recognise their own race privilege, racism and ethnocentricity.

In the following sections of this chapter, I explore several themes which I consider central to anti-racist and culturally aff rming practice, but which remain relatively underdeveloped in the literature. These include: the importance of cultural knowledge—of self, of the cultural bases of theories and practices, and of other culturally based pathways for practice; understandings of race relations, especially of white privilege and power; and how these understandings are most effectively learned.

The place of cultural knowledge in anti-racist practice

Substantial and particular cultural knowledge and an understanding of one's cultural self are critical to all aspects of anti-racist practice. Cultural ignorance and ethnocentricity of people within the dominant cultural and racial group perpetuate cultural and racial oppression. Ignorance results in the cultural meanings, values, beliefs and ways which are at the centre of the lives of people within dominated cultural groups being marginalised, not recognised, valued or accepted. Cultural domination results, whether it is intended or not. Although very important, goodwill, good intentions and f ne skills of empathy are not suff cient mitigating factors on their own.

Informed and sensitive cultural knowledge is essential to processes of healing and recovery from the devastating community, family and personal effects of race-related oppression, and therefore to anti-racist practice. Waldegrave and colleagues from The Family Centre, Aotearoa (New Zealand) have made a signif cant contribution to this area of theory development and practice (for example, see Waldgrave 1990). Their family and community work involves carefully listening to people's stories for the articulation of meanings and hopes, and assisting in various ways with the weaving of new and liberating meanings and opportunities. It is probably the cultural context, more than any other factor, which determines underlying meaning systems, so an informed and particular cultural knowledge is essential for 'just' and healing practice.

Wahiri Campbell, a Maori therapist/community worker from The Family Centre, illustrates these points from their work with families (personal conversations, 1993). The Centre was asked by a young Maori family to help them decide on custody and care arrangements for their children who had been in state care and were now to be returned to their family. The parents had separated, and the mother was unable to assume care for them at the time because of illness. A Pakeha (white New Zealand) worker and the family were endeavouring to make the decision together. They considered at least two possibilities, including the father caring for the children, and the maternal grandmother doing so. After much discussion, the worker and the family were tentatively agreeing that the father should take custody of the children when Wahiri, the Maori cultural consultant involved, suggested: 'In our culture the closest family relationship is between grandparents and *mokopuna* (grandchildren); these *mokopuna* should be with their grandmother.' The family members immediately recognised this as the right way for them and made their decision accordingly. Wahiri went on to explain that in the Maori cultural context if the former course had been adopted the deep sensibilities of people would have been fractured, extended family relationships weakened, the *mana* (status or position) of the family in the community lowered, and therefore the usual supports for the care of the children would have been seriously eroded. Clinical knowledge based in Western understandings would have supported a decision for the father to assume care, but Maori culture indicated another way, which was immediately recognised by the family as the right way for them. This experience was a critical one for The Family Centre in forming the principle that 'cultural knowledge must take precedence over Western clinical knowledge'.

Cultures give rise to particular understandings and patterns of relationship which are not simply different conf gurations of the same component parts. They are not readily or automatically recognisable from one culture to another. However, they provide a very signif cant context for the development and maintenance of the sense of identity, of belonging and of wellbeing, and they will be threatened rather than aff rmed by workers operating from different and sometimes contradictory cultural values. Theories and practices utilised in the human services need to take account of people's culturally based pathways to healing and growth. This does not imply that all cultural understandings and ways are liberating or just—they are not—but it respects the principle that change must evolve from within rather than being imposed from outside.

Theories and practices most commonly adopted in Australia come from Western cultures and ref ect those underlying values, meanings and arrangements. They involve an emphasis on individualism and nuclear families; particular gender arrangements, and patterns of marriage, partnering and child-rearing; higher esteem for youth than for eldership; democratic processes of participation and authority; and secular and materialistic approaches to life. Individual self-worth is often regarded as a primary goal. However, people from communal and extended family cultures do not relate easily to such concepts, f nding them confusing and alienating. Personal identity is expressed in extended family and places of belonging, not in individualistic concepts.

Spirituality is another dimension of personal, family and community life where particular knowledge and understanding are critical to aff rming and working with people's meaning systems. In many non-European cultures, spirituality is a fundamental value integrated into every aspect of life. An integrated spirituality is centred on the essential quality of relationship and connectedness—between people, between people and their ancestors and descendants, between people and the land and environment, between people and the creator spirit. These understandings will be profoundly relevant to the ways in which people see their identity and belonging, their relationships, and cultural processes of recovery, healing and change. The denigration of spirituality by much of Western scientif c, clinical and technical knowledge, the dualistic separation of spiritual and physical, linear and logical ways of thinking, and values of materialism and consumerism all mean that workers socialised within these Western meanings struggle to understand this more central and integrated spirituality. Such failure to understand can lead to disrespectful and dismissive responses to people where the meanings of life they bring, and their issues and pathways to healing, are not recognised. This results in a form of cultural racism, and social work practice becomes another forum for domination.

Cultural knowledge is therefore central knowledge. There are many contentious questions concerning how human services respond to this assertion. Sometimes, for example, it is considered important that the worker (or the organisation) hold similar cultural understandings to the family or group concerned. This may be particularly important for Indigenous peoples because human service work can so easily become a further site for domination. Language, and f uency in English, might be another consideration supporting such responses. However, workers in the mainstream also need to take up the challenge of this assertion that cultural knowledge is central knowledge, and f nd ways of developing suff cient cultural knowledge to facilitate healing, growth and change. This is a big challenge and Waldegrave (1990) sounds a warning against what he terms 'cultural tourism'—that is, the tendency for workers 'to move around culture' with about as much sensitivity and cultural understanding as a tourist. He suggests that inadequate knowledge unwittingly involves those workers in cross-cultural collisions, and f nally causes a retreat back to the known, in the belief that the approach will not work, and that people are 'resistant' or closed to help. My experience supports this observation.

It follows, then, that the place of cultural knowledge requires more emphasis than it gets in social work and anti-racist literature. It also follows that workers, particularly from the standpoint of the dominant racial and cultural context, need more resources and direction for developing the necessary knowledge and skills than are readily available. This knowledge-seeking will involve: acknowledgement of the cultural base of theories and practices, and critique of their claims to be international and intercultural; development of principles for culturally based practice by and with people from marginalised cultural communities; and self-learning—about our own cultural meaning structures and our location within the power relations of race and culture.

Learning about culture

The literature concerning cross-cultural practice is extensive and diverse, particularly as it relates to counselling. Some of this literature fails to integrate the understanding that, in working with cultural diversity, we are not just dealing with difference, but with the social processes of racism, of privilege and oppression at both the structural and personal levels. A second concern relates to the approaches taken to this learning. Two broad approaches are evident, the 'etic' and the 'emic'. Etic approaches study culture from the outside in the light of categories and concepts which are external to the culture but are universally applied—categories that easily become reduced to mechanistic conceptual constructs. This approach relies heavily on cognitive processes of learning. Other literature and my own experience suggest that cultural meanings are not best learned this way. Emic approaches are those where learning is undertaken from within and where understandings generated are seen as specif c to that cultural context. Geertz (1973) suggests that the analysis of culture 'is not an experimental science in search of law but an interpretive one in search of meaning' (1973: 5). He advises students to immerse themselves in observation and reading, weaving from the particular through the general narratives (the larger social contexts) and back (Geertz 1995). He is critical of etic approaches as he considers that it is not helpful to conceive of culture as a massive causal force shaping belief and behaviour to an abstractable pattern, that we are not faced with a set of abstractable themes which can be summarised and somehow put together. In considering gender relations, for example, he says one cannot simply identify dimensions such as sex, status, boldness or modesty and conf gure them together. Cultures are more complex and contradictory f elds of action than this, involving as they do the interplay of the local and the broad, the f gure and the ground, the particular and the general narrative. He considers emic approaches to be more propositional and dynamic, and more constructive approaches to learning culture.

Learning about cultural meanings and ways, and also race privilege, from 'within' often involves personally confronting experiences, and moving away from familiar places of belonging, position and culture in order to provide an opportunity for viewing oneself with something of an outsider's view (see, for example, Manning 2007). I have found that, in the course of this learning, it is very important to accept the position of learner, which involves deep respect and humility. It is important to 'stand under' more than to understand. This is a stance which involves giving up the power of dominance, together with a preparedness to relinquish one's own cultural ways of making meaning and to learn and value new ones; it cannot be achieved without a process of transformation of self. It involves acceptance of, and engagement with, uncertainty and discomfort. The art of listening and looking is important and the approach of observer/inquirer often preferable to that of questioner/inquirer. The learning process is not simply about learning facts or frameworks, but about gaining a deeper awareness of diverse culturally based meanings of life, relationships and communication. I have learned that, for me, the deepest enlightenment and learning comes from exposure to, and immersion in, particular cultural contexts.

Learning about race relations and 'white' privilege

Closely intertwined with learning about culture and culturally based theories and practices, and learning about oneself as a cultural being, is learning about oneself within the relations of race. Frankenberg (1993), writing about race relations in the United States, was one of the f rst to discuss her awakening to the impact of colonisation and oppression on black people and especially to her own white race privilege. She, like other writers since (see Sue 2003), considers that recognition of white race privilege in the relations of race is more diff cult than the recognition of the oppression of others, and that white people tend to conceptualise themselves as neutral in the relations of race (1993). She concludes that seeing oneself as a culturally specif c being may require moving away from one's usual situation. In the Australian context, Denborough (1996) discusses his confronting experiences while working with Indigenous people in prison. It was their challenge to him in relation to being white and middle class that led to his awakening regarding race privilege. He also observes that it is easy to avoid acknowledging the inherent benef ts that come with being white, where cultural practices can remain unmarked and unnamed and yet be the benchmark for all.

In a similar way, I can identify particular experiences which have been very signif cant in my own learning. I have been very personally and profoundly confronted with my own race privilege as I have encountered and listened to people who have experienced the devastating effects of racism: colonisation, extreme poverty and hunger, war, imprisonment, detention, torture, rape, refugee experience, exploitation, exclusion and the persisting day-to-day experiences of racism. Often their experiences have been amplif ed for me by their startling personal honesty, courage, hope, strength, hospitality and generosity of spirit, little known in Western acquisitive society. Examining and understanding the operations of white privilege and power, and f nding ways to challenge and resist these in ourselves, our professions and at the wider level of society are at the centre of anti-racist practice.

Conclusion

Terrible oppression, violence and tragedy linked to racial and cultural difference are evident in various parts of the world today. On the home front, following the national apology to Indigenous Australians we are challenged to continue together to redef ne and reshape their place within Australian society, and at the same time to determine a more just response to immigrants, refugees and people seeking asylum. We have an urgent need to better understand the operations of racism and cultural difference in order to help build a more just and peaceful society, and world. This chapter has canvassed some ways in which critical theories can be expanded to assist the development of anti-racist and culturally aff rming theories and practices for social work and the human services. It has encouraged us as students and practitioners to identify and challenge racism at all levels. This includes the challenge to create opportunities to explore and examine our own position within the relations of race and culture, so sharpening our capacity to recognise and resist white domination and privilege—within ourselves where relevant, and in our professions and workplaces. The challenge is also to make explicit the cultural bases of theories and practices and to open more spaces for the documentation of new theories and practices based on relevant cultural meanings.

8

reversing colonial practices with Indigenous peoples

Christine Fejo-King and Linda Briskman

Australian social work has some way to go in understanding Australia's Indigenous peoples across the dimensions of culture, policy and history. In order to contribute to policy and practice debates, social work must f rst and foremost examine the theoretical and policy constructs upon which its practices are based. It is important to be cognisant of the admonishment of Aboriginal social worker Stephanie Gilbert, who provides a timely reminder that social workers continue to hold central roles in areas where injustices have been carried out against Indigenous peoples, including child protection and health (Gilbert 2001).

To further traverse the complex terrain, it needs to be understood that social work operates within a political context that aims to 'close the gap', an uncritical 'practical reconciliation' notion[1] premised on Western-style aspirations of economic gain, home ownership, education and employment. This represents a disjuncture with Aboriginal aspirations that go further to include sovereignty, land justice, cultural recognition and spirituality. Indigenous knowledge has been subjugated, discarded and denigrated in solution-seeking, and problems need to be seen as amenable to solution and not intractable (Crawford et al. 2007). Many of the issues still confronting Indigenous Australians can be attributed to the colonial process and ongoing colonialism in the structural and policy arrangements that f lter down to human service practice.

In addition, social workers, like other community members, are confronted with a media barrage that focuses on dysfunction in Aboriginal communities and evades stories of strength and resilience. This then presents Indigenous communities as 'victims' rather than 'survivors'. In policy terms, this detracts from goals of liberation, instead emphasising social control, law and order and paternalistic responses.

In exploring the dilemmas, we turn to a critical social work lens to establish whether some selected paradigms—whiteness, colonialism and racism—can forge understandings that work towards achieving the human rights of Indigenous peoples. Drawing on the examples of the 2008 government apology to Indigenous Australians and the 2007 Northern Territory 'emergency response', we provide a critical social work analysis of ongoing policy imposition and how this critique can assist social workers in formulating critical practice, a practice that can be derived from a commitment to critical social work education.

The inclusion of a critical perspective in policy directions is a challenge that confronts social work with Indigenous communities. Such a challenge asks the critical social worker to adopt a ref ective approach to understanding their own values and beliefs, and those of the profession, and to interrogate the application of value systems in policy and practice applications.

The context

At the time we write, there have been some important changes for Indigenous Australians. First, there was a change of government from a conservative coalition to Labor in November 2007. In early 2008 the new prime minister, Kevin Rudd, offered an apology to Indigenous peoples for past wrongs, ending years of frustration with the previous Howard government's failure to do so, a dereliction of moral responsibility that resulted in disappointment, hurt and anger among many Indigenous Australians. Second, the Declaration on the Rights of Indigenous Peoples was, after a long and bumpy road, adopted in 2007 by the United Nations General Assembly, although a number of Western governments, including Australia, stood in opposition to it. The Rudd Labor government has signalled that it will now support the declaration, another measure that provides some optimism.

For Aboriginal and Torres Strait Islander peoples, the apology offered by the Australian government was seen as a possible beginning of a new chapter in the relationship between Indigenous and non-Indigenous Australia, and a long-awaited actioning of one of the recommendations of the *Bringing Them Home* report (HREOC 1997).

For the Stolen Generations, the apology inspired the prospect of renewal and healing where there had previously been pessimism and sadness, as many had believed that they would not live to see the day when the symbolism of an apology would be offered for the anguish and sorrow resulting from their forced removal from family, community, culture, language and country, or the resulting abuses they experienced for no reason other than their race.

The apology was also seen as a f rst step into a blank page where history, or 'theirstory', could become 'ourstory'. An example of the concept of ourstory can best be illustrated through the Aboriginal and Torres Strait Islander view of the apology being important not just for them, but for the broader Australian population, as it provided an opportunity of healing for the nation as a whole. These thoughts have been vindicated through many emails that have been received by the Stolen Generations Alliance with comments about how Australians, both Indigenous and non-Indigenous, feel they can now hold their heads up and be proud of being Australian for the f rst time. The two-way healing can best be illustrated through a story related about events following Apology Day.

As the Stolen Generations who had come to Canberra to hear the apology in person congregated at Canberra Airport to return to their various homes, they noticed something different about themselves and about others who were not part of their groups. They felt a great weight had been lifted from their shoulders. They were happy, and this happiness was ref ected in the way they saw themselves, held themselves, and communicated with those around them with smiles and an openness that they would not previously have offered. As they looked into the faces and eyes of the 'other', they saw the same happiness, hope and acceptance ref ected back at them for the f rst time in their lives.

Another important issue for Aboriginal and Torres Strait Islander peoples that received attention through the process of the apology was the recognition of Indigenous Australians as the First Nations of this land. This recognition is an important step forward in acknowledging something that may not necessarily have been the intent of the prime minister and the leader of the opposition—that is, the recognition of the sovereignty of Aboriginal and Torres Strait Islander peoples, which has never been ceded. This recognition of the First Nations of Australia supported the very public yet apparently unrecognised and unspoken notion of sovereignty, which was enacted through the historic welcome to country which occurred for the f rst time ever in the Australian Parliament. Prime Minister Rudd stated that the welcome to country would occur at each sitting of the Parliament and this was agreed to by the leader of the opposition.

These actions and their possible implications are sure to attract attention and discussion in the future. It will be interesting to see how this is handled, and whether the Australian government will keep its pre-election promise to ratify the United Nations Declaration on the Rights of Indigenous Peoples and how, if at all, there will be substance and action, or if these were only hollow words and empty promises.

Theoretical leads

There is not one body of theory that enhances our understanding of Indigenous issues in Australia, nor is there one body of knowledge that helps in formulating solutions. What is clear is that some theories from which practice has been derived are clearly against the interests of Indigenous families and communities. These include some in the psycho-dynamic realm that advocate a form of child care based on Western models of attachment, and that ignore the extended family and the holistic approach to children and families that permeates Indigenous world-views. Mental health is another area in which Indigenous people have attacked Western paradigms of knowledge and their application, as they frequently ignore Aboriginal constructs of emotional wellbeing, fail to consider the impact of colonialism and ignore the strength of spiritual connections in healing. Indigenous academics, activists and practitioners are at the forefront of challenging conventional Western approaches and formulating new knowledges that have their basis in Aboriginal cultural practices.

Turning to critical social work pointers, one of the most powerful constructs to f nd its way into theorising Indigenous issues is that of 'whiteness', stemming from the work of Ruth Frankenberg (1993, 1997) in the United States and applied increasingly to the Australian context. As discussed in the previous chapter, examining the social construction of whiteness assists in understanding the dominance of monocultural concepts that fail to consider a diversity of world-views and ways of being. Proponents of a whiteness framework tell us that being white is not questioned, as it is the standard against which everything is measured and is hence invisible (Briskman 2007).

For non-Indigenous social workers, this can mean a blindness to their own race privilege whereby a 'colourblind' approach to practice may reproduce racist practices (Mullaly 1993). Once we begin to recognise that white is a colour, we can begin to question the assumptions that strip white people of their ethnicity (Macedo & Bartolome 1999) and reverse the assumption that race is 'the prison reserved for the Other' (Moreton-Robinson 2000: xix). It is through such recognition that we can adopt a stance that interrogates the privilege and power of dominant groups which becomes normalised and not scrutinised (Quinn 2003).

Constructs of whiteness need to be considered within the ongoing colonialist discourse that stemmed from the Enlightenment period of the eighteenth century that included a belief in progress. This belief resulted in the proclamation of superiority of those deemed to be at a more 'advanced' stage on the journey of progress (Briskman 2007) and permitted the colonial domination of nations considered less civilised through the imposition of Western ways (Ife 2001). In order to challenge ongoing colonialism, social workers need to shed their position of seeing the world through a dominant lens (McLeod 2000) and cease to promote the values they espouse on those with whom they work (Ife 2001).

A third construct, closely related to the two above, which social workers need to consider in formulating theory and practice responses is that of racism, and particularly the manner in which this is enacted in policy and practice in organisations where social workers are employed. Racism is a tenet not often acknowledged by practitioners, but it still underpins the way people are dealt with, including the way Australia treats its First Peoples. Although former constructions of race based on biological and social Darwinist assumptions have thankfully disappeared from the Australian landscape, the 'new racisms' that emerge, like constructs of whiteness and colonialism, mask social work practice. Broadly, racism can be def ned as beliefs, statements and acts that render certain groups inferior on the basis that they do not belong to the culture of origin of the dominant ethnic group within the state apparatus (Hollinsworth 1997).

How this applies to social work practice with Indigenous peoples does not necessarily manifest in overt acts that we often associate with, for example, sporting f xtures and racist taunts; rather, it is the embedding of racism, often so subtle that it may be unrecognised, in policy and in organisational practices (Briskman 2007). In this, the language is often deceptive, as it is enshrined in notions of inclusivity and equality as opposed to recognition and acclamation of diversity in all its manifestations. This pits groups against each other, as underlying the policy dictates can lurk notions of inferiority underpinned by assimilation constructs that endeavour to 'elevate' Aboriginal people to Western paradigms of being and fail to acknowledge the strengths of their own society. This was particularly evident in the policies and practices of forcibly removing Indigenous children from their families (see, for example, HREOC 1997; Briskman 2003a) and has re-emerged in the federal government's 'emergency intervention' in the Northern Territory, which we will be discussing in this chapter.

Beyond closing the gap

Understanding the gap in wellbeing between Indigenous and other Australians is an important starting point for critical social workers. Alongside this, it is important to understand the premises that government calls on in its endeavours to bridge the divide. This Closing the Gap policy example highlights the dilemmas that face social workers in working with imperfect policy constructions.

Solution-f nding is f lled with contradictions. Indigenous communities are beset with problems which black and white Australia aspire to rectify. These include remaining at the bottom of the socioeconomic ladder, including dire health status, serious alcohol and substance abuse, over-representation in the criminal justice system and under-representation in the employment market (Briskman 2008). For Indigenous academic Judy Atkinson (2008), societal systems have functioned abusively and, in the main, as colonising tools.

Within the context of ongoing disadvantage in every socio-economic sphere, it is hard to dispute the desire to enhance Indigenous wellbeing. However, there exists a number of fundamental assumptions that require challenging, and the Close the Gap campaign enables a consideration of the assumptions and alternatives.

The 'close the gap' thrust emerged following concerns about Aboriginal life chances that were expressed by Indigenous and non-Indigenous people throughout the country. In its *Social Justice* report of 2005, the Aboriginal and Torres Strait Islander Social Justice Commissioner, Tom Calma, called for Australian governments to commit to achieving Aboriginal and Islander health and life expectation equality within 25 years.

The goals of the campaign are seemingly sound, as they highlight the fact that Aboriginal and Torres Strait Islanders have a life expectancy that is up to twenty years less than that of other Australians (Neill 2002), a national scandal. Among the methods advocated are increasing Indigenous Australians' access to health services, addressing issues such as poor housing, nutrition and education, and building Indigenous control and participation in the delivery of health and other services.

Reminiscent of the policy of practical reconciliation of the Howard government, Close the Gap focuses on specif c areas of 'dysfunction' such as health, housing and education, as opposed to a rights-based approach. Such measures are conceptually premised on a paradigm of liberal individualism and feed into the prejudices of those who focus on micro-issues as opposed to simultaneously advocating for land justice, sovereignty and self-determination. It harnesses the views of those Indigenous and non-Indigenous spokespersons who advocate dealing with problem areas in their own right, with a perhaps unintended consequence of shifting the blame to communities, which are then asked to provide their own solutions with minimal resources, rather than examining underlying causal factors that have created them in the f rst place. There is a legacy of similar failed attempts over many decades and across different political regimes.

Such examples of policy demonstrate the need for social workers to avoid populist discourses and to examine the legacy of past and continuing policy impositions, drawing on their knowledge of theory, practice and community. Alongside this is the need to consider how measures to bring about change are implemented, by asking questions about participation, resourcing, punitive impositions and outcomes.

This may be best understood by considering the question of education, for at the centre of the Closing the Gap initiative of the Australian government is education for Indigenous children. There is no doubt that education plays an important role in the future of Aboriginal and Torres Strait Islander children and will impact on the social determinants of health. However, there must be a recognition of the importance of two-way education that will continue to aff rm the Aboriginality of the children, or these children will have entered a fast track to assimilation. This will create another generation of Aboriginal children who have lost their connection to their homelands, law and culture. These factors have been identif ed as being important to the development of identity, resilience, self-esteem and the capacity to walk safely in two worlds, which is the expectation that is being placed on these children.

The importance of two-way education: Christine Fejo-King explains

I f rst became aware of the writings of Freire (1972) as a young social work student in the 1970s, while attending the South Australian Institute of Technology—Aboriginal Task Force.

The works of Freire and Saul Alinsky (1971) became the 'Bible' that many of us studied and internalised. This was the basis of practice that saw the birth of Aboriginal organisations such as the National Aboriginal Community Controlled Health Organisation, the Secretariat of National Aboriginal and Islander Child Care, the Aboriginal and Islander child-care agencies and the Indigenous Social Workers Association. This learning was instrumental in the development of the Aboriginal Child Placement Principle (later changed to incorporate Torres Strait Islander people), and the call for an investigation into the Stolen Generations that led to the *Bringing Them Home* report, and ultimately the recent apology to the Stolen Generations by Prime Minister Kevin Rudd (2008).

The importance of the internalisation of the teachings of these two writers was foundational to the progression of Aboriginal and Torres Strait Islander social activism and critical social work practice. However, I believe that the time has come to challenge Freire's teaching and the way that Western knowledge has been privileged over Indigenous knowledge, ways of knowing and being in Australia. It is time for a shift to privilege two-way knowledge-sharing.

This is a concept that recognises that both parties in an exchange of knowledge have valued information to share and that both parties can learn from one another; it does not privilege one set of knowledge above another. This is not a new concept; however, it does go some way to illustrating the work of Freire (1972) as being a two-edged sword for Indigenous social workers. On the one hand, Freire's (1972) teaching about 'changing the consciousness of the oppressed' (1972: 47) was an important step forward. However, speaking from experience as an Indigenous social worker, I know that once you become aware of your oppression, you seek to emancipate and empower yourself, your family and your people. This was where the work of Saul Alinsky became prominent in my mind and in the mind of others, as it offered a way forward.

For Freire, the importance of education in emancipation was fundamental, and by developing the skills to read and write, the peasants of South America were able to 'develop their power to perceive critically the way they exist in the world with which and in which they f nd themselves; they come to see the world not as a static reality but as a reality in process of transformation' (Macedo 2000). This should be the vision of critical social work and of education rather than as a tool of colonisation and genocide of the mind (Hill 2003) which is the ultimate result that occurs when young people learn to accept, internalise, privilege and own Western knowledge. Our languages could be lost, or spirituality and connection to land eradicated, and the loss would be too great to bear in the long run. Those with the vision to see this possibility in the future must take action to ensure that this does not occur.

Critical social work practice must be visionary, and learn from those practitioners who have gone full circle in their embracing of Freire's teachings to naming them as deeply Western and undermining, 'the forms of intergenerational knowledge that are the basis of the diverse approaches to sustaining local commons as sites of resistance to economic and technological globalization' (Bowers 2005: viii). Positive intergenerational knowledge is the foundation of good mental health and self-esteem, and is the buffer that prevents many of the issues Aboriginal and Torres Strait Islander peoples are combating today.

Ethical practice demands that the social workers of Australia critically ref ect on their practice and the way that they embrace and support government policies with which other nations have experimented, who in turn warn us of the consequences of good intentions gone wrong.

Policy exemplar: Northern Territory emergency response (NTER)

The question arises of how does critical social work assist in understanding, critiquing and inf uencing policy? By way of a further example, we turn to the Commonwealth government's 'emergency response' intervention in the Northern Territory. There is a pressing need to engage in robust debates about such policy developments in order to recognise that the imposition of discriminatory measures, shrouded in 'good intentions', demonstrates the ongoing inability to recognise the power of dominant groups in society, an ongoing form of colonialist practice and covert institutional racism that singles out specif c groups for policies that are not meted out to others in the society. Support for the human rights of Indigenous peoples is limited. There is at least a rhetoric of affording the First Peoples the rights of other citizens, such as the right to good health. However, there is a negation of the collective rights that Indigenous people hold in high regard. Moreover, social workers may be charged with implementing policies that are inconsistent with Indigenous cultural values and with the values and ethics of the social work profession.

With the introduction of the NTER, the paradox is that there was general consensus within the Aboriginal community of the Northern Territory that action needed to be taken to assist families and communities to address the issues that they were facing. However, there is debate around the quasi-military (Ife 2008b) response by the Howard government which has remained in place under the current Rudd government. In this whole response, what is missing is the historical context and the questions of how the Aboriginal communities found themselves in the situation that brought about the 'emergency response' and the role of power, and government disengagement (Dillon & Westbury 2007).

As social workers, we are very aware of how power may be maintained by providing only a subsistence existence to the people to be controlled. On ref ection, this theory can be seen in practice by government against Aboriginal peoples for generations. The land, the most valuable economic resource, was removed, then the children were taken away through the Stolen Generations. International trade and internal trade routes that extended as far as the Northern Territory to Victoria were blocked off with the appropriation of the land by non-Indigenous peoples who put up fences. Control of the movements and interactions of Aboriginal people occurred through the power of the Chief Protector of Aborigines. Over the years, there was disengagement of government and the non-recognition of Aboriginal law. When the nations, communities and families became dysfunctional, the blame for the situation that the people found themselves in, with the clashing of the two cultures and the disempowerment of the very blocks that kept Aboriginal society intact, the 'great disremembering' of the strength of Aboriginal society became the norm. The 'blame' for the dysfunctional results of the disempowerment of Aboriginal peoples was and is placed at the feet of the Aboriginal peoples, rather than at the feet of those who instigated this disempowerment, who controlled and manipulated and who did not have the skills or the political will to make real and meaningful change and to re-empower the people they had subjugated.

For years, Aboriginal peoples in remote communities have been ignored or identif ed as an economic drain in neo-liberal thinking in Australia, where the economic bottom line is all important and where individual ideology is privileged over the group ideology that is an intricate part of the Aboriginal world-view. The substantial role that Aboriginal peoples have played with regard to border security in this time of international security concerns around terrorism, drug running and people smuggling, and the care of the land and animals through Indigenous knowledge (Dillon & Westbury 2007), have become a 'part of the "cult of forgetfulness" and the "cult of disremembering" in mainstream Australian society' (Stanner 1969: 25, 35, cited in Dillon & Westbury 2007: 1).

A part of the unseen impact of the 'emergency response' has been the view that child sexual abuse is an Aboriginal issue, which those working in child protection know not to be true. This perception, however, has had the effect of demonising Aboriginal men and families within the eyes of the wider Australian community. It has resulted in the dumping of child sexual abuse upon the Aboriginal and Torres Strait Islander peoples with a huge negative psychological, emotional and social toll. The NTER can be and is viewed by many as cultural abuse, which has been def ned as:

> when the culture of a people is ignored, denigrated, or worse, intentionally attacked. It is abuse because it strikes at the very identity and soul of the people it is aimed at; it attacks their sense of self-esteem, it attacks their connectedness to their family and community (Bamblett 2007).

An important question to ask is where is the evidence of this 'cultural abuse'? The National Coalition of Aboriginal and Torres Strait Islander Social Workers Association (NCATSISWA) has received reports from around the country of Aboriginal children, especially the boys, telling their parents that they didn't want to be Aboriginal anymore, as they fear they will grow up to be an Aboriginal man and 'Aboriginal men do bad things to their children and beat up their wives' and they then turn to their fathers and ask, 'Dad, are you going to hurt us?' The pain and anguish of the grandfathers, fathers, brothers and uncles have gone to the very heart of Aboriginal men, attacking their very being. Social workers of Australia, how will you respond, and how are you responding to this human crisis?

In the f rst year of the 'emergency response', children all over the Northern Territory did not receive presents for birthdays and Christmas as their parents were not able to access their funds. This may seem a trivial matter; however, the psychological impact on both the parents and children should not be underestimated. With a view to rectifying this situation, the National Coalition of Aboriginal and Torres Strait Islander Social Workers, in partnership with a number of Aboriginal communities across the Northern Territory, the Rotary Clubs of South Australia and the Northern Territory and the Northern Territory Registrars Association, have been working to address this issue. They have gathered presents for children up to the age of sixteen that will be delivered across the Northern Territory over the next holiday season.

At the time of writing, a review of the 'emergency response' had taken place with the Labor government announcing that it would maintain the core features of the previous policy.

Social work education

The question that must be asked of social work educators and curriculum developers is simply this: How are you preparing upcoming social workers of Australia? An analogy that is often used is that of a person going to see a medical practitioner. If you are ill, would you go to see a medical practitioner who is sensitive and aware of medical practice or would you go to see someone who is a capable and competent practitioner? Of course you would go to someone who is capable and competent, and yet critical, capable and competent social work practice with Aboriginal and Torres Strait Islander peoples is not the current standard or the baseline to be achieved prior to enabling practice with this population group in a range of human services areas. Where does the capacity to undertake this form of critical social work practice begin? It must begin in the Schools of Social Work where Aboriginal and Torres Strait Islander competency in practice must be an integral part of the curricula. This must be supported through placements that enable social work students and educators to interact, build capacity, and gain experience and understanding of Aboriginal ways of knowing, being and doing.

For a number of years, the National Coalition of Aboriginal and Torres Strait Islander Social Workers Association has been calling for the Partnerships and Community Empowerment (PACE) initiative to be implemented by Schools of

Social Work and the Australian Association of Social Workers in partnership with it. Now the Australian government, in an effort to close the gap in life expectancy between Indigenous and non-Indigenous Australians in a generation, is calling for exactly this kind of practice. Partnership and empowerment have been identif ed by the World Health Organization as being the most productive and successful way of achieving this goal (WHO 2008a).

The Australian government is so committed to this goal that Reconciliation Australia has been funded to assist corporate Australia, the education sector, peak bodies, and any other Australian organisation which supports positive practice and win-win situations, to develop a Reconciliation Action Plan (RAP) that will assist them, through relationships of respect, to identify and develop opportunities to rectify the gulf in the socio-economic conditions between Indigenous and non-Indigenous Australians. There is certainly an opportunity for Australian social workers and other professional groups to take up this opportunity and show leadership within their spheres of inf uence.

The future

Although a somewhat bleak picture has been presented in this chapter, there has been progress in the last decade in the social work response to Indigenous theorising and to practice improvements. The invisibility of Indigenous Australians in social work curricula is slowly being redressed, and social workers are gaining critical awareness through relationships with Indigenous organisations, through the burgeoning Indigenous writing on social work, and through f lm, music and other forms of artistic representation by Indigenous Australians. From a basis of understanding and critical ref ection, social workers can adopt a role as policy advocates and critical practitioners.

As outlined in this chapter, there are some basic elements for the advancement of a critical social work approach, including a critical understanding of history, the application of relevant theoretical constructs, an awareness of policy and its impact, and a revamping of social work education.

9

reconstructing social work practices with families

Susie Costello[1]

Families are the basic units of identity, connection and care in Australian society. Families can be nurturing, validating, confusing and damaging. Many people spend much of their time trying to make sense of their own family experiences and relationships. Vulnerable family members often experience oppression within their own families. Family forms that diverge from the traditional nuclear family live with discrimination, homophobia, racism and other forms of oppression. This chapter explores critical approaches to conceptualising, critiquing and working with vulnerable families.

What do we mean by 'family'?

'Family' is a contested term. Despite the diversity of families, the notion of 'familism' prevails in the Australian culture (Mason 2001: 70), the dominant view being that 'family' refers to a white, heterosexual, nuclear household, with a breadwinner husband and homemaking wife taking care of their children. Yet the two-parent family with dependent children[2] only represents about a third (37 per cent) of Australia's families (ABS 2008a) and a minority of households worldwide. Some people consider their families to be only the relatives with whom they live; others include extended family members and for some the notion of family includes people who are unrelated. In many parts of Africa and Asia, people typically live in extended families (Baker 2001), yet migrants are disadvantaged by familist def nitions that exclude entry to multiple family members. Australian Indigenous people often live with extended families, particularly in rural areas, with poverty and overcrowding affecting their living conditions (ABS 1996).

The Australian Bureau of Statistics (ABS 2005) def nes family as:

> Two or more persons, one of whom is at least 15 years of age, who are related by blood, marriage (registered or de facto), adoption, step or fostering, and who are usually resident in the same household. The basis of a family is formed by identifying the presence of a couple relationship, lone parent–child relationship or other blood relationship. Some households will, therefore, contain more than one family.

The concept of family evokes the emotional connectedness of families, emphasising patterns of, or lack of, caring and intimacy (Baker 2001). Our identity evolves within the experiences and contexts of our family's position within the class, gender, racial and cultural structures of our society. Family membership and culture are transferred through generations with legacies of expectation, obligation, guilt and pride. With the aim of transforming oppressive structures and practices that discriminate and marginalise families and family members, critical social work has a signif cant role in family work.

Critical social work practice with vulnerable families with children

Children are the youngest, smallest, least powerful citizens with minimal opportunities for decision-making. Yet our culture does not make children a priority of care, as evidenced by people's ranking of child abuse signif cantly lower than concerns such as government rates and charges (Tucci et al. 2006). The UN Convention on the Rights of the Child def nes a child as a person under eighteen years of age. Being under eighteen, children do not vote so their opinions do not inf uence governments' allocation of funding and policies. The underresourced, overwhelmed children's services, education, child mental health, early childhood services and child care indicate a societal lack of concern for the wellbeing of children (Perry 2005).

The Australian Association of Social Workers (AASW 2008) identif es social workers' signif cant role in promoting the wellbeing and ensuring the safety and protection of all children and young people—especially those who are most vulnerable. Fulf lling this responsibility requires a foundational knowledge of the social, economic and environmental factors that render families vulnerable, plus a capacity for ref exive thinking about practice and power. Practice responses require theoretical knowledge specif cally related to working with families and children.

Vulnerable families

Who are the vulnerable families and what makes them vulnerable? Vinson's (2004) research shows that location indicates and determines vulnerability. Families growing up in Australia's poorest postcodes are up to seven times more at risk of child abuse and neglect, and likely to suffer from low incomes, long-term unemployment, early school leaving, physical and mental disabilities and prison admissions. The state intervenes predominantly in poor families' lives, particularly in sole-parent households with low incomes, f nancial stress, social isolation and little support from their immediate family (AIHW 2007a). Aboriginal and Torres Strait Islander children are seven times as likely to be on care and protection orders or in out-of-home care (AIHW 2007a). This makes Indigenous children the most vulnerable of the vulnerable. Structural factors such as poverty, unemployment and domestic violence are factors in this overrepresentation (Stanley et al. 2003), with 42 per cent of Indigenous families experiencing domestic violence compared with 23 per cent for others (AIC 2001).

Increasing numbers of families with children have both parents in the paid workforce. Overworked, overstressed parents struggle to relate to, much less supervise, their children and teenagers who are establishing a 'second family' with peer groups, virtually and in reality (Taffel 2001). Many children feel disconnected from adults. They perceive that adults do not listen, respect or believe them, or take their views into account (Tucci et al. 2008).

Families that can afford to, consult private counsellors or psychiatrists who discreetly 'respect' the privacy of the family. Others require, or have imposed on them, social workers with minimal experience of the forms of oppression facing families in the public welfare system. In their work in public housing estates, detention centres or prisons, workers are exposed to many of the same risks faced by these clients: crime, abuse, violence, discrimination, health risks and vicarious trauma through bearing witness to the awfulness of some people's stories and lives (Costello 2004). Critical ref exivity can alert workers to the responsibility and blindness of their privileged middle-class status as educated, employed professionals, regardless of their family background (Healy 2005a).

Understanding and using power

Inevitably, practitioners make assumptions based on their own experiences, which may obscure the impact of oppression arising from racism, sexism, classism, abilism, urbanism, racism, homophobia, familism and other forms of power or oppression. Social workers' commitment to human rights and anti-oppressive philosophies does not guarantee inclusive, consultative, respectful responses to unexpected diverse practices and viewpoints. Power operates in complex ways within families and between the social worker and family and other professionals and institutions. Foucault (1984) identif ed the following:

- Power is exercised, not possessed: it is something people create and use.
- Power is both repressive and productive; a person can use power *over* someone to subjugate, control and restrict or use power to inform, support or transform.
- Power comes from the bottom up. It derives from the lived experiences of everyday life; we all have the potential to create some form of power (cited in Fook 2002a: 52).

In the face of oppression, the critical social worker's task is to analyse and negotiate a change of power relations and structures in ways that empower everyone. The idea is not to *not have* power, or be powerless, but to use and share power by ref ecting on and being transparent about the practitioner's role and obligations and the processes and operations of power (Healy 2005a). Social workers can go home after 'helping' families who live with violence and oppression. Through critical ref exivity, social workers question their taken-for-granted assumptions (Taylor & White 2000) and examine the origins and operations of power.

Lack of awareness or misuse of power can be dangerous for vulnerable family members and social workers, particularly when there is violence and abuse. Without awareness of patriarchal power, for example, workers are blind to familist discourses that excuse male violence and prescribe women's submission to their partners' and children's needs (Lenore 1994). Stanley and Goddard (2002) found that workers' fear and lack of training regarding how to respond to violent men led them to unconsciously avoid or collude with perpetrators' power (O'Hagan 1997), resulting in children being removed from their homes rather than the perpetrator being challenged to take responsibility for his behaviour and/or removed.

Avoiding the dynamics of power by ignoring perpetrators of abuse is ineffective but common. It is easier for workers to advocate for victims and avoid rather than engage empathetically with the struggles of perpetrators (Pyles 2005). Engagement does not mean excusing, forgiving or compromising. Critical engaging includes identifying, naming and working to transform injustice, rather than avoiding or escaping it. Case study 9.1 considers ways of attempting to engage and transform power dynamics in an interaction with an aggressive man.[3]

Gina and Bruce's family f ts the dominant construction of the nuclear family. Patriarchal, racist and familist discourses bind their 'ideal' family system in silence until the status quo is challenged from elsewhere (Wadsworth 2007). Finding the pivotal point of leverage through which to enter the isolating barriers of violence and control is the challenge for the critical social worker. Assessing the impact of psychological damage is often the point of entry in terms of child protection. Psychological theories are key discourses drawn on by practitioners to assist vulnerable families such as this one. The next section critiques discourses around the psychological theories of attachment, trauma and development in relation to child protection.

Protection and the law

The extent to which the state intervenes in families' lives is contentious. The notion of social parenthood (Edgar 2000: 31) or 'socially distributed parenting' (McGurk 1996) considers children the responsibility of all citizens with minimal intervention by the state. Yet children clearly need laws and policies to protect them from their families: thousands of children live with domestic violence each year; the majority of child homicides are committed by family members, with the under f ves at highest risk; and the number of children removed from their families for their own protection in Australia has more than doubled over the last decade (Tucci et al. 2008).

In the Australian state of Victoria, the *Children, Youth and Families Act* 2005 has reduced the 'intrusion of the state', devolving responsibility instead to community organisations. The impetus to provide evidence of child abuse and neglect, without which the state will not act, places community social workers in an invidious position. Sandwiched between the hard-to-reach power of the state to protect and the pain of witnessing children suffering in increasingly complex family situations, these workers can become burnt out and lost in bureaucracy. In the project of meeting the enormous bureaucratic demands of their job, while trying to assemble evidence of cumulative harm, they can lose sight of basic social work values of respect for human rights and social justice. While the rhetoric of choice and respect continues, the formalised risk assessments and monitoring by community workers render them quasi-child protection workers.

Case study 9.1

Sylvia[4] works as a school student welfare coordinator. She met with twelve-year-old Talia and her pregnant Filipina mother Gina after Talia's induced vomiting at school indicated her anxiety about what was happening at home. Talia nervously admitted that her father Bruce hit her mother but Gina insisted he was a good man who provided for their two children well. Sylvia informed Talia and Gina of their rights to safety, prepared a safety plan and gave them the number of the police. Talia was fearful of the consequences for herself and her mother if Bruce knew they had spoken to anyone.

Sylvia was in her office when Bruce arrived angrily, asking if she was the social worker 'who filled my wife with bullshit ideas'.

As Bruce entered the room, Sylvia felt far from powerful. She was unprepared and alone and intimidated by Bruce's aggression, his strong physical presence and his personal power as breadwinner and head of his family. Sylvia's power (and safety) depends on her knowledge and training of how to manage herself and the angry client. This reveals a contested layer of power between the worker and manager. Workers are often unsupported in stating their fears to their managers, resulting in assault, threats and other forms of intimidation (Stanley & Goddard 2002). Managers are responsible for ensuring a safe workplace, including providing training and debriefing for dealing with dangerous situations; however, without awareness of rights or the support of a union, workers may not feel confident in naming their fears and needs for safe work practices.

In terms of direct practice with aggressive clients, Matsakis (1998) suggests practitioners speak slowly and gently, explain their role, listen with empathy, let them talk and affirm clients' anger as legitimate. Searing (2003) suggests workers respond to clients' material needs if possible and appear confident, even if they do not feel it. Yet clients want 'authenticity' from social workers rather than professional or textbook responses. Young recommends a 'no-bullshit' approach (Findlay 2007) to name and confront inappropriate behaviour by 'telling as it is', using conversational, respectful language. Identifying strengths and options invites dialogue. Fine and Turner (1991) suggest 'closing space' conversationally on socially unacceptable actions while 'opening space' about underlying feelings so as not to tyrannise clients who have less positional or ascribed power: Sylvia's response to Bruce may go something like this (not all at once):

»

> Yes, Bruce, I did meet with Gina and Talia and it sounds like there is a lot of stress at home for you all. What's going on for you? Gina tells me you work hard and are very involved in your children's lives. Would you like to sit down and tell me what's going on for you? It's hard for me to hear what you have to say when you shout at me. I'm interested to hear as I don't understand how come you think it's alright to hurt Gina, who you say you love. That can't go on, as you would realise. Are you surprised to hear that Gina and your children want more of your caring father side than your violent side? There are obviously times when you can manage your violence, but it sounds like it's taking you over. What's that like for you?

Seeking Bruce's explanations and strengths may open space for him to reveal his shame and fear. Sylvia can invite him to take responsibility for his behaviour (Jenkins 1991) through a narrative approach that separates 'the person' from 'the problem' by 'externalising' the problem as a separate 'thing'—violence—over which some control can be exercised.

Regardless of explanations, however, nothing excuses violence. In attempting to renegotiate the power imbalances, the worker must not lose sight of the rights and safety of the children and Gina as the priority. The critical goal is to identify and aim to transform unequal power dynamics to benefit everyone. If Bruce does not choose to acknowledge or change his behaviour, other parts of the system need to be mobilised. For the children, this may mean the involvement of child protective services. For Gina, who as a migrant woman with little economic, positional or personal power has little sense of her entitlement to safety, it is important to keep the door open through ongoing contact and support, perhaps disguised as practical or child-focused assistance. The process of developing a safety plan of how to call the police and where to hide money and keys to escape can sow seeds for later self-protection.

Best Interest Principles from the UN Convention on the Rights of the Child are implemented in legislation for workers in the front line of work with vulnerable children. Social workers are expected to have specif c working knowledge about parenting, children's rights and developmental needs, attachment, trauma and the impact of 'cumulative harm', law (family, mental heath, protective and child-care), social policies, organisational and interdisciplinary contexts and resources

(Iwaniec 2007). Without a critical lens, these bodies of knowledge can become singular technologies imposed instrumentally without ethical decision-making or contextual or cultural considerations.

The place of psychological theories

In advocating for the least powerful members of families, child welfare workers must navigate 'incommensurable' discourses (Marcus 1994). The scientif c psychological discourse is alien to critical social work's interpretative analysis of language and power. Critical ref exivity is particularly useful here as a vehicle for the practitioner to ref ect on what is excluded by a particular theoretical structure or discourse to reveal their internal locus and operations of power, and to remain vigilant to the dynamics of power between the organisation, workers and clients.

Through a critical lens, psychodynamic perspectives may enhance practitioners' understanding of their own subconscious responses and behaviours triggered by clients' pain and aggression. Waddell (1989) argues that social workers avoid emotional pain by responding only to clients' immediate material needs through 'servicing': providing or referring to services, rather than 'serving' or emotionally 'being with' a client in emotional distress. In bearing witness, social workers risk feeling powerless, paralysed, withdrawn and numb, along with feelings of fear, outrage and anger at perpetrators, political regimes, the victim, themselves and their own inadequacies (Perlesz 1999). Full acknowledgement of the knowledge/power dimension and their own positioned subjectivities through ref exivity assists practitioners to combine alternative practice approaches (D'Cruz et al. 2007).

Trauma theories

Conventional trauma theory attributes feelings of vulnerability, helplessness, and loss of safety and control to a single shock or series of events such as disasters, violent events, divorce, assault, bullying, serious accidents or losses (Jenkins 2004). Children who witness or experience regular and persistent violence are said to undergo alterations to their brain development with detrimental effects on their capacity to learn or form relationships and possible chronic, lifelong mental health problems such as post-traumatic stress disorder (Perry 2005). 'Diagnosis' and 'treatment' of post-traumatic stress disorder are prescribed through the American diagnostic tools and involve reassociating cognitions, feelings and behaviours.

Limitations of conventional trauma theory include the medicalised language and processes of diagnosis and treatment that can be disempowering for people who have developed their own coping strategies to manage unbearable psychological memories (Burstow 2003). Not everyone wants or needs trauma recovery treatment that revisits the pain. Trauma theory may attribute blame to the families and overlook physiological explanations (Nicolson & Fawcett 2007; Goodman & Williams 2007) or critical explanations. Trauma theory has been limited to individual, single events. There is a lack of understanding, for example, about the impact of transgenerational trauma on Holocaust survivors, Indigenous people from the Stolen Generations, refugees and abused children. This can leave victims in, and blamed for, their circumstances. Yet, without understanding trauma, workers may prescribe speech therapy or special education, or diagnose generalised 'developmental delay', leaving the child in a violent or neglectful environment.

Attachment theories

Bowlby's (1951) research into the mental health of parentless children in postwar Europe concluded that, to grow up mentally healthy, 'the infant and young child should experience a warm, intimate and continuous relationship with his [*sic*] mother (or permanent mother substitute) in which both f nd satisfaction and enjoyment' (1951: 13). Attachment discourses claim that interruptions to early processes of attachment between a child and their primary carer can cause permanent psychological damage (Rossiter 2005).

The dangers of using this theory without considering history and context are obvious in their potential to blame the carer—usually the mother—for failing to establish the correct attachment with her child. Insuff cient knowledge of, or over-reliance on, attachment theory can distort its value. A critical perspective validates theories about human connection *and* considers the structural oppressions and multigenerational inf uences impacting on the family's capacity to form healthy attachments (Caffery & Erdman 2003). Strength-based writers focus on resilience and the capacity of infants and children to form multiple attachments, moving away from discourses that emphasise the biological mother as the primary attachment f gure (Rolfe 2004; Streeck-Fischer & van der Kolk 2000).

Developmental theories

Developmental theories focus on the changing physical, psychological and/or social characteristics of children over time. These theories state that children progress through a succession of stages, each with certain developmental tasks to be completed. This takes place 'only in the context of signif cant emotional relationships . . . [of which] the most signif cant . . . are family relationships whether by blood, adoption, marriage or commitment' (Carter & McGoldrick 1999: 5). Family life-cycle models identify stages for families, such as young people leaving home, coupling, child rearing, separation, divorce, repartnering and retirement, each of which involves tasks and emotional challenges for the whole family (Carter & McGoldrick 1999) and has contextual and cultural particularities.

Through critical ref exivity, practitioners can be aware of the risks of developmental frameworks being applied too rigorously from a familist perspective that assumes all people progress through similar stages (Baker 2001). Discourses about child development have been used to classify, discriminate and control disadvantaged people (Rose 1990). The signif cance of rules around transitions can be overlooked without a cultural lens. Used with a critical analysis of power, conf ict and diversity, a developmental model can be useful for normalising the behaviours, beliefs and emotions people feel at transitional stages in families.

Social workers need a critical knowledge of psychodynamic theories, yet may be vulnerable to the lure of 'professional' recognition and status of the 'psy' (Healy 2005a) discourses. Case study 9.2 considers the use of some of these theories in the situation of an Indigenous family brought to the attention of the statutory government department for child protection.

Social action and political change

Lacking a critical understanding of diversity or culture, social workers have played a signif cant part in removing Indigenous children from their families, colluding with the discourse of the time that living with non-related, white people in children's homes or foster families was better for these children than living with their own families. Since the last edition of this book, Australia has elected a new government, with some positive implications for families: the Rudd Labor government swiftly asserted a National Apology to Indigenous People, a commitment to address the causes and incidence of homelessness and to coordinate national integrated responses to domestic violence and child protection.

Responding to disrupted attachment and its consequent grief and trauma can be addressed through collective processes that help people realise their power, take control of their lives and solve their own problems (Saleebey 2006). In consultation with Aboriginal elders, the Dulwich Centre brought together several Aboriginal communities in participatory research gatherings around campf res to yarn and exchange stories about problems facing their communities, such as breakdowns in mutual respect, grief and loss, and parenting. The process focused on the

Case study 9.2

Darlene, aged 37, is caring for her six children on a supporting parent's benefit. She loves her children and would do anything for them. Darlene is finding it hard caring for the children since Robert, the father of the youngest three children, was locked up for non-payment of parking fines. The school reported concerns to Child Protection Services about the 'sexualised' behaviours of the youngest two girls, Kirrae (6) and Taylah (9). The girls have been simulating sexual acts in the playground. School staff are also worried that Bindi (4) has undiagnosed and untreated foetal alcohol syndrome.

Three years ago, Child Protection Services investigated reports that Darlene's alcohol and *yarndi* [an Aboriginal word for marijuana] problems were affecting her ability to care for her children. There were reports about unhygienic and chaotic conditions in the house, with acquaintances coming and going throughout the day and night. Darlene's mother is a respected Elder in the Aboriginal community and is affectionately known as Aunty Beryl. She has moved in to help Darlene as she is very caring with her grandchildren. Aunty Beryl is a member of the Stolen Generations. Her own life experiences make her very suspicious and hostile towards 'the welfare'. Darlene's oldest sister and two children recently moved in after her husband was killed in a car accident. Various adult cousins stay with Darlene when they visit from the country.

The case was referred to the community organisation for assessment.

The task for the social worker in this case is complex: to seek evidence to substantiate or dismiss the allegations of sexual abuse and neglect. Child protection workers aim to interview children in the most appropriate and sensitive manner, sometimes at the child's school. The principles of respect, transparency, honesty and caring are paramount in this process. Workers are ascribed with enormous power in this task, power that has a history of misuse resulting in intergenerational transmissions of trauma, oppression and discrimination for this family and others.

Indigenous children are frequently placed in out-of-home care due to issues of neglect. As in the wider population, neglect is often the result of poverty and a breakdown of parents' capacity and capability to meet the needs of children and ensure their safety and wellbeing. However, for Indigenous families these issues are more complex as the practical realities of oppression are exacerbated by the legacy of past policies of forced removal of children, intergenerational effects of previous separations and cultural differences in child-rearing practices (HREOC 1997; AIHW 2007a).

»

Contact by a non-Indigenous social worker is likely to trigger deep-seated fear, grief and trauma, as aggressive defences against the repetition of child removal. Racist, familist assumptions may bias a non-Indigenous social worker entering this situation: the house is overcrowded and may be untidy; the father is absent, not 'winning the bread'; and the mother is neither cleaning nor caring, according to the reports. Darlene may be alcohol or drug affected and abusive.

How might a non-Indigenous worker establish a good relationship with the family, the most important factor in protecting children (Darlington Social Research Unit 1998)? Aboriginal and Torres Strait Islanders' styles of helping include 'tuning in and sussing out', starting with 'a yarn, a joke and a cup of tea' (Lynn 1998). But a visit by an outsider will not be seen as 'helpful' until trust and credibility can be established.

In the state of Victoria, the Lakidjeka [Aboriginal word for child] Aboriginal Child Specialist Advice and Support Service (ACSASS) has been profiled as a best-practice model for Indigenous responses to child protection issues (Higgins & Butler 2007). The Lakidjeka caseworker works with the child protection worker investigating the report. Lakidjeka provides an Indigenous perspective on risk and safety assessments, and cultural and case management advice to DHS. The service supports families by advocating an Indigenous perspective on all significant child protection decisions; improving the engagement of Indigenous children and families under statutory investigation processes; providing advice on culturally relevant support services for Indigenous children and their families; and encouraging involvement of extended family and community members in the support of the family.[5]

Together with the Lakidjeka worker, the social worker needs to tell the family members why they are there in a respectful, honest and caring way. In facilitating this process, the Indigenous co-worker puts herself on the line in vouching for a non-Indigenous worker and can be caught between professional and cultural expectations and boundaries (Bennett & Zubrzycki 2003). The situation calls for the 'no bullshit approach' (Findlay 2007), where the worker is upfront about the surveillance and monitoring role, advising the family *not* to trust them and giving them as much choice as possible (Kagan & Schlosberg 1989), while apologising for the lack of choices, citizenship, rights or dignity afforded to Indigenous people by non-Indigenous Australians, including social workers. Such an apology implicitly implies responsibility to transform the injustices.

Even with an Indigenous worker present, 'bearing witness' to families' fury and pain is hard (Perlesz 1999). Workers' defences may invoke 'cultural relativism' »

(Gillingham 2006) or white guilt, preventing non-Indigenous workers from naming and acting on abuse and injustice for fear of replicating past policies. Here, workers can use their position of responsibility and power to close space on unacceptable practices in ways that open space for Indigenous realities and involvement.

How do you talk with and assess four-, six- and nine-year-olds? How do they think? How do the indicators of foetal alcohol syndrome compare with those of developmental delay, abuse and trauma? The Child Development and Trauma Guide (DHS 2008) indicates that Kirrae, at six, may be anxious to please and to gain adult approval but lose interest in a conversation that she does not enjoy, whereas at nine, Taylah may 'think in complex ways for long periods of time' and like to have her opinion respected. When affected by trauma, children at all stages may display reduced eye contact (DHS 2008).

A critical appraisal of trauma theory takes the worker beyond the prescriptive level to consider the cross-cultural context wherein lowered eyes indicate respect in some Indigenous communities. A stance of working alongside the family respects their expertise about their children and, unless there are obvious signs, practitioners would get to know the family and children over several visits (DHS 2008). Considering the dynamics within Aboriginal communities, the Indigenous worker may know the family and can yarn about common friends and activities. The workers might engage the children by using puppets, art materials or other visual resources such as Koori Strength Cards (SNAICC 2008) to encourage the child to depict their family, an event or a dream. Children may hold loyalties that cannot be spoken about. Symbolic communication offers avenues for conveying fear without disclosing facts or breaching invisible loyalties. Protective Behaviours statements are a useful way to convey that 'We all have the right to feel safe all of the time', that bodies give warning signs when feeling unsafe—'Nothing is so awful we can't talk with someone about it'—and to identify someone that children feel confident talking to when they are unsafe (KAMSC 2008).

Assessment evolves over several meetings. During this time, the workers' goal is to support and strengthen the family emotionally ('serving') through listening, exchanging stories and spirituality with knowledge of cultural and community norms (Lynn 1998); and practically ('servicing': Waddell 1989), providing information, referral, in-home support, material aid, life skills training, parenting education skills development and advocacy (Wise 2001; AIHW 2007a). Social workers are guided by ethical (professionally directed) judgement and codes of conduct, and given power to ensure minimum standards of wellbeing for vulnerable people »

> and themselves (Healy 2005a). The workers must assess Darlene's ability to tune into and prioritise her children's needs, and assess whether she and her family can keep them safe. If a relative is found to have sexually abused the children, will the family be able to confront and stop him or are there family and cultural rules that prevent that? Can they assist the children's recovery from the abuse? Assessment should locate the family's strengths and capacity to care for their children within the broader structural factors (oppression, patriarchy, relevant dominant discourses and their impact) and identify ways of transforming racist, colonialist practices.

strengths and resources, and honoured the knowledge held by, the communities. The communities decided that: 'Despite the injustices of the past and all that has happened to separate us from our children, we are now taking a stand to turn things around so that the future is better for our grandchildren and great grandchildren.' There was a decision to reclaim the parenting skills that were taken from them, to f nd ways that would work to give young people a sense of pride and responsibility (Narrandera 2002; Denborough et al. 2006).

Direct work with families is not enough to transform unjust systems of power beyond the local level. The stories of oppressed people need to be told and heard. The Dulwich Centre's free online access to narratives of their consultative work extends the critical project of transforming discourses to a broad readership. Similarly, the social work-led Australian Childhood Foundation (ACF 2008) combines research, campaigns, education advocacy and counselling for children, young people and their families in their child abuse-prevention programs. As an independent children's charity, the ACF performs an independent monitoring function by listening to and publishing children's feedback about protective, therapeutic and support services, evaluating the impact of child abuse on children and conducting discourse analyses of media depictions and community perceptions of children and child abuse. Its aim is to produce evidence-based advice to government, and to child health and welfare organisations.

Conclusion

Families are the key site of identity, connection and care in our society, with multiple forms contesting the prevailing discourse of the nuclear family. Individual families' access to power and choice is limited or enhanced by their location within dominant or subordinate structures of power, the analysis and transformation of which are central to critical social work. As decision-makers in families' lives, social workers need to be critically ref exive about where power lies, and how it operates to oppress or empower people, particularly those who are vulnerable.

Indigenous families remain the most disadvantaged, with the highest rate of poverty and child protection intervention, and children are the most vulnerable of all citizens. There are enormous pressures on social workers in family support and child protection when it comes to assessing risk and ensuring children's safety. Current legislation requires a working knowledge of attachment, trauma and developmental theories that have the potential to stigmatise and oppress when used without a critical analysis.

Workers can experience powerlessness through intimidation and abuse and being in an unsupported work situation, despite their privilege as employed educated professionals. Family workers have a crucial role in identifying the beliefs, assumptions and prejudices affecting families, while raising families' and other workers' consciousness about structural impediments to participation.

Families require a continuum of services which are strengths based, culturally sensitive and inclusive, and which enhance cultural and family wellbeing and build families' capacity to keep children safe, to build healthy relationships and to access available support. Participatory research and social action can validate families' 'lived experiences' and generate bottom-up solutions to challenge policies and practices that oppress families and family members.

10

examining the meaning of childhood in critical social work practice

Heather D'Cruz

This chapter aims to make explicit the complexities of critical social work practice with children in different f elds—for example, in schools, child protection, or family support and counselling (Dupper 2003; Alston & Mckinnon 2005a). Assumptions about children and childhood inf uence organisational policies and social work practices in those contexts.

I aim to critically engage with these underpinning assumptions by drawing on social theories that explore questions about the identity of 'the child', and the legal, social and cultural contexts in which the identity of 'the child' is constructed (Kessen 1983; James & Prout 1997; Gittins 1998).[1] The chapter also considers how the identity of 'the child' is related to complementary identities of 'parent' and 'adult' (D'Cruz 2004: 51–3; 194–237).

While critical social work practice aims to challenge the structural inequalities and forms of oppression that are seen to cause many social problems, including child maltreatment, family violence and dysfunction, it is also the case that the sociology of social problems takes a critical approach to how something becomes a social problem (Foucault 1965, 1977, 1978a; Hacking 1991; Best 2004). That is, there is a political process whereby social actors, including social workers, participate in def ning and debating the reality of a social problem, its boundaries and what is to be done. The different claims-making processes are associated with discourses whereby language as a way of representing versions of knowledge is also a device of power that is deployed by different participants in struggles over what is true and legitimate and what is not (Potter 1996; D'Cruz 2004). The sociology of social problems therefore also fundamentally challenges the normative bases for claims and counter-claims by which a problem emerges and how, through 'dividing practices' (Foucault 1965, 1977, 1978a), identities of normal and abnormal subjects are produced, with particular consequences.

Social workers are inextricably bound up in such processes because social work is a normative profession. That is, the purpose of social work is to make decisions based on moral claims—for example, attending to the different needs and rights of individuals identif ed as 'children' and 'parent(s)', and the power dynamics between such identities within a grouping called 'the family' (Frost & Stein 1989; Charles 2000; Baker 2001). A sociology of social problems does not preclude engagement with professional aims and ethics through critical social work practice. Instead, there is an argument to be made that social workers should be simultaneously open to critique our own normative assumptions about what we are doing, why we are doing it and the consequences, including for the clients we aim to help.

For example, the placement of children into foster care as a protective intervention is associated with many negative outcomes, although it may be argued that we cannot know the consequences if children had remained in the care of their parents (Erera 2002: 46–7). Investigations of 'child sexual abuse' may generate or increase the trauma for the child—for example, the Cleveland crisis in the United Kingdom in 1987 (Campbell 1988; Corby 1998: 29–38; Parton 1991; Richardson & Bacon 1991). Parent education programs are criticised as context-free parenting techniques taught to parents, which do not take account of their particular circumstances or the dynamics of parent–child relationships (Millei & Lee 2007). Therefore, as social workers working with children in the care of their families, we need to critique our relationships with families (parents and children) as expressions of state knowledge/power, whereby we exercise judgements as legally and ethically justif ed, while also questioning the normative assumptions underpinning such judgements.

This chapter addresses these theoretical and practical questions by setting out ideas of 'the child' and 'childhood' from a sociological perspective that allows us to critique the 'social' that social workers take for granted as justif able and uncontentious, given the ethical and legal implications of social problems related to children's general wellbeing. To achieve these aims, the chapter considers these normative questions from the sociological perspective of social constructionism.

Before we engage with the sociology of the 'child' as a socially constructed identity, we present Case study 10.1, which has been reworked for this chapter as an

Case study 10.1

Mary, a senior social worker at an Australian state child protection office, received a phone call one Friday afternoon from a school principal, Mr Smith, saying that the parents of Henry, a six-year-old boy at the school, had made contact to say that the day before their son had been taken into the toilets by Simon, who sucked his penis and licked him. Simon told Henry: 'What I'm going to do will make you a big boy.' Henry told his parents and they contacted Mr Smith asking to see him. Henry otherwise seemed to be fine. Mr Smith requested Mary to look into this. In the meantime, he asked the class teacher, Ms Jones, to keep an eye on both children.

Mary consulted with her team leader, Sally. They decided that this report was not urgent and could be followed up the following week. They categorised the principal's report as 'Child Concern', and wrote a file summary that the report involved 'Two six-year-old boys behaving in a sexually inappropriate manner at school.'

On Monday afternoon, Mr Smith phoned again. This time he said that Simon had again approached Henry. Ms Jones noticed that Simon was leading Henry away. The school was becoming quite anxious.

This time Mary and Sally decided that they needed to look at it there and then as it wasn't a one-off incident. They changed their case category from 'Child Concern' to 'Child Maltreatment—sexual abuse' and began their investigation.

However, rather than treat Henry as the victim of sexual abuse by Simon as the perpetrator, as reported by the school, they decided to investigate *Simon* as a possible victim of sexual abuse. Mary said that she 'had difficulty calling this six-year-old boy, Simon, a perpetrator of sexual abuse'. Instead, Mary and Sally interpreted Simon's statement to Henry, 'What I am going to do will make you a big boy', as something that someone else had said to him. Thus the workers transformed Simon's identity from possible perpetrator of sexual abuse to a victim of someone else, an unknown abuser in a different unreported incident. Mary and Sally's aim was 'to investigate the child Simon who had perpetrated the act to find out if anything was happening to him'.

The workers discovered that the children at this school had received a form of instruction about childhood sexuality that used language familiar to children, while prohibiting certain practices. They were told that games, touching and 'doing silly things'—also known as 'rudies'—in the toilets and in relation to 'bums and doodles' were all bad and naughty. 'Rude games are things that you don't do.'

»

While the workers believed that Simon had been exposed to something, Mary said that he became 'more and more cagey . . . *I'm not going to tell you anything . . . about anything*. He was the innocent child, as having nothing to do with the rude games. He emphatically denied that anybody had touched him, ever.'

Later, Simon's mother told Mary and Sally about the time she 'dealt with' Simon and his girl cousin of the same age, when she found them experimenting: 'Simon would know his actions were wrong.' Mary said: 'I agreed with her. I also said I think this is why Simon will not tell us anything.'

The workers had no choice but to record 'sexual abuse—unsubstantiated' as the outcome of their investigation of whether Simon had been sexually abused. One might regard the outcome in this case as unsatisfactory, because the workers could not find out what had happened to Simon.

However, this case study has shown how workers' assumptions about children and their sexuality influenced how they approached the initial report made by the school principal. If different workers were involved, they may well have investigated Simon as the perpetrator and Henry as his victim, and the case outcome would have been 'sexual abuse—substantiated', with a six-year-old boy recorded as a perpetrator of sexual abuse.

example of critical social work practice involving 'children' that also illustrates the process of social constructionism in practice. It has previously been analysed using discourse analysis to examine how child protection practitioners constructed what happened to 'children' who were the subjects of reports that 'something happened' (D'Cruz 2004: 144–7).

In the following sections, I set out the sociological dimensions related to the identity of 'the child' and the meaning of 'childhood'.

The 'child' as a socially constructed identity

The idea of the 'child' as a socially constructed identity and the meaning of 'childhood' are discussed in this section according to four dimensions: the identity category of 'the child'; the 'child' in relation to the 'adult' and the 'parent'; the 'child' as a social, legal and cultural identity; and images of the 'child'. Each of these explores different aspects of how the 'child' as an identity may change depending on context, with implications for social work policies and practices with actual children and their parents and carers.

The identity category of 'the child'

While we often talk about children as if they were all the same, the sociology of the child and childhood argues that the 'child' as an identity-category is not homogeneous. That is, there are considerable differences *within* the identity of the 'child', not least of which is the wide age-range covering from birth to eighteen years in most societies and certainly as embodied in the UN Convention on the Rights of the Child (UNCROC) (United Nations High Commissioner for Human Rights 1997–2003). There is also continuing unresolved debate in the f eld of reproductive health that includes abortion and assisted reproduction through technologies such as IVF, as well as what to name the biological entity before birth, because the naming as 'child', 'foetus', 'embryo' and similar also constitutes debates about when the 'child' as a legal and social identity actually exists (Charlesworth 1989; Moore 1996; Albury 1998).

Simple ref ections on our own experiences as children, or on the children we know in our personal and professional lives, would tell us that there is considerable complexity in the lives of the actual individuals who are grouped over such a wide range of ages into a single legal category. These differences related to age and stage inform professional practices when we assess children's wellbeing and needs for care and protection, as we are likely to intervene differently depending on whether the child involved in a referral of maltreatment is an infant or a teenager, without trivialising the signif cance of potential harm to the individual child involved. For example, a report of a parent shaking a child may be investigated differently if the 'child' is an infant or a teenager, as the consequences will be quite different.

In addition to the differences related to age and stage, children and their experiences of childhood would also differ according to their social class, race, ethnicity, culture, gender, (dis)ability and language, as well as the place and time in which they live (Jenks 1996; James & Prout 1997).

As social workers, our greater familiarity with a 'forced commonality of an ideological discourse of childhood' (Jenks 1996: 122) has tended to inf uence policies and practices that regulate or rescue children, often in the name of their welfare, care and protection, with consequences for 'being a child as lacking responsibility, having rights to protection and training but not to autonomy' (Jenks 1996: 122). This ideological discourse of childhood fundamentally relates to how the identities of the 'child', 'adult' and 'parent' articulate with each other.

The 'child' in relation to the 'adult' and the 'parent'

The UNCROC def nes a 'child' as being younger than eighteen years (United Nations High Commissioner for Human Rights 1997–2003). While eighteen years is generally accepted as the age of majority in domestic law in most countries, there is still some variation. For example, fourteen years is the age of majority in Uzbekistan, twenty in Japan, and 21 in several other countries, including Monaco, Lesotho and Argentina (Age of Majority n. d.). In Australia until the 1970s, 21 years was the legal age of majority. As can be seen, the dividing line between 'child' and 'adult' is quite arbitrary and is a consequence of social, political and cultural contexts ref ected in laws and policies.

An individual who reaches the age of legal majority is granted civil, social, legal and political rights; yet within this there are differences in regard to what is allowable at ages younger than the legal age of majority—for example, getting a driver's licence, enlisting in the armed forces, drinking alcohol, voting and age of consent to sexual activity, which may further be differentiated between heterosexual and homosexual practices (AVERT 2008). Overall, however, this legal def nition of the identity of the 'child' and the experience of 'childhood' inf uences social work professional practice with children and families, so that an individual aged anywhere between birth and legal majority can be the subject of referrals related to their wellbeing as a 'child'.

The legal (and social) demarcation of the identity of the 'child' from that of an 'adult' implicitly creates a binary relationship between these two identities as being mutually exclusive. That is, if you are legally a 'child', you cannot at the same time also be an 'adult', and therefore you cannot participate in some activities, roles and responsibilities that are demarcated as strictly being 'for adults'. Some of these legal boundaries have been mentioned above, and children may be charged with offences if they engage in activities deemed to be 'for adults only', such as drinking alcohol or driving a car.

Furthermore, there is also an implicit binary between the identity of 'child' and 'parent' (mother and/or father). The relationship between these identities is based on biology, where a child is born to a parent through natural or assisted pregnancies (White & Woollett 1999: 31–3), or a psycho-socio-legal relationship conferred through adoption, fostering or similar arrangements (Erera 2002: 20–57, 59–98). Space does not permit a discussion of the arrangements between individuals known as a 'family', where there are critiques of the normative assumptions of heterosexuality of parenting/partnering (Benkov 1994; Hicks 1996; Erera 2002: 13–16), and as a benign 'haven in a heartless world' (Frost & Stein 1989). These critiques that conceptualise the dynamics of 'the [nuclear] family' include a 'political economy' (Baker 2001), a 'patriarchal relation' (Charles 2000; Baker 2001) and 'the politics of gender and generation' (Frost & Stein 1989); all emphasise power and inequality of relations, even where there are no concerns about maltreatment of children, because the fundamental normative arrangement in 'a family' is that children remain under the paternalistic, decision-making authority of their 'parents' (Fox Harding 1991). This paternalism is extended as a feature of all relationships between 'children' and 'adults'—for example, in schools, child and family welfare, or child protection (Wattam & Parton 1999; Scott & Swain 2002).

Now consider the practice problematics that disrupt the normative assumptions that the identities of 'child' and 'adult', and 'child' and 'parent' are mutually exclusive. One very common practice problematic that becomes a reason for social work intervention is when a 'child' is simultaneously a 'parent'. The 'child' (usually an adolescent girl) may become pregnant and suddenly she disrupts the apparently mutually exclusive identities of 'parent (mother)' and 'child'. The breach of this normative differentiation between 'child' and 'parent' may precipitate reproductive health services, family counselling, advice about education and career, and in more extreme cases, child protection intervention (Voydanoff & Donnelly 1990), partly due to *cultural* assumptions about age, stage and competence to 'mother' a child. Furthermore, child protection may be involved if the 'child/parent-mother' is seen as a victim of sexual abuse as the cause of her pregnancy (D'Cruz 2004: 220–3).

Another practice problematic is associated with the 'child' who is simultaneously an 'adult', and in a relationship with their own (ageing) 'parent'. Hockey and James (1995) discuss the complexities associated with the 'cultural stereotypes of ageing as "second childhood"' (1995: 137), where the aged parent returns to 'dependency', a 'child's status', 'previously relinquished on becoming adult' (1995: 138). 'By linking old age with childhood the hegemony of adulthood remains unchallenged' (1995: 138). Furthermore, the relationship between the 'adult/child' and the 'adult/(aged) parent' is complicated by changing expectations about rights, duties and responsibilities, even where elders are culturally valued (Harris 1990: 241–8; Vincent 1999: 9–10).

The 'child' as a social, legal and cultural identity

The 'child' as a social, legal and cultural identity has not always existed as we understand it in contemporary Western society. While Ariès (1962) was initially associated with the concept of the 'discovery of childhood', Pollock (1983, 1987) argues that 'childhood' may not have been discovered in the sense of being a sudden differentiation between people called 'adults' and those called 'children'. However, Pollock (1983, 1987), Jenks (1996) and James and Prout (1997) discuss how the 'child' as an identity and the associated meaning of 'childhood' are contingent on time and place. The subsequent changing images of the child are related to social, political, legal and cultural contexts.

For example, Hendrick's (1997) 'interpretative survey' of British childhood from 1800 to the present proposed that there were different dominant constructions of 'the child' at different times, related to changing policy agendas about the place of 'the child' in 'the family' and in the wider society. Some of the changing policy agendas have included the factory child, the delinquent child and the welfare child, and were associated with different ways in which the child and family related to each other, and to the wider society. Similarly, Scott and Swain (2002), whose history of child protection in Australia examined how cruelty to children was confronted in Victoria, discuss the changes over time, as 'various stages . . . each . . . posing different questions' (Scott & Swain 2002: xii–xiii).

In my own research on child protection in Western Australia, in which I investigated how meanings of 'child maltreatment' and identities of responsibility were social constructions by child protection practitioners (D'Cruz 2004), I also explored how assumptions about the identities of 'the child' and 'the parent' were fundamental to the processes and outcomes of practice. As part of this study, I used a 'genealogical method' (Foucault 1971, 1978, 1980) to examine policies about protection of 'children' as 'shifting meanings and identities, embedded in power relations, and contingent in time, place and socio-political and cultural institutions' (D'Cruz 2004: 18). This analysis showed 'how the concept of "protection" was associated with the identity of "child" in a particular place (Western Australia) over time, from colonisation [in 1829] to "the present", and was differentiated by "race-as-Aboriginality"' (D'Cruz 2004: 19). The implications and consequences for policy and practice (D'Cruz 2004: 105) were that 'race-as-Aboriginality' has been an organising feature that has generated different discourses and different effects for members of Aboriginal and non-Aboriginal communities. This feature has inf uenced different meanings of 'protection' as it applied to different groups, divided along racial lines:

> 'Protection' for the non-Aboriginal population differentiated between 'protection' of (good) children/protection from (bad, female) carers', and 'protection from (bad) children/protection of the (non-Aboriginal) community'. For the Aboriginal population, 'protection' meant surveillance, discipline of (abnormal, black) bodies and protection of the (white non-Aboriginal) community (D'Cruz 2004: 105).

Contemporary protectionist discourses espouse racial equality that minimises differences, including Aboriginality. Furthermore, hierarchies of maltreatment that give greater emphasis to sexual or physical maltreatment and less to neglect have created unexpected complexities in the ways in which Aboriginal children and families are engaged in child protection services that are less inclined to intervene in problems related to poverty and disadvantage (D'Cruz 2004: 105).

The above examples (Hendrick 1997; Scott & Swain 2002; D'Cruz 2004: 75–105) show in various ways that the identity of 'the child' is contextual, contingent on time and place. That is, there may be changes over time in the same or different places, and there may be changes related to different places, within the same timeframe. Within these changes in identity, the *image* of 'the child' (as opposed to *actual* children who live in those contexts) also changes. This does not mean that one image completely replaces another, although it might. Instead, new images may emerge that compete with or dominate others.

Images of the 'child'

Social workers who work with children in different f elds of practice may f nd one or more of these images of the 'child' implicitly inf uencing organisational policies and expected practices—the conf icts with parents, carers and the children themselves, as well as controversies of what should (or did) happen in some cases that become public for different reasons.

Thus contemporary 'child protection' (and some earlier 'child welfare') policies and practices have tended to construct 'the child' as a 'waif' or 'vulnerable victim' (Eekelaar et al. 1982; Scott & Swain 2002). The related policies and practices have been described as 'child centred', but have been criticised as 'child rescue' or 'paternalism' (Fox Harding 1991; Wattam & Parton 1999), where an external, protective adult saves the child from bad or dangerous parents. This is an adversarial relationship, where the perspectives of the protective adult/professional are dominant, and in which the child is also silenced in what ought to happen in regard to his/her care and protection.

A more recent image of the 'child' is conceptualised by Donahoo (2007) as 'idolising children'. By this, Donahoo means that in contemporary Western societies, children are to be revered and protected from every possible disadvantage and problem. At the same time, parents are expected to be superheroes: to be 'perfect parents' to 'extraordinary children'. An example of the idolisation of children may be seen in the title of a recent report on 'child sexual abuse' in the Northern Territory (Anderson & Wilde 2007): *Little Children are Sacred*. While the purpose of the inquiry and its recommendations are not in dispute, one wonders whether it is necessary to idolise children as sacred before we can attend to a signif cant problem of 'child sexual abuse'.

The idolisation and sacredness of children resonate with a more particular image of childhood vulnerability: their innocence (Kitzinger 1997; Callery 1998: 5–9; Gittins 1998; Pryjmachuk 1998: 45–6; Davis 2005). This image is primarily associated with sexualities and sexual practices. 'Children' are constructed as asexual, with sexuality as a set of practices associated with 'adult' identity and prohibited to 'children' as a 'crime against childhood' (Kitzinger 1997: 165–89), perpetrated by 'dangerous adults'—for example, 'stranger danger' (Think Safe 2008; Childnet International 2008).

Davis (2005) argues that contemporary constructions of 'children' as asexual and innocent have generated particular ways of being '(legitimate) victims of sexual abuse'. These expectations may complicate *actual* children's accounts of sexualised experiences that may involve 'adults' or other 'children', where there may be ambiguities in the meanings of consent and coercion (Bell 1993). Children's accounts that do not f t these images of innocence may be dismissed, or the children may be inf uenced to give accounts that f t the appropriate image of innocence (and believability) (Davis 2005). Furthermore, children's own inculcation into images of the 'good child' as asexual and innocent may prevent them from disclosing sexual practices, as this may contradict the preferred identity of goodness (D'Cruz 2004: 144–7). While the overwhelming image of 'sexual dangerousness' is the adult, male, paedophile, practice is more complicated if differentiating between play and abuse when all the participants are 'children' (Lamb & Coakley 1993).

The images of the child discussed above have tended implicitly to idealise the 'child' as the embodiment of goodness and therefore deserving of care and protection, either by parents/carers or by the state. However, images of some children as savages or community threats (Eekelaar et al. 1982; Scott & Swain 2002) that have persisted over time in various places change the emphasis from care and protection of 'the child', to protection of the community, with consequences for the severity of the treatment of such children by parents or the state—for example, corporal punishment, institutionalisation and in some places capital punishment (Amnesty International 2002).

For example, there is considerable research which shows that black teenage boys in Britain are more likely to be stopped and searched compared with white teenage boys (Bland et al. 2002a, 2002b), with similar experiences found among Indigenous Australian boys (Davis & Watson 2006). Boys as young as six years old may lose their rights as 'children' if they are categorised as perpetrators of sexual abuse because they are seen to have 'lost their innocence' or to have 'become dangerous' to other children in the community (D'Cruz 2004, 144–7, 196–8).

Another image that may be associated with policy and practice controversies is that the child is parental property (Brennan & Noggle 1997). The ownership of the child as private property is an expression of power associated with gender and generation in the (heterosexual) nuclear family (Frost & Stein 1989), and is justif ed by claims of parental autonomy and family privacy (Donzelot 1980, 1988).

Finally, a more recent image of the child is that of an individual with rights. Children's rights as a global issue were f rst articulated in the United Nations Convention on the Rights of the Child (UNCROC) (United Nations Commissioner for Human Rights 1997–2003), although ideas about children's rights (Freeman 1983; Franklin 1986) and liberation (Fox Harding 1991) have been proposed by children's advocates for some time. While the lack of rights accorded to children was recognised as contributing to their extreme disadvantage and lack of social and material power in most contexts, the UNCROC has also been criticised as an expression of Western imperialism towards developing countries (Boyden 1997), and because the achievement of the stated ideals for children's lives is conditional on the national contexts in which they live.

The idea of 'children-as-citizens' has emerged internationally as a form of children's rights. This approach refers to extending citizenship in terms of participation, equal and equitable access to resources, opportunities and outcomes, and choices in their lives (Lister 1990; Lister et al. 2001; Willow et al. 2004; Balen et al. 2006).

Children's rights and the 'child-as-citizen': participatory and child-centred professional practice

The idea of 'children-as-citizens' differs from other child-centred approaches discussed above. As citizens, children are seen as active subjects, able to make decisions and exercise choices for themselves. This approach to children's rights and citizenship is ref ected in contemporary developments internationally of participatory and child-centred professional practice, and ref ected in many countries—including Australia—through the appointment of Children's Ombudsmen, Children's Commissioners, Children's Advocates, and Bureaux, Off ces and Commissions for Children.[2]

Researchers have been advocating the inclusion of children's perspectives on policies that affect their lives—for example, on poverty (Middleton et al. 1994; Davis & Ridge 1997; Roker 1998, cited in Ridge 2002: 5), as 'active members of households'

(Shropshire & Middleton 1999, cited in Ridge 2002: 4), family economics (Jensen & Saporiti 1992; Qvortup 1997, in Ridge 2002: 3), as survivors of sexual abuse (Wattam & Parton 1999) and custody/access in family law (James & James 2004).

If one considers extending to 'children' citizenship rights normally seen as applicable only to 'adults', we need to consider the questions of which rights we extend, and to which 'children', if we accept that the identity of 'child' is heterogeneous and complicated as argued in the sections above.

For example, should 'children' have the right to vote? If so, which 'children'? Can 'children' have a voice in the society and represent themselves in formal institutions such as courts? If so, which 'children'? Are there any 'children' who would have to rely on 'adults' to represent their views? If so, which 'children' and in what circumstances? Should 'children' have access to conf dential medical care? If so, which 'children'? At what age should 'parents' no longer have the right to know about their 'children's' medical care? At what age should a 'child' be allowed to seek conf dential advice about contraception or abortion? In cases involving concerns about 'children's' wellbeing, especially reports of harm, are all 'children' able to make decisions about their immediate and future safety on which professionals must act? Or does the professional weigh up a variety of considerations in which the 'child's' views are included but do not carry special weight? What might be the ethical implications for professionals who act on 'children's' wishes if there is subsequent harm to the 'child'? What might be the legal implications in terms of professional liability and duty of care towards the 'child'?

Researchers who accept the ideal of 'child-as-citizen' and who can also engage with these sorts of practice complexities are exploring these questions (McLaughlin 2005; D'Cruz & Stagnitti 2008). As yet, there is no answer that is expected or even possible, because the question is as complicated as the individuals and their circumstances that create the conditions for social work practice with children and their families.

Conclusion

This chapter has discussed, from a social constructionist perspective, the idea of 'the child' as a social, legal and cultural identity that inf uences policies and practices towards actual children in 'family' contexts. This perspective engages with the sociology of social problems that acknowledges the moral imperatives of critical social work practice while at the same time asserting the importance of engaging critically with the normative assumptions of social work which are not politically or ethically neutral in their consequences. Thus it has been argued that 'the child' is a socially constructed, dynamic identity that must be located in place and time, and that has consequences for how actual children's lives, problems, needs and circumstances are understood. The dynamics of power must be appreciated and understood in relations between 'children' and 'adults' (parents and carers in 'the family', and also social workers and other professionals). It is therefore important that social workers in various practice contexts that provide services directly or indirectly to 'children' must critically engage with the structural forms of oppression of children, and also their own normative assumptions about 'children', 'adults' and 'parents', and that such engagement should inform the policies in their organisations in order to lead to political, ethical and effective practice.

11

using critical reflection to improve feminist practice

Christine Morley

Historically, feminist theorists and practitioners have used modernist, emancipatory ideals to guide their work. While there is a multiplicity of feminisms, principles such as acknowledging women's rights as human rights, freedom from gender-based violence and oppression, rejecting the uncritical acceptance of traditional gender roles, critiquing ostensibly 'natural' social arrangements and challenging patriarchal structures to facilitate greater gender equity unite many feminists (Marchant & Wearing 1986a; Fook 1993; Bell & Klein 1996; Dominelli 2002). Women's experiences and gender power relations are central to feminist analyses (Dominelli 2002; Weeks 2003). Feminists have convincingly highlighted the gendered inequalities entrenched in social institutions and policy, resulting from the relegation of women to the private sphere (Segal 1995; Bryson 2002; Dominelli 2002; Morley & Macfarlane 2008).

While feminism as a social movement emerged in many Western industrialised countries—including Australia—in the 1960s, it was in the 1970s that feminist practice started to be articulated in social work. Feminist social workers criticised the 'gender blindness' apparent in radical social work, which initially failed to adequately acknowledge the impact of gender inequality (Healy 2005c: 176). This remains an important issue for social work, considering that the vast majority of service users and practitioners are women (McCormack 2001, cited in Weeks 2003).

Feminist values and commitments remain constant; however, the practice context in which feminist practitioners work is always changing. Consequently, some commentators argue that feminist ideals have lost their contemporary relevance (Graham 1992; Lawrence 1992; Seidman 1994; Wise 1995; Featherstone 2005). Over the past two decades, feminism has been subjected to harsh backlash (Bell & Klein 1996; Weeks 2003) and a conservative neo-liberal context that has been hostile to feminist values, practices and services (Featherstone 2005; Phillips 2006; Morley & Macfarlane 2008).

Given this context, feminist activists have conceded that many of the gains made by the women's movement are actively being dismantled (Corrigan 2006). This has raised questions about whether theorising social issues exclusively from modernist feminist perspectives may be limiting and inadvertently compound the dominant power structures and social problems that we seek to challenge (Healy 2000; Featherstone 2005).

While feminist practice has become more specialised in recent years, in that it has largely been conf ned to particular issues such as sexual assault or domestic violence (Featherstone 2005), even these spaces are now being colonised by clinical, individualised and essentially degendered approaches to policy and practice (Morley & Macfarlane 2008). In addition, it has been argued that, 'despite the relevance of these contemporary theories within the social work literature, their inf uence on social work, particularly day to day practice . . . is limited' (Healy 2000: 37).

Given these concerns, how has feminism developed to benef t from drawing upon a postmodern informed critical ref ection? And what does contemporary feminist practice look like? This chapter highlights the continued importance of feminist analyses to critical social work, and explores how feminist practices have adapted to respond to changing, more complex and uncertain practice contexts, through engaging with critical postmodernism. Case study 11.1 provides an example of how critical ref ection can be used to enhance contemporary feminist practice.[1]

Critical reflection

Research indicates that there are often disparities between the theories practitioners believe are informing their practice, and the theories that are actually implicit in their actions (Argyris & Schön 1976). Critical ref ection is integral to critical practice because it challenges dominant power relations and structures by 'pinpointing the ways in which we might unwittingly aff rm discourses that work against us, and the people we are working with', and emphasises practitioners' own personal agency to respond (Fook 2000: 133). It has been described as self-ref ection on how

Case study 11.1: initial construction of my practice

Context and background

I had been working for approximately six years as an after-hours counsellor/advocate for a sexual assault service. In the early hours of the morning, I was paged to attend a crisis care unit for a young Anglo-Australian woman who had been assaulted. On arriving, I negotiated with the police to meet with Lee (aged twenty) privately in order to ascertain whether she wished to make a police report, and/or have a forensic examination.[2] Lee was exhausted. She said she felt numb and that she wanted to go home.

Despite her exhaustion, Lee decided to have a forensic examination and to brief two members of the police about her experience, with the understanding that she wasn't prepared to make a formal statement at that stage (given her level of shock, tiredness, lack of faith in the legal system and fear of retribution from the perpetrators). Due to the nature of the assault, a number of police units from different regions were involved. Just as Lee was about to leave the hospital, another five detectives entered the crisis care unit. Major difficulties arose in relation to one of the detectives from the rape squad.

The critical incident

Without any consultation, the detective burst into the crisis care unit and demanded that Lee go to the crime scene with him immediately. We explained that Lee felt traumatised and exhausted. This appeared to be of little consequence to the detective.

He stipulated that he 'required' Lee 'to cooperate'. While Lee was clear that she did not want to return to the public place where she had been violently assaulted by three Anglo-Australian male strangers earlier that evening, the detective dominated her by invoking legal relevancies, raising his voice, invading her personal space and threatening to charge her with false reporting, if she was not prepared to 'back up her allegations with action'. I continued to advocate for her right to leave, and tried to convince the detective to commence investigations without her. I believed his response towards Lee to be offensive, aggressive, inappropriate and in breach of the Police Code of Practice.

My interaction with this detective became intensely conflictual and lasted for several hours, which I believe upon reflection severely exacerbated Lee's emotional trauma. Ultimately, I was able to resist his bullying, but the process » had resulted in Lee becoming more withdrawn and distressed. He eventually conceded to investigate the crime scene without Lee, while she went straight home from the hospital.

Despite this, I was particularly concerned about the impact of the detective's conduct on Lee's emotional wellbeing, and felt that the adversarial process with the detective may have worsened her experience. Ultimately, I felt powerless because I believed there had been an element of luck involved in the detective's decision to retreat from his position. I didn't feel confident that my advocacy and resistance practices would necessarily result in a favourable outcome for the victim/survivor should a similar situation arise in the future. This led to feelings of vulnerability, and doubt about my feminist practice and its capacity to appropriately support victims/survivors in the context of oppressive systems.

Theorising my practice: explicit/intentional feminist assumptions

Much of how I conceptualised my role in working with Lee fitted comfortably within my espoused feminist framework. This included trying to empower Lee through the provision of information and discussing the legal and medical options available to her; trying to create a safe and confidential space for Lee to discuss how she was coping and to reflect on her emotional responses to the sexual assault; validating and normalising her feelings about the sexual assault, rather than pathologising her responses (Weeks 2003); resisting any suggestion of self-blame for the assault; and contextualising her sense of self-blame within a socio-political context and consciousness-raising about the social myths which dominate this context (Hurst 1995; Scott et al. 1995; Weeks 2003). I let Lee know that my role was independent from that of the police and medical practitioners, and that I was there to support her, listen to her needs and decisions, and ensure that what she chose to happen in this process would be respected. This stance also reflects a feminist commitment to minimise power disparities that may exist between myself as a service provider and Lee as a service user (Healy 2005c).

When conflict with the detective arose, I drew upon feminist critiques of the legal system to understand how the insensitive response of the detective was probably informed by the misogynist culture that is embedded throughout much of the police force (Easteal 1996a, 1996b; Hovdestad 2001), and the social mythology which functions to either blame or disbelieve victims/survivors and/ »

or to exonerate perpetrators (Corbett & Larcombe 1994). To counteract this, I approached the situation from an unequivocal position of believing Lee's account of her experience, rejecting manifestations of social mythology that transfer responsibility for the assault from the perpetrators to her (Weeks 2003). Hence my work was political in that at no time did I position myself as neutral, given that neutrality just bolsters the power of the oppressor (Dominelli 2002). My overt support for the victim/survivor against oppressive systems and their representatives was therefore intentional, due to locating the sexual assault in the socio-political context of the inequitable power relations produced by patriarchal structures (Yurchesyn et al. 1992; Allen 1996; Townsend 1996; Easteal 1996b; Mack 1998).

In order to minimise the impact of the detective's behaviour on Lee, I situated myself as a buffer between Lee and the police. Consistent with a feminist framework, which recognises that an experience of sexual assault denies the person who has been assaulted even the basic right to control what happens to their body, there was a clear intention embedded in my approach to position myself as a resource to facilitate Lee having as much control over the process as possible through the creation and respect of her choices (Weeks 2003).

These intentional aspects of my practice were entirely unproblematic for my espoused feminist theoretical framework. However, critical reflection on my practice revealed a number of parallel unconscious assumptions which had a variety of unintended consequences. Without detracting from the valuable contributions that modernist feminist analyses make to practice, in developing feminism for contemporary contexts, it is necessary to acknowledge that feminist frameworks, like all deductive, modernist theories, have gaps and limitations, which benefit from being interrogated and deconstructed (Lister 2003).

internalised dialogue has been constructed, and can therefore be deconstructed, changed and reconstructed to improve practice (Fook 2002). The remainder of this chapter uses critical ref ection, informed by postmodernism, to scrutinise the unconscious and unintentional aspects of my practice, and to demonstrate how reconstruction of this practice may enhance the implementation of feminist values and principles into practice.

It should be acknowledged that postmodernism, with its rejection of universal and totalising ways of knowing (Kermode & Brown 1996; Ife 1997; Macey 2000; Parton & O'Byrne 2000a) and related critiques of modernist perspectives that are based on 'f xed, universal explanations of reality' (Sands & Nuccio 1992: 492; Featherstone & Fawcett 1995; Macey 2000; Parton & O'Byrne 2000a), presents a number of tensions for social work (Weedon 1987; Giroux 1990; Taylor-Gooby 1993; Seidman 1994; Healy 2000; Hancock & Taylor 2001; Fraser & Briskman 2005) and also for feminism (Bulbeck 1994; Hare-Mustin & Marecek 1994; MacDonald 1996; Stromquist 2000; Holmes & Warelow 2000). Indeed, from a postmodern perspective, patriarchy itself can be considered a modernist universal construct. This has led some feminists to criticise postmodernism for failing to adequately take account of the material realities associated with the social disadvantage experienced by women, given that, used in isolation, postmodernism inheres a sense that all values are lost (MacDonald 1996; Stromquist 2000).

However, far from sacrif cing the modernist ideals of equity, community, social justice and human rights, in drawing on *both* critical and postmodern theories to inform practice, I understand this theoretical combination to preserve the progressive social change commitments and emancipatory visions of modernist feminisms (Sands & Nuccio 1992; Fraser & Briskman 2005). Critical postmodern theories extend feminism by recognising and reconstructing the limitations of modernist conceptions of power, identity, dichotomous categories and universal narratives (Fook 2002). Therefore, in using critical postmodern ideas (Fook 1996; 2002; Ife 1997; Leonard 1997; Pease & Fook 1999a; Allan et al. 2003; Hick et al. 2005) to enhance feminism through critical ref ection, the commitments to challenge feminist constructions of the consequences of patriarchy and contribute to the transformation of a more socially just society (Van Den Bergh & Cooper 1986; Marchant & Wearing 1986a; Dominelli 2002) are preserved.

Critical reflection on my account of the story

Positioning my account as a social construction

Ref ection on my initial account indicated that I originally perceived my representation of the incident to be an objective description. This ref ects a modernist view that there is one singular truth (Featherstone & Fawcett, 1995; Macey 2000; Parton & O'Byrne 2000a).

In deconstructing these assumptions, I began to realise that my account was not a factual representation of the 'truth', but a series of interpretations, which had marginalised other constructions—a socially constructed version that was inf uenced by my own social, cultural and political lens, and mediated by my own biography and social positioning (Fook 1999). Using critical ref ection to understand the construction of my story involved acknowledging the impact of myself on this process, and unravelling the ways in which my interpretations had actually distorted aspects of my recollection (Fook 1996).

Extending the feminist emphasis on structural factors

My initial belief about my story being an objective representation of reality was partly formed through my understanding of the issues in structural terms. While feminist thinking quite legitimately identif es the structural and institutional dimensions of the problem (Dominelli 2002; Healy 2005c; Payne 2005), drawing on this analysis exclusively appeared to have a number of unintended and disempowering consequences. For example, in theorising Lee's personal experience with the detective as political, in that patriarchal structures such as the legal system often fail to respond in appropriate and socially just ways (Stuart 1993; Gilmore 1995; Easteal 1996a; Taylor 1996; Scutt 1998), I constructed the problem in abstract, external and inaccessible terms, as if the solution was out of my hands as a practitioner, and out of reach of the victim/survivor (Healy 2000; Fook 2002).

This is perhaps why it has been suggested that feminism, as a modernist emancipatory project used in isolation, may unintentionally contribute to a sense of powerlessness (Healy 2000; Fook 2000; 2002; Morley & Macfarlane 2008). While feminism remains vital for critical practice, critical ref ection on my practice demonstrates how some of the modernist constructions in my thinking undermined my use of feminist theory and practice.

Rethinking the assumption that counselling is ineffective in responding to structural issues

Related to the feminist contention that social problems are structural and external, the assumption that individual work is somehow less important or effective was hidden by my broader feminist commitment to structural interventions and macro social change (Fook 1995). Many feminist theories emphasise collective action implied by the unity of women to transform dominant patriarchal forces and produce social change (Marchant & Wearing 1986a; Sands & Nuccio 1992; MacDonald 1996; Thorpe & Irwin 1996; Forcey & Nash 1998; Stromquist 2000; Weeks 2003). Arguably, without feminist efforts to raise consciousness about legal injustices in relation to sexual assault, we would not have seen the reforms that have been achieved (Weeks 2003). However, are greater gender equity and the empowerment of women only possible through large-scale social change? Ironically, the emancipatory, transformative aims of feminism may inadvertently construct social change as a practical impossibility (Healy 2000).

For example, this assumption which privileges macro interventions invoked an implicit belief that my role as a counsellor/advocate was not effective in responding to the structural issues embedded in the detective's response. This was evident in my narrative given that, despite successfully advocating to achieve the needs of the victim/survivor, my initial assessment of my practice was simply that is was not good enough. I felt as though the level of conf ict had not justif ed the outcome, that the process was disempowering for all concerned, and I was deeply concerned that the experience might have further exacerbated Lee's trauma.

Modernist feminist discourses suggest that structural, institutional and historically entrenched belief systems should be targeted for change (Allen 1996; Dominelli 2002). Given that much our work as feminist practitioners is with individual women, or groups of women at a relatively micro level (Weeks 2003), this discourse has the potential to alienate practitioners from the means of change and devalue micro-level critical practice. Deconstructing these assumptions highlights how the macro issues have artif cially been separated from individual practice that happens at the micro level, in a way that unnecessarily devalues the individual counselling in which practitioners engage with victims/survivors. Obviously, it was not my intention to buy into this dichotomy, as I f rmly believe individual counselling can potentially be of immense benef t to victims/survivors, thus enabling me to validate smaller, local acts of resistance in practice, as well as structural change.

Resisting being drawn into oppositional power relations

Implicit within my story was a binary 'us and them' construction which assumed that my counsellor/advocate role was completely separate from those of the other professionals involved. Making this distinction more pronounced, I had understood the situation dichotomously as one in which I was faced with the option of either aligning with the detective, whom I saw as an oppressor, or aligning with the victim/survivor, whom I was committed to supporting. I indicated that I felt I needed to situate myself as a buffer between the victim/survivor and the police. This similarly hides an implicit assumption about two mutually exclusive sides, in which I was united with the victim/survivor in opposition to the police.

Thinking about the world in dichotomous categories is another feature of modernist thinking (Featherstone & Fawcett 1995; Parton & O'Byrne 2000a; Fook 2002). Feminism utilises the gendered categories of masculinity and femininity to determine in the context of a patriarchal society that, for example, men are powerful and women are powerless; men are privileged, women are oppressed. The construction of dichotomous categories establishes, or is ref ective of, hierarchical power relationships. Locating our experiences within the construction of these dichotomies arguably operates to bolster dominant power relations (Fook 2002; Fook & Morley 2005; Morley 2005).

The ways in which feminist practitioners conceptualise the advocacy component of our roles is also indicative of perpetuating this dichotomy. Advocacy, from a modernist, feminist perspective, is assumed to involve two polarised protagonists, and aims to represent the interests of the least powerful person or group to the more powerful side (Fook 2002). This assumption was embedded in my work, and I unwittingly located Lee as the weaker party, in opposition to the detective whom I assumed was not concerned for the victim/survivor. These power dynamics are assumed to be f xed, and therefore constitute 'deterministic views [which] fail to account for contradictions' (Fook 2002: 9) in terms of how, despite an experience of victimisation, 'victims' can and do display tremendous amounts of strength and courage, and may have other experiences in different contexts, and at different points in time, which are powerful.

Reconstructing the notion of professionalism

Paralleling this, within a feminist analysis service users are often implicitly assumed to be powerless in relation to workers and systems. Yet, paradoxically, research indicates that most counsellor/advocates, despite having their own professional education and status, assume that other professionals have more power than they do, particularly if they are social workers. This arguably ref ects a broader devaluing of social work, particularly when contrasted against other professionals, who have closer alignments with scientif c and medical bodies of knowledge that are socially constructed as superior (Pardeck & Murphy 1993). The status issue is something with which social work seems to struggle in general, but this is particularly the case for feminist practitioners who, perhaps unlike other professionals, deliberately aim to reduce power disparities between ourselves and our service users (Healy 2005c). We respect our service users as the expert on their experiences (Weeks 2003), and often feel reluctant to acknowledge our own expertise because there is a sense that this might create inequitable power relations (Hurst 1995; Scott et al. 1995). In addition, given that many women's services have grown out of grassroots histories of community development and social activism (Weeks 2003), many feminist practitioners aim to create an anti-professional culture, with the assumption that professionalism may alienate the women with whom we work, and again contribute to uncritical power relations (Fook 2002). A by-product of this commitment, however, may be that some feminist social work practitioners feel less worthy or valid in relation to other professionals.

The assumptions that professionalism and expertise, as they are def ned in dominant discourse, contribute to hierarchical power relations between ourselves and our service users may be linked to beliefs that power is inherently oppressive (Rees 1991). Indeed, feminist analyses, in the context of understanding violence against women, convincingly highlight the links between gender, power and violence, through examining the structural power disparities between men and women, and the impact of patriarchal institutions and relations that characterise dominant social arrangements in Western society (Dominelli 2002). Such an analysis, however, may reinforce a perception that power is something that feminist practitioners do not have, and actually would not want to have, because power is constructed as the domain of the dominant groups, which is on the other side of the dichotomy. This separateness may produce a complicity with oppression within and among feminist practitioners, adding to a sense of powerlessness for both practitioners and the service users we seek to support (Fook 2002b).

Reconstructing modernist notions of power

This analysis ref ects additional modernist assumptions that conceptualise power as a tangible commodity or possession. Power, from a feminist perspective, is often seen to be f nite, hierarchical in nature and embedded in formal structures, or accorded to people through professional status (Rees 1991; Parker et al. 2000; Fook 2002). However, these modernist notions of power might lead feminist practitioners to believe that they experience a reduction of power when they work to equalise power relations with service users because the giving of power, from this perspective, always occurs with a def cit, at the expense of the person or group giving it (Fook 2002b; Healy 2000).

Yet drawing from critical postmodernists enables feminist practitioners to recognise that power is also inscribed within discourse, rather than exclusively residing in social structure (Purvis & Hunt 1993; Pease et al. 2003a). Power in this sense can also be conceptualised as the capacity to inf uence, manipulate or exercise control over discourse (Foucault 1987, cited in Featherstone & Fawcett 1995; Rees 1991; Parker et al. 1999; Fook 2002b). In this way, power is embedded in social interactions and contexts (not just limited to social structure), and can be productive because what is important about power is how it is utilised (Fook 2002b).

Such a reconstruction enables feminist practitioners to develop greater agency—that is, 'the capacity to be actively involved in the process of social change' (Always 1995, cited in Pease et al. 2003a). This agency enabled me to rethink the ways in which I had unwittingly bought into oppositional power relations with the detective. For example, recognising the artif cially constructed nature of the binary categories (for example, us versus him) and how my acceptance of these dichotomies ironically bolstered the perceived power of the detective in relation to myself and Lee (Fook 2002b) highlighted how my *intentions* to empower militated against my *capacity* to empower. In this sense, although the stated principles of modernist feminism are clearly emancipatory, the intentions do not automatically translate into emancipatory practice (Fook 2000, 2002b).

Reconstructing modernist notions of identity

In relation to my case study, critical ref ection highlighted the gaps, missing discourses and exceptions to the dominant discourse surrounding Lee as a powerless victim being oppressed by a dominating detective. Modernist feminist narratives are not only implicated in constructing identity in dichotomous terms, but also in ways that are static. Deconstructing this assumption elucidates how people occupy multiple subject positions at different points in time. For example, while Lee's experience as a victim/survivor was privileged in my original account, at the same time she was also a mother, a daughter, a musician, a neighbour, partner, friend, employee, and so on.

This enables a more holistic account of Lee's identities, in which we can acknowledge her multiple, changing and sometimes contradictory subjectivities. While in one sense Lee was desperate and exhausted, she concurrently displayed tremendous strength and resistance. Drawing on the thinking of some postmodernists, identity can be interpreted as an evolving construction that can change from one context to another, creating opportunities to privilege different aspects of Lee's identity, thus reconstructing her in more empowered and enabled terms.

Postmodernism abandons grand narratives around identity through conceptualising identity as situational, socially constructed and discursively produced. This enables a more complex and sophisticated practice response, and may provide a means of acknowledging women's relative disadvantage without contributing to it by how we theorise and respond to it.

As an example of this, when I initially ref ected on my practice, part of my disappointment with it emerged from my assumption that the conf ict that occurred between myself and the detective was damaging and detrimental for Lee. Yet in developing a more holistic narrative about Lee's experience, I also needed to acknowledge that there were times during the process when she started to advocate for herself by expressing some of the resistance toward the detective that I had been modelling. This process of resistance could also be interpreted as quite empowering, and certainly challenges the construction of her as a powerless, passive victim. Conversely, this reconstruction creates the opportunity to discursively relocate Lee within the discourse as an agent of change who challenged dominant power relations.

Similarly, in recognising that I had constructed the detective as a one-dimensional character whose problematic behaviours were permanent, f xed and unchanging from one context to the next, I utilised postmodern ideas about multiple, relative and f uid identities to reconstruct his identity by considering other factors and interpretations (Sands 1996; Fook 2002b). While not wanting to minimise or excuse his poor conduct, recognising that there could have been a myriad of reasons for his behaviour (instead of just concluding that he was abusive or incompetent) frees me up to consider, for example, that personal issues may have been impacting on his practice. Alternatively, his boss might have been pressuring him to proceed. There may have been other legal demands imposed on him of which I was unaware. In addition, he may not have been provided with appropriate education and training regarding awareness of gender issues. This particular interpretation enables me to take an educative role rather than a defensive position, and any of these other possible interpretations assist in diffusing my anger towards the detective which, on ref ection, contributed to the oppositional power relations between us.

Challenging oppositional practices

Challenging my f xed constructions also assisted me in repositioning the detective in less oppositional terms and developing an interpretation which is more valuing of his contribution. For example, rather than seeing police involvement as a problem, I could reinterpret that the police were trying to assist Lee and help facilitate her access to resources. Using postmodernism to reconstruct the differences between what the police offer and I offered as a feminist practitioner means that these differences do not have to be constructed as a threat to equity. In fact, this variety could be benef cial for the service user.

Given that feminist practitioners are working to facilitate progressive structural change and greater gender equity through challenging dominant power relations (Weeks 2003), an unintended manifestation of feminist practice may be that it can encourage practitioners to be at loggerheads with systems and their representatives. Modernist feminist discourses construct two oppositional sides in which those on the other side of the dualism are the enemy. Therefore, there is sometimes a sense that to not operate in confrontational or adversarial ways would almost be tantamount to conforming to preserve dominant power relations, or betraying our united position. Deconstruction of my account of the case study revealed my use of warlike language such as 'battling', 'threat' and 'enemy'. These constructions not only legitimated my defensiveness, but contributed to the perhaps unnecessary oppositional and adversarial relations between myself and the police that I believed were detrimental to Lee.

This need to be united in sisterhood is a cornerstone of feminism, and this has raised signif cant questions in terms of how we challenge dominant power relations without buying into dichotomous hierarchies which inhibit our capacity to challenge. Within the feminist organisations in which I worked, one of the ways dichotomous power relations were maintained was through a culture of discussing the atrocities, as we saw them, that other professionals and systems had enacted. While this unites feminist practitioners in solidarity, it does so in a way that is oppositional to other systems professionals, such as the police, and locates us in a marginalised position in relation to these systems and professionals.

Ref ective of this, my original account indicated that the problems we experienced during the crisis care unit lay solely with the detective and everything that he represented structurally: being white, professional, middle class, and benef ting from patriarchal norms, structures and institutions which accord him male power and privilege (Dominelli 2002). Constructing him by his difference from us, and emphasising his aggression and domination, validated my construction of him as the enemy.

Yet deconstruction suggests that one of the consequences of this is that each time practitioners construct themselves as separate from other professionals, and shift blame to other professionals, they contribute to their own sense of powerlessness. Blaming the detective and feeling justif ed in my response cast the problem as external from myself, which exonerates me, yet locates him as being in control, powerful and active. Failing to examine my contribution to the situation was actually more disempowering for me, because it is the taking back of responsibility for my part in the struggle that reconstructs me with the agency to create a different, and more empowering, response (Ellermann 1998; Alberti 2000; Fook 2002b; Morley 2004, 2007; Rossiter 2005).

Critical ref ection enabled me to acknowledge that my own responses to the detective were somewhat oppositional, and at times inf ammatory. Recognising my contribution to the conf ict provides me with the agency to change my part in it, which liberates me from my initial sense of powerlessness and uncertainty regarding how to respond should a similarly conf ictual situation arise again in the future (Ellermann 1998; Alberti 2000; Fook 2002b; Morley 2004, 2007; Rossiter 2005).

This creates new practice opportunities which might include, for example, talking to the detective about Lee's wishes, and asking him what *we* are going to do about this situation. This approach aims to cultivate more complex alliances, positioning him as part of the solution rather than constructing him as the problem, and challenges the oppositional power relations that permeated my initial presentation of the scenario. Positioning the detective as an ally, and engaging him to act in the victim/survivor's interests, may increase the likelihood of this occurring. While this is uncertain, at least this construction creates possibility, whereas conf ict proved not to be conducive in eliciting an effective or cooperative response from the police on this occasion. Ultimately, this reconstruction removes me from of a position of powerlessness, and situates me in a better position to support the victim/survivor, thereby improving how feminist values are enacted in practice.

Embracing diversity

Yet my initial sense that it was a problem that the role of the police was different from mine appears to be another limitation of modernist feminist thinking: How can we acknowledge difference without it becoming a threat to equity? Related to this consideration: What are the possibilities to continue the feminist tradition of universalising the experiences of women, for example, without disenfranchising women who consider other dimensions of their identities as more signif cant than gender (Parton & O'Byrne 2000a)? For example, some Indigenous victims/survivors may experience issues related to colonisation and racism more profoundly than gender discrimination (Pettman 1992; Pine 1996). How do we account for, and respond adequately to, diverse experiences? Could it sometimes be unhelpful or limiting to privilege gender as the primary dimension of difference?

While the postmodern emphasis on celebrating diversity has been interpreted as a challenge to the universal gendered analysis of oppression (Sands & Nuccio 1992; Bulbeck 1994), and therefore implicated in fragmenting universal, feminist arguments, feminism's emphasis on sameness and commonality has been criticised for excluding women with diverse experiences and backgrounds (Hare-Mustin & Marecek 1994). Because postmodernism 'presents itself as a celebration of the multiplicity of individual experiences' (Kermode & Brown 1996: 376; Parton & O'Byrne 2000a), it does not need to conceptualise women (or indeed victims/ survivors) as an homogeneous group in order to respond appropriately to women's experiences, both shared and diverse. This recognises that women experience various layers of intersecting oppressions, both through gender and other categories of difference, and creates the 'conceptual space' (Rossiter 2005) to legitimate a variety of stories, voices and cultural experiences that have unintentionally been disenfranchised by modernist feminist discourses. This 'offers empowerment to women who can otherwise be smothered . . . by the idea of a sisterhood' (Pine 1996: 6), which has the capacity to meaningfully put into practice the espoused emancipatory aims of feminist frameworks by improving their capacity to be inclusive of all women (Mullings & Schulz 2006; Weber 2006: 24).

Conclusion

This chapter has largely explored the ways in which a postmodern informed critical ref ection may enhance feminist theory and practice, and the implications that this may potentially hold for contemporary critical social work practice with women. While still considered vital to social transformation, modernist feminist frameworks, like all theories, benef t from being positioned as 'incomplete process[es]' which can be extended towards the aim of constructing more inclusive, creative, emancipatory and intentional practices (Eisler 2004).

A critique of the grand narratives associated with feminism does not require an absolute retreat from its principles (Lister 2003: 89). Instead, the goals of contemporary feminism may be to resist participating in unhelpful and dichotomous discourses and learn to value 'everyday' acts of resistance, at the micro and collective levels, by 'courageously engag[ing] in acts of deconstructing and reconstructing practice, to learn what is required in various contexts to achieve critical emancipatory aims' (Morley & Macfarlane 2008). Contemporary feminist practice therefore continues to strive for social transformation to produce social justice and greater gender equity while f nding meaningful ways to relate the universal to the particular. This may involve: reconstructing power relations and possibilities for agency; acknowledging contextual uncertainties and contradictions; responding more effectively to complexities around identity; advocating by building more complex alliances; and valuing a diverse range of knowledge systems that contribute to emancipatory and critical practices (Fook 2002; Morley & Macfarlane 2008).[3]

12

challenges and directions for profeminist practice with men

Bob Pease

In this chapter, I explore the implications of critical theory for social work practice with men. Such a perspective recognises structural inequalities in men's lives but also emphasises the importance of dominant discourses in shaping men's diverse subjectivities. This means that we must locate men in the context of patriarchy and the divisions of class, race, sexuality and other forms of social inequality, while at the same time exploring the ways in which patriarchal belief systems become embedded in men's psyches. This dual perspective draws upon the theoretical frameworks of Connell (1995), Hearn (1998), Kimmel (2000) and Kimmel et al. (2005) in the critical studies of men, and some of my own recent writing and practice in profeminist masculinity politics (Pease 2004–05; 2006b; 2008; Rees & Pease 2007).

I have written elsewhere about the limitations of traditional approaches to working with men in social work, and the importance of adopting a critical theoretical framework and a profeminist commitment among men to challenge sexism in the human services (Pease 2001). In this chapter, I extend that analysis by examining men's practices in personal and public life, in the context of social difference and inequality in men's lives. I also outline the practice implications of a critical approach to men in the areas of male social workers' social location, and in working with individuals, groups and communities.

Profeminism as a basis for practice with men

A critical approach to working with men necessitates an explicit profeminist commitment, and this is consistent with structural (Moreau 1990; Mullaly 2007), anti-oppressive (Baines 2007a; Clifford & Burke 2008) and postmodern critical (Leonard 1997; Pease and Fook 1999; Fook 2002a; Davies and Leonard 2004) approaches to social work practice. For men, profeminism involves a sense of responsibility for our own and other men's sexism, and a commitment to work with women to end men's violence (Douglas 1993). It acknowledges that men benef t from the oppression of women, drawing men's attention to the privileges we receive as men and the harmful effects these privileges have on women (Thorne-Finch 1992). Profeminist men also recognise that sexism has an impact on men as well as women. To oppress others, it is necessary to suppress oneself. Systemic male dominance dehumanises men too, as evidenced in stress-related illnesses and emotional inexpressiveness. Furthermore, not all men benef t equally from the operation of the structures of domination. Issues of race, sexuality, class, disability and age signif cantly affect the extent to which men benef t from patriarchy.

Over twenty years ago, Tolman et al. (1986) articulated eleven principles for a profeminist commitment among men in social work: develop a historical, contextual understanding of women's experience; be responsible for themselves and other men; redef ne masculinity; accept women's scrutiny without making them responsible; support the efforts of women without interfering; struggle against racism and classism; overcome homophobia and heterosexism; work against violence in all its forms; do not set up a false dichotomy between oneself and other men; act at individual, interpersonal and organisational levels; and attend to process and product. They noted at the time that very few men had been proactive in promoting feminist values such as these in social work and that men had contributed very little to ending sexism (Tolman et al. 1986). Dominelli (1999) made a similar observation thirteen years later. Writing in 2008, little has changed. However, I believe that men in social work have an important part to play in challenging sexism. This chapter builds upon other initiatives in developing a new agenda for profeminist practice with men in social work (Pease and Camilleri 2001; Christie 2001b; Scourf eld 2003; Featherstone et al. 2007).[1]

Understanding men's practices

McMaster (2000) argues that issues associated with masculinity underlie the problems that men present with at human service organisations. The general consequences of traditional masculinity that have been identif ed include emotional inexpressiveness, poor health, distant fathering, family breakdown, stress associated with competitiveness and overwork (Brooks 1998), the over-representation of men in substance abuse, high-risk behaviours, homelessness, suicide and criminality (Lichtenberg 1999).

A number of writers have suggested that men will change when they consider these costs of masculinity for themselves. I have argued previously, however, that the focus on the problems facing men has placed too much emphasis on the costs for men associated with patriarchal relations and given insuff cient attention to the costs to women and children of men's practices (Pease 2000). In this regard, Cowburn and Pengelly (1999: 198) make the distinction between 'men with problems' and 'men as problems'. The latter include rape and sexual assault, violence against women in the home, sexual harassment and sexual misconduct as a group norm. Brooks (1998: 2) refers to these practices as 'the dark side of masculinity'.

Hearn (1996) has developed a critique of the concept of masculinity itself, however, arguing that it may divert attention away from gendered power relations between men and women. He prefers the concept of 'men's practices' to describe what men do, think and feel. This is consistent with Pringle's (1998a) central principles for critical social work practice with men: (1) maintaining a focus on the relations between men and women rather than on men alone; (2) examining the complexities of masculinity while grounding these in the materiality of men's practices; and (3) maintaining the issue of power at the centre of one's analysis of men's practices.

I have been guided by Hearn and Pringle on this matter, in arguing that men's practices should be the focus of critical social work with men. This focus enables us to move beyond the dichotomising portrayal of men as either 'victims' or 'perpetrators'. I suggest here that there are six main arenas in which men's practices are enacted: sexuality; intimacy and emotional expressiveness; health and wellbeing; family and care of others; paid work; and violence against women.

Sexuality

Objectif cation and f xation are key processes in many men's sexual relationships with women, in which often a part of the woman is seen to represent the whole

(Kaufman 1993). Some writers argue that there is a connection between the construction of men's sexuality along the objectif cation, f xation and conquest lines and the prevalence of sexual assault and rape (Schacht & Atkinson 1992). Male heterosexual socialisation leads to the assumption that men should take the initiative in sex and be dominant. Sattem et al. (1984) argue that it is male sexual socialisation that helps to predispose some men to rape. Lisak's (1991: 243) research demonstrates 'an association between rape myths, stereotypical sex role beliefs and attitudes, the culture's misogynist messages and both the propensity for and actual perpetration of sexual aggression'. Thus, culturally supported attitudes and norms foster sexually aggressive behaviour.

If this is so, male sexual coercion can be prevented by challenging the cultural values that promote aggression and male domination over women as a natural right. This involves confronting the mythology that sees sexual coercion as an inevitable product of male needs. Otherwise, there is a danger of unintentionally endorsing the 'naturalness' of men's urge to dominate women, rather than challenging the way in which our society condones male coercive sexuality.

Changing the basis of men's sexual desire will require challenging men's sense of entitlement through consciousness-raising and therapy (Segal 1990). In order for men's sexuality to be non-oppressive, it would have to incorporate getting aroused without exerting power over the other (Plummer 2005). The centrality of male power within heterosexual relations is not static or unchangeable. Sex does not have to be about domination and submission. Eisler (1996) has outlined a model of partnership sex that constructs new images of men's sexuality encompassing passivity, sensuality, joy and generosity. While many men appear reluctant to relinquish control in heterosexual relations, partnership sex is possible (Plummer 2005).

Intimacy and emotional expressiveness

Many women have expressed dissatisfaction with their intimate relationships with men. One of the constant requests from heterosexual women is for men to express themselves more than they do. Most men have been constantly challenged for not giving enough of themselves in their relationships (Muller 2007). Men's inability to express emotions has serious consequences for men's relationships with women, their friendships with men and their capacity to provide for the nurturant needs of their children, and it also has consequences for men themselves because men are robbed of potentially rich emotional experiences.

But is men's emotional inexpressiveness a tragedy, as many writers suggest (Balswick 1982), or is it a way in which men maintain their social power? Sattel

(1989) argues that inexpressiveness is a strategy for men to maintain their positions of privilege. To exercise organisational power, one must be able to guard against one's own emotional investment in the consequences of the decision. One must be blinded to the potential pain one's decisions inf ict on others. Inexpressiveness validates the rightness of one's position. The social positions of highest power demand veneers of inexpressiveness. In this view, men are inexpressive as a defensive strategy enacted by them to maintain their power (Sattel 1989).

Men's primary model for relationships tends to be hierarchical. Men have a tendency to either dominate women or withdraw from them in their intimate relationships (Rabin 1996). If men have diff culty giving up power and control in their relationships, it will hamper their capacity for intimacy (Dienhart 1998). Hooks (2004: 41) argues that only when men repudiate 'the will to dominate' will they be able to experience love and intimacy. Thus men's relationships with women will be impoverished as long as they continue to control and subordinate women (Sattel 1989). In recent years, men have been under greater pressure from women for both equality and emotional closeness (Johansson 2007), and they will need to adapt to the demands for intimacy that is connected to gender democracy.

Health and wellbeing

The issue of men's health started to surface publicly in Australia in the early 1990s. Numerous studies have drawn attention to sex differences in health status between women and men (Fletcher 1997; Mathers 2000). According to gender group averages, life expectancy for men in Australia is six years less than for women. A signif cant number of commentators draw attention to these and related statistics to indicate that, on average, Australian men die from nearly all non-gender-specif c causes at higher rates than women (Smith 2007).

Men's health status is used by some segments of the men's movement to claim that men are a disadvantaged group and are discriminated against in health services compared with women. However, men's health conferences and men's health policy documents often ignore the social divisions between men and the relationship between men's health status and their relationship to gender-based power. A profeminist approach to men's health emphasises diversity and difference in men's lives, and the costs of men's adherence to forms of social domination. Thus we must encourage men to develop a critical consciousness of the material and ideological factors that impact on their health and acknowledge the circumstances of men marginalised by class, race and sexuality (Pease 2009).

Family and care of others

Research conducted over the last ten years consistently demonstrates that women's involvement in the paid labour force does not signif cantly affect the amount of unpaid work they do at home. Wives continue to do considerably more housework than husbands (Dempsey 1997; Bittman et al. 2003; Breen and Cook 2005; Craig 2007). This includes the invisible work of thinking about and planning meals and other psychological responsibilities for domestic life that women carry more than men. Resentments and disputes over various forms of marital inequality such as these are among the factors that men and women cite as contributing to the breakdown of their marriages (Dempsey 1997). Many women want their husbands to do more housework and child care, they want more opportunities for leisure and they want a greater say in decision-making (Dempsey 2000; Mannino & Deutsch 2007). It would seem that marital breakdown may be related to continued gender inequalities in marriage, and to men's sense of male entitlement and their sexism.

There is a prevalent view in the contemporary literature about men in families that greater involvement of men in child care is important to heal the 'father wound' which is caused by fathers' remoteness and absence (Diamond 2007). However, while this literature advocates greater involvement of men with their children, it also encourages clear distinctions between men's and women's roles. For example, fathers are expected to be the main transmitters of culturally approved masculinity to their sons. McMahon (1999) pointed out ten years ago in his analysis of 'new father' writing that only a minority of such texts argue for equity in child-care work. This is still the case today.

Women's sense of personal and relationship wellbeing increases and their depression decreases if husbands share the housework (Dempsey 1997). Men can also gain from an improved relationship and from a sense of partnership by being equally involved in domestic work (Pease 2002b). When fathers take on signif cant responsibility for children, they develop sensitivities associated with women. Such men report that the experience of child care makes them more complete people, and that it enables them to develop the more caring and emotional dimensions of themselves (Marsiglio & Pleck 2005). It is thus important that critical social work with men in families emphasises gender equality in household work.

Paid work

Men have been socialised to pursue work as the central life interest, and consequently regard child rearing and domestic responsibilities as secondary. Work-related behaviours inf uence men's personalities and carry over into the home setting. The competitive world of work encourages men to estrange themselves from their feelings as a way of surviving. Furthermore, given the masculinised nature of some men's work, the aura of masculinity is sustained by keeping women out, or 'keeping them in their place' if they get in.

Some men are 'now less willing to spend endless hours at work, to subordinate their family life to the interests of the corporation; to lead an unbalanced life in which personal well-being comes last' (Edgar 1998: 3). Thus there is pressure on workplaces to become more family friendly. In response to these issues, in recent years we have seen the development of anti-sexist educational programs targeted at men in the workplace. The purpose of these workshops is to encourage male managers to work more cooperatively with people and to place a higher value on family issues (Russell & Hwang 2004).

If more egalitarian relationships between women and men are to emerge, however, signif cant alterations to the nature and structure of paid employment are required. Such alterations should include the f exible restructuring of work to take account of child-care needs, increases in government-subsidised child care, paid parental leave which leaves either partner the option of selecting child care as a priority, increased availability of job sharing and part-time work, and changes in the nature of career values (Hobson 2002; Ranson 2007).

Men's violence

It is widely acknowledged that almost all of the perpetrators of violence are men. However, while most violence is male, not all men are violent. In contrast to the socio-biological arguments that explain men's violence by reference to testosterone and hormonal patterns (Turner 1994), there is nothing inherent in men that leads them to be violent.

Cross-cultural research shows that the greater the level of gender inequality in a society, the higher the level of violence there is against women. Studies of societies in which there was little violence 'found that the def nition of masculinity has a signif cant impact on the propensity toward violence' (Kimmel 2000: 245). Those societies where gender inequality was highest were those where masculinity and femininity were seen to be polar opposites. This analysis has signif cant implications not only for preventative approaches to men's violence but also for the establishment of gender democracy across all levels of society.

Intervention with perpetrators of violence is too often aimed at men's abuse of authority in the family, and not at the nature and constitution of this authority itself. The organisation of the family is untouched by this approach. Interventions may help the man control his violence while leaving the basic power structure of the family unaltered (Pease 2004–05). Thus, in the longer term, we must eliminate the imbalance of power between men and women if we want to eliminate violence. Until the power inequality of the relationship is altered, there is greater likelihood of male coercion and domination remaining.

Social difference and inequality in men's lives

Men are not a homogeneous group, and variations among men are central to the understanding of men's lives. This diversity entails differences between men in relation to class, ethnicity, age, sexuality, bodily facility, religion, world-views, parental/marital status, occupation and propensity for violence (Pease 2000). It is always important to consider which men we are talking about.

Class

Power is not shared equally among men, and men's class locations influence the nature of their dominance over women. Most working-class men do not experience work as a satisfying or rewarding experience, and the promise of masculine independence and power is not fulfilled (Leach 1993). Many aspects of working-class men's work erode their sense of masculinity. The pressure of production targets, being controlled by foremen and supervisors, and having to put up with constant noise and dirt are common experiences for workers. Because of how it is socially organised, the experience of manual work poses a constant threat to masculinity (Morgan 2005). As working-class men lack social power in the class hierarchy, it is claimed that they are more likely to treat women as underlings in order to compensate. They are quicker to resist changes in the balance in sex roles at home and at work (Flood & Pease 2006). Having women to dominate can partly be seen as compensation for having to put up with the indignities and oppressions of the workplace.

Pyke (1996) argues that working-class men's masculine identity and self-esteem are undermined by their subordinate position in the social order. As their jobs do not provide satisfaction or social power, they need to maintain their dominance in other ways. This may result in asserting their power and reproducing their masculinity through more extreme methods of controlling women. Working-class masculinity becomes strung between the contradictory poles of the powerlessness of men's wage labour and the power and privilege they have over women of the same class. As most male social work clients are likely to be working class, this contradictory location in relation to power needs to be considered in developing strategies for challenging sexism (Pease 2004–05). Those of us who are white middle-class professional men must recognise more than just our gender privilege. We need to understand our class and race privilege as well when, for example, we challenge abusive and controlling practices of men from marginalised backgrounds.

Race and culture

The writings of African American men in North America emphasise the role of racism in the development of white masculinity. Due to their exclusion from satisfying paid work, most black men do not expect to attain the benef ts of traditional masculinity. As prevailing def nitions of masculinity imply power, control and authority, these attributes are seen as having been denied to most black men since slavery (Mercia & Julien 1988). Black and white men differ in terms of their power relations with women because of their tenuous position in the relations of production. According to Staples (1989), black men's subordination as a racial minority has more than cancelled out their advantages as males in the larger society.

Issues of culture and race have played little part in Australian men's literature. There has been no attempt to analyse the changing modes of masculinity resulting from migration to Australia and we know little about the effects of migration on men's work, leisure and domestic relations (Hibbins & Pease 2009). The research of Poynting et al. (1998, 2009) with Lebanese young men in Sydney, however, points to some of the key issues. They found a highly developed solidarity against 'Aussie' males that took forms of what Connell (1995) calls 'protest masculinity'. This protest masculinity involves exaggerated claims of potency and hypermasculinity, as a result of marginalisation. The link between masculinity and ethnicity has implications for critical social work practice with men from culturally and linguistically diverse backgrounds. (See Rees & Pease 2007 for the implications of this analysis for working with refugee men who commit violence against their intimate partners.)

There has been very little analysis of the changing modes of masculinity among Indigenous men, including the implications for gender identity of the move of many away from traditional societies to an urban, capitalist society. Studies of Indigenous men tend to not address masculinity and sexual identity, although obviously they have lost their traditional power and authority since white settlement. Many have embraced alcoholism and become the recipients of welfare (McCoy 2008). Historical processes have devalued the Indigenous male role in both the family and the community. When Indigenous men were conf ned to reserves, many lost respect and self-esteem (Atkinson & Pease 2001).

Within this context, it is claimed that Indigenous women in contemporary society are not characteristically subordinate. Atkinson (Atkinson & Pease 2001) argues that 'Aboriginal men not only had unequal relationships with dominant mainstream culture but also with Aboriginal women, particularly those who forged dominant roles in family and community affairs' (Atkinson & Pease 2001: 187). There are, however, conf icting views about the impact of colonisation on Indigenous women and men, the extent of Indigenous men's violence against Indigenous women, and the extent to which this is a product of colonisation (Larson & Peterson 2001; Daly & Stubbs 2006; Nancarrow 2006). White social workers need to be aware of these debates, and they need to be sensitive to the separate areas of men's and women's business when working with Indigenous men.

Sexuality

Heterosexual masculinity is a privileged masculinity that is created and maintained by homophobia at the expense of homosexual men and women (Robinson 2007). As homosexuality is not the norm, gay men have had to question the association of masculinity with heterosexuality. In response to this equation of homosexuality with femininity, some gay men have attempted to create alternative gay masculinities (Graham 2007).

As gay men do not dominate women sexually, they do not benef t in the same way from the oppression of women. On the other hand, while gay men are in a subordinate position in the institution of heterosexuality, at the same time they stand with straight men in the privilege of being in a dominant position in relation to women. Gay men are known to dominate lesbians in activist groups and women generally in workplaces, which can either be seen as a compensation for their own oppression or as a ref ection of their masculinity. Ward (2000) challenges the view that gay men have a special understanding of sexism simply because they are gay men. She argues that while gay men have a shared experience of gender-related oppression, they can still be sexist. Rather, she suggests that sexism takes on specif c forms in gay communities—what she calls 'queer sexism'.

Many writers have emphasised the importance of understanding the ways in which class, race and sexuality inf uence men's commitment to gender equality. Men do not have the same resources or motivations to promote an end to male privilege. The fact that men are divided among themselves along the lines of class, race, ethnicity and sexuality makes the task of analysing men's power more diff cult. However, these differences among men also open up possibilities for gay, working-class, non-white or disabled men to f nd points of contact with feminist women.

An intersectional analysis of privilege makes it clear that almost everyone experiences both privilege and subordination. Multiple forms of social difference shape both unities among and differences between men. Thus men do not share uniformly in the benef ts of gender inequality (Flood & Pease 2005). Such an analysis provides a framework for designing interventions with men that take into account their different positionings in relation to privilege and oppression.

Critical social work practice with men

Pringle (1995) identif es four levels at which male social workers should engage in anti-oppressive practice: one's own behaviour; individual work; group work; and structural change at the community and societal levels.

Working on one's own social location and behaviour

Many writers have drawn attention to the gendered patterns of employment in social work (Christie 2001a, 2006; Camilleri & Jones 2001; Scourf eld 2003). The starting point for men's profeminist practice with men must involve a critical ref ection upon the privileges associated with one's own position in the gender order and the gendered division of labour within social work. Christie (2001a) has stressed the importance of male social workers critically ref ecting upon and challenging their gendered privilege and the gendered nature of their work. Pringle (2001: 45) similarly argues that male social workers 'have a particular responsibility to engage in challenging those oppressive structures of power from which they may benef t directly'. This requires male social workers to monitor and challenge their own behaviour. It also means that male social workers need to recognise the contradictions and dilemmas arising from their position.

Cree (2001) has suggested that men in social work should consider engaging in consciousness-raising work. Anti-patriarchal consciousness-raising with men can clarify the social dimensions and historical shifts of masculinities. It can provide a link between personal experiences and the wider social context of men's lives. Men can come to understand their own sexist behaviour, to develop emotional support with other men and encourage their anti-sexism.

Individual work with men

As previously discussed, when gender issues facing men are noted in social work, the tendency is to focus on how men may be oppressed by traditional masculinity and sex roles. Longres and Bailey (1979) f rst drew attention to this issue in their review of social work journals in 1979, and little has changed since then. Men will not construct a profeminist practice by focusing solely on the costs of sexism for men.

Men often want things to change but they do not want to relinquish their power. A profeminist approach encourages men to rethink their power. It involves what Cree (2001: 161) calls 'critical engagement'—how to 'build open connection with men while at the same time not being seen to condone their behaviour or attitudes'.

Many of the beliefs men hold are the cause of the troubles in their lives. Thus the starting point for work with men is to assess their beliefs. What beliefs does the man hold about masculinity? What are the sources of these beliefs? What are the potential harmful effects of these beliefs? How are these beliefs associated with the diff culties the man is experiencing (Allen & Gordon 1990)?

Men's socialisation leads to individual beliefs that can promote abusive behaviours (Russell 1995). Men need to be helped to acknowledge their tendencies to act oppressively and they should be assisted to devise strategies for avoiding those situations and changing their behaviour. They should also be encouraged to develop wider repertoires of behaviour and models of masculinity not associated with violence, control and objectif cation (Pringle 1995).

Mary Russell (1995), in her work with men who hold abusive beliefs, has articulated a set of respectful beliefs and behaviours. A respectful belief system about heterosexual relationships is seen to involve: a belief in one's connectedness and interrelatedness with one's partner; a belief that the partner is an equal person whose differences are valued; and a belief in the necessity for mutual exchange. To reconstruct masculinity means that it is possible for men to feel good about being men without the negative repercussions of traditional patterns of aggressive masculine behaviour.

Group work with men

There are many positive claims made for men's groups. Andronico (1999) argues that men's groups are ideal forums in which to raise issues relevant to men in the twenty-f rst century. He suggests that the sense of community fostered by groups leads men to feel less isolated and alone. Brooks (1998: 104) similarly argues that, because 'men learn to be men in front of other men', then it is in front of other men that men 'can unlearn some of the more unproductive lessons about manhood and relearn and reinforce some of the more positive lessons'.

The psychological and therapeutic literature on men's groups, however, tends to ignore the dangers and problems associated with such groups. Profeminist writers have drawn attention to a range of issues that need to be addressed in group work with men. Funk (1993: 130) cautions us 'to be careful not to get caught in the habit of focusing on the support and on feeling good about being men'. Similarly, Rowan (1997) notes that, whatever the intentions, men's groups have a tendency to 'slide into some kind of warm self-congratulation' (1997: 222). He says that, while such groups can provide moving experiences for the men, they seem to contribute little to challenging the patriarchal arrangements between men and women. McBride (1995: 89) has argued that any therapeutic benef t for men meeting in groups needs to be 'set against and indeed counter the history of male dominance, collusion and violence' experienced in such groups.

As I have written previously (Pease 2003a), I believe that anti-patriarchal consciousness-raising group work with men can clarify the social dimensions and historical shifts in masculinites. Anti-patriarchal consciousness-raising in men's groups can provide a link between personal experiences and the wider social context of men's lives. Men can come to understand their own sexist behaviour and develop emotional support from other men to encourage their anti-sexism.

Over the last twenty years in Australia, we have witnessed a dramatic increase in the development of education and counselling programs for violent men. The provision of services to violent men has proved controversial. While they have been seen by some as constituting a viable alternative to legal sanctions, they have been condemned by others as psychologising and decriminalising men's violence. Many of the early programs focused on childhood precedents of violent behaviour, anger management and communication in relationships, and failed to adequately address issues of gender inequality, women's safety and accountability. More recently, explicitly profeminist educational programs that challenge patriarchal belief systems have predominated.

Profeminist group work emhasises the importance of working in groups with men who oppress and disempower others, where men's prejudices and oppressive behaviours can be challenged (Pringle 1997). As Hearn (2001) comments, profeminist models educate men about the oppressiveness of their beliefs and behaviours, and involve them in analysing their use of power and control tactics to enable them to move towards more equal relationships with women.

While profeminist men's behaviour-change programs are now recognised by governments as a key intervention into men's violence, I have raised questions about the extent to which feminist analyses of men's violence have been incorporated into the principles, theories and strategies for working with violent men (Pease 2004–05).

I have argued that the emphasis on the capacity of men to change their violent and abusive behaviours has not adequately examined the cultural and structural limitations on the process of change in individual men's lives. Thus such programs have not incorporated the key feminist insights about men's violence as a political problem requiring social transformation.

Creating change at community and societal levels

Feminist and profeminist writers in social work emphasise that personal change does not go far enough, and advocate the importance of connecting personal change with cultural and structural change (Cree 2001; Pease 2004–05). Work with men should be one aspect of a broader strategy for changing unequal power relations between women and men.

Over twenty years ago, Eisler (1987) distinguished between dominator societies and partnership societies. A dominator society ranks the male above the female, has a high degree of institutionalised social violence, including wife-beating and rape, and has a hierarchical and authoritarian social organisation. A partnership society values the sexes equally, and has a low degree of social violence and an egalitarian social structure (Eisler & Loye 1990). The model of a partnership society remains an inspiring vision for profeminist men to work towards.

In working towards this goal, we need to raise consciousness, especially among men, about the human costs of men's violence and how the eroticising of such violence reinforces men's domination (Eisler 1996). We also need to develop collective political actions to challenge institutional violence. Feminism has been the underlying foundation of social movements against men's violence. In an earlier version of this chapter (Pease 2003b), I argued that if such movements are to succeed, they will need to involve signif cant numbers of men as well as women.

I still believe that men need to become more actively involved as partners with women in social movements against violence towards women. However, as the involvement of men in men's violence prevention has become more widely supported, I have become concerned that the tensions, dilemmas and dangers of such involvement have not adequately been addressed. These dangers include: reducing funding for women's services and programs; weakening the feminist orientation; silencing women; taking over the campaign; colluding with violent men; gaining more praise; and failing to earn women's trust (Pease 2008).

I have argued that, in developing alliances between women and men, particular conditions need to be met and specif c principles need to be adopted to address the potential problems associated with such partnerships (Pease 2008). The theoretical premises underpinning men's involvement in violence prevention need to be based upon feminist theory and the critical scholarship on men and masculinities. We have to ensure that, in involving men in men's violence prevention, we do not replicate the same structures and processes that reproduce the violence we are challenging.

Conclusion

Working with men to eliminate sexism and violence against women is an emerging f eld of practice for critical social work. Such a practice needs to be informed by a profeminist agenda that recognises both the institutionalised power that men hold over women, and the way in which many men are also marginalised by class, race and sexuality. Analysing men's practices in key sites of sexual politics provides the best starting point for social workers to challenge the reproduction of patriarchal relations and to work towards gender equality with women.

13
empowering and rights-based approaches to working with older people

Barbara Black

This chapter will examine critical social work with older people specifically as it relates to the area of the abuse and mistreatment of older people. Several critical theoretical approaches familiar to social workers will be discussed, including feminism, structural social work, and human rights-based advocacy and empowerment. These integrated frameworks aim for positive outcomes for the individuals or groups identified, and are important for developing ways of responding to older people, particularly regarding elder abuse, both at the micro and macro levels. In exploring critical social work with older people, the diversity of the older population will be highlighted and the social context discussed. An elder abuse case study is analysed, highlighting the effectiveness of rights-focused advocacy and empowerment interventions.

The role of critical theory

Critical theory has its foundations in social critique tied to consciousness-raising and the possibility of positive and liberating social change (Lincoln & Guba 2000). It is useful in promoting a broad understanding of the ways in which current policies and procedures may impact on older people. It may also be used to take a wider focus and look at the effects of societal factors, such as ageism, contemporary views and responses relating to aged care services, human rights and the forces of global capitalism. Critical theory leads to consideration of dimensions of inequality and appropriate social theory with which to critique and understand the abuse and mistreatment of older people.

In the twentieth century, gerontology emerged as a distinct perspective that sought to bring together a variety of theories and methods from several different disciplines and professions to address the 'problem' of old age (Achenbaum 1997). The critical theories which developed in relation to older people have been termed 'critical gerontology'. This stream of critical theory is seen as having a role in critically examining the social and cultural production of ageing and gerontological knowledge, while giving consideration to factors such as class, generational, gender and racial/ethnic divisions as well as ideological forces embedded in their production and reproduction (Estes 1991, in Achenbaum 1997: 22). Several strands of critical gerontology exist, ref ecting the diversity of the older population and the multifaceted nature of gerontologic inquiry, and these theoretical perspectives facilitate 'the weaving together of disparate intellectual ideas into a powerful critique of prevailing gerontological ideas' (Achenbaum 1997: 23), ideas which are implicit throughout this chapter.

Elder abuse

This chapter gives some attention to the question of elder abuse, as it is important that critical social work perspectives give attention to this relatively invisible area.

Elder abuse has become an issue of growing prominence due to increasing societal awareness of interpersonal violence and abuse of the human rights of vulnerable or minority populations, linked with issues raised by the ageing of the population. There are varying def nitions of elder abuse. Some def ne it as any act which causes harm to an older person and occurs within an informal relationship of trust, such as that of family or friends (APEA:WA 2006), while others include abuse by institutions and paid carers in this def nition (McDonald & Collins 2000; UNESCO 2002; Sadler 2006). Abuse may be carried out by an individual, a number of people or an organisation. For example, the entire workforce of an organisation may be guilty of abusing all clients due to attitudes and practices which fail to recognise basic human rights, such as the right to privacy, the right to make choices, and the right to be considered and treated as an individual (Sorensen & Black 2001).

International elder abuse prevalence studies estimate that between 4 and 6 per cent of the older population have experienced some form of abuse, when all types of abuse are considered (Sadler 2006). However, the prevalence of elder abuse is diff cult to establish given that taboos about this issue are likely to result in under-reporting. Forms of elder abuse include f nancial or material abuse, emotional or psychological abuse, physical abuse, sexual abuse, social abuse and neglect (APEA: WA 2006). Financial and psychological abuse are the most reported types of abuse in some studies (Boldy et al. 2002; Faye & Sellick 2003), while others report psychological and physical abuse as the most common forms (Sadler 2006).

A critical theory social work perspective may assist in providing structural and historical insights into the nature of the issues being examined in relation to elder abuse, paving the way for suggestions and recommendations for positive change. Several critical theory perspectives may be adopted for this purpose, including feminism, structural social work and human rights. Advocacy and empowerment may also be used, and these perspectives will be explored later in the chapter.

Feminism

It is important to consider the inf uence of gender in regard to the older population. As women tend to live longer than men, there is a larger proportion of women over the age of 65 in Australia. Work in the welfare sector in general, and in aged care in particular, is a highly feminised industry; the majority of welfare workers are women and it is mostly daughters or female relatives who are the 'next of kin' or the point of contact for aged care services. Thus this area lends itself to examination under a feminist perspective, including from the diverse strands of feminism that include liberal, Marxist, radical and cultural feminism (Porter 1998). Ageing may marginalise the experiences of women through interconnected oppression in terms of gender and ageing (Powell 2006). Adopting a feminist perspective allows examination of whether a patriarchal discourse acts to dampen human rights claims for older people as well as increase the effects of ageism, and to consider whether the situation would be different if there were more men involved.

Structural social work

As noted in other chapters in this book, social institutions or structures are an inherent, inbuilt part of our society (Mullaly 2007). Structural social work looks at the structures of society as a focus for change, and not solely the individual. Traditional critical social theory emphasises social structures as the major source of social problems (Mullaly 2007). Because these structures are generally established and operated by a particular social group, such as white, middle-class males, they may ref ect and reinforce the assumptions, views, ideals, culture and interests of this group (Mullaly 2007). Social structures may be imbued with sexism, racism and ageism, in that there is a dominant group within each that has more social, political and economic power than the subordinate groups. The domination of the powerful over the powerless has often been so internalised into the structures of society that it has become an intrinsic part of the workings of these social institutions (Mullaly 2007). Consider, for example, the poorly funded and highly regulated environment of residential aged care and the impact this institutional context has on the rights of its residents.

Human rights

The human rights discourse has gained prominence and widespread recognition over the last half-century. Human rights have been def ned in various ways. A simple way to describe them is as universal rights that belong to all people, regardless of national origin, race, culture, age, gender or anything else (Ife 2001). The idea of human rights has a broad visceral appeal to our sense of fairness and equality. It is a powerful discourse which seeks to overcome divisiveness and sectarianism, and unite people from all walks of life into a single movement asserting human values and the universality of humanity (Ife 2001).

Human rights have been def ned and understood in different ways throughout history, shifting and changing in response to changes in society and different social movements. Over time, perceptions of human rights have changed to encompass an ever-expanding demographic. However, there are still individuals and groups of people at the margins whose rights are not fully protected or realised. The utility of focusing on rights rather than care and service provision is that a rights focus is more inclusive, as it views older people as part of humanity, and therefore as being entitled to the same rights as everybody else. A human rights approach may also serve to highlight the fact that older people are often discriminated against, 'infantilised' and treated as if they do not know what is in their own best interests.

Key to understanding the phenomenon of abuse and mistreatment of older people is an examination of social context. The next section explores ageing issues in Australia, including the ageing of the population and age discrimination, known as ageism.

Older people in Australia

In common with those of most Western countries, Australia's population is ageing. This has largely come about as a consequence of increasing longevity and declining birth rates (Off ce of Seniors Interests 1997). Over the last century, male life expectancy at birth has increased from 55 to 79 years, while female life expectancy has increased from 59 to 83 years (ABS 2008). The current generation of older people is the largest that Australia has ever experienced, and as such has considerable political inf uence (Legge & Cant 1995).

Disability

Disability and illness are not necessarily associated with the ageing process; however, the risk of developing a debilitating illness or disease does increase with age (Sax 1993). As a consequence, the use of health and aged care services generally also increases with age (AIHW 2007b). As people get older, they are more likely to be affected by chronic illness, such as rheumatism or arthritis, as well as physical deterioration.

The most frequent effects of this are impaired mobility and diff culty with self-care. Communication diff culties may develop in relation to deterioration in sight and hearing. Impaired mental functioning may also be an issue, with conditions such as dementia affecting older people. Small changes in physical capability can have major social effects, and often tip the balance between relative independence and dependence for individuals. Injuries caused by falls can have drastic consequences, including the loss of the ability to live independently and a loss of conf dence (Bishop 1999).While there is a large increase at older ages in the number of people requiring assistance with activities of daily living, it is interesting to note that the majority of these people continue to live in the community rather than in residential aged care (AIHW 2003).

Dementia

Dementia is a term used to describe the symptoms of a range of illnesses that cause a progressive decline in a person's mental functioning. Impairment may be caused in multiple higher cortical functions, including memory, intellect, rationality, social skills and normal emotional reactions (Alzheimer's Association 2005). Dementia is not a normal part of ageing, but a pathological condition, and there are a number of different forms of dementia, each with its own causes. The most common is Alzheimer's disease. Of particular concern associated with the ageing of the population is the increase in the number and proportion of the older population with dementia, as well as the associated need for care in the home and in residential care facilities (AIHW 2003).

Aged care services

A range of aged care services is available to provide support and assistance to older people. A large proportion of these services are community based, such as meals on wheels, home nursing and domestic assistance, and are provided in the older person's home. Otherwise, if unable to be supported to live at home, older people may move into residential aged care. The issues mentioned earlier, including increasing rates of disability and dementia that occur with age, make older people receiving aged care services quite dependent on other people for assistance. This renders them vulnerable to rights abuses, and often means they are less able to support and maintain their own rights and best interests. People who live in residential aged care are potentially disadvantaged by many factors, including disability, mental incapacity and living in a somewhat restricted, regimented institutional environment where their lives are largely regulated by the staff and management of their facilities. It is also important to understand that while some people move into aged care facilities as the result of choice and planning, many people move into facilities quite suddenly, as a result of a fall or accident. This relocation can be a stressful experience accompanied by multiple losses, including the loss of independence, home, possessions, family relationships and pets (Nay 1993).

As sites for change and action in relation to elder abuse, consider institutions such as aged care facilities and hospitals. The very nature of institutional care serves to multiply the impediments to residents exercising their rights. This may also be exacerbated by the fact that residents may have lost the capacity or will to exercise their rights as a consequence of illness, disability or adaptation to the strictures of the institutional environment. Although there are many complaint, monitoring and accountability measures available, there are several obstacles to their effectiveness. One diff culty is the vulnerability of many older people. Often the people most in need of having their rights protected are those who have little way of accessing complaint mechanisms and communicating their needs due to physical limitations, communication diff culties or a lack of knowledge of their rights, entitlements and the complaint mechanisms available (Black 2004). There are also the social barriers of feeling too intimidated to complain, not wanting to be seen as a 'whinger', not wanting to damage their relationship with staff and management, and feeling grateful for the care they do receive (Black 2004).

Institutions are protective and often paternalistic by nature, and this may place restrictions on people's rights where there is a conf ict with the institution's duty of care. Older people's rights are also often of lower priority to other concerns, and rights issues may give way under strictures such as limited funding. For example, residents may not be able to have showers whenever they wish because there is not enough money to employ enough staff for this purpose. For these reasons, it is imperative that there are strong monitoring, accountability and complaint mechanisms in place in order to support people's rights with these structures (Black 2004).

Ageing and ageism

When working with older people, it is important to have an awareness of the impact of different societal views of older people. This feeds into an awareness of critical social work theoretical frameworks highlighting the links between experiences, material conditions and the dominant ideologies in society (Pease et al. 2003a). Having an awareness of these ideologies and educating people about them allows us as social workers to challenge those affected by oppression to take appropriate action to transform their situation.

There are varying views and stereotypes of older people in our society. These range from comforting images of the 'rocking-chair granny' to views of older people as frail and vulnerable. Older people are often stereotyped as being incapacitated by illness and disability, 'clogging up' the health system and dependent on others for care. Ageing is commonly associated with stereotypes of deterioration, disability, dementia and death, with the effect of stigmatising older people (Legge & Cant 1995). Such negative stereotypes and denigration may translate into lack of societal concern for older people, and place them at greater risk of marginalisation and denial of equality in accessing opportunities, resources and entitlements (UNESCO 2002). This is known as 'ageism', and in the context of this chapter references to the concept of ageism refer to age discrimination against older people. The term 'ageism' was f rst used to describe the process of 'systematic stereotyping and discrimination against people because they are old' (Butler 1975, in Sax 1993: 2). However, more recently ageism has also been used to refer to any form of discrimination or stereotyping on the basis of age, whether the person is old or young (Sax 1993).

Ageism has served to legitimate the use of chronological age to systematically deny resources and opportunities to people based on age, and older people may suffer variations of this, ranging from well-meaning patronage to unambiguous discrimination (Blytheway 1994). Many positive stereotypes of older people also exist. These images include that of the caring grandparent as well as the sage of all wisdom and experience. However, these images are relatively weak in comparison with existing negative stereotypes. Society's preoccupation with youth and beauty, combined with the dominant stereotypes which imply that ageing equals debility, have largely eroded the images of wisdom, power, benevolence and respect which were once associated with elders.

Ageism has had many negative consequences for older people in our society. It has generated and reinforced fear and denigration of the ageing process, and given rise to negative stereotypes and presumptions regarding the competence of older people and their need for protection (Blytheway 1994). These negative stereotypes may inf uence attitudes and decisions concerning older people. They may also inf uence older people's images of their own self-worth (Westhorp & Sebastian 1997). In this sense, ageism is comparable with sexism and racism, as all of these ideologies depend on prejudice, which justif es forms of inequality (Blytheway 1994). Where ageism differs is that the whole of society has an interest in it, as it is something which will eventually affect us all—should we live long enough—unlike issues of race or gender.

The notion that the vast majority of older people are a burden on the community and are being 'looked after' has been challenged by much research data. Older people today are more visible, active and independent than ever before. The overwhelming majority of older people live in private accommodation—only 6 per cent live in non-private dwellings, which include aged care homes and hospitals (AIHW 2007b). Even among those aged 85 years and over, 74 per cent live in private dwellings. Almost a quarter of men aged 65–69 years participate in the workforce, along with 13 per cent of women in the same age group. Also, despite having relatively low average levels of income, research data shows that 24 per cent of all older Australians provide direct or indirect f nancial support for adult children or other relatives living outside the household (AIHW 2007b).

Ageism, when combined with dimensions of disadvantage, such as poverty, disability, and cultural and linguistic diversity, may place some older people at risk of marginalisation and denial of equality in accessing opportunities, resources and entitlements. It may also contribute to some forms of elder abuse. As ageist attitudes become entrenched in our culture, older people may internalise them and believe that they deserve to be treated in a lesser manner than others.

Diversity in the older population

It has been proposed that the strongest stereotype in relation to older people is that they are all the same (Victor 1991, in Vincent 1999: 142). A key aspect of countering ageism lies in establishing the diversity of old age and the different ways of living (Vincent 1999). It is important to note that older people are not a homogeneous group. They are a diverse population with signif cant variation in factors such as age, income, health, living arrangements and past experiences (Sax 1993). As is the case with most Western countries, current populations of older people in Australia are healthier, better educated and more likely to be f nancially independent than ever before (Sax 1993). However, some sections of the older population are disadvantaged in comparison with the general population due to factors such as cultural and linguistic background, disability, mental health issues (including dementia), sexuality and economic factors.

One area of difference which needs to be considered is that of economic diversity, or differences in class. Major changes occur in the sources and levels of income as people get older, and declining participation in the workforce contributes signif cantly to these changes (McLennan 1999). The aged pension is the main form of income support for older people, with nearly 80 per cent of the older population in receipt of it or the equivalent service pension (ABS 2008). The living standards of older people are also supported through continued participation in the workforce and retirement benef ts provided by superannuation (AIHW 2002). Although average incomes of older people are relatively low, average wealth is relatively high (AIHW 2007b), with older people likely to have accumulated assets during their working lives. However, it must be acknowledged that there are great differences in assets and income across the older population, with those older people who have managed to accumulate assets enjoying a comfortable retirement, while others with few or no assets struggle on income support pensions. Also, as women are more likely to marry men older than themselves and have a longer life expectancy than men, the gender disparity in the older population has resulted in older women being more likely to live alone and be on limited incomes (Finch & Groves 1985; Gibson 1998).

The older population is quite culturally diverse as a consequence of Australian immigration policy. Around 35 per cent were born overseas, with 39 per cent of these coming from English-speaking countries, and 61 per cent from non-English speaking countries (AIHW 2007b). However, Indigenous Australians aged 65 years and over comprise only 0.5 per cent of the older population, a much smaller proportion than their representation among the population generally, at 2.5 per cent (AIHW 2007b). This is the result of Aboriginal people having a life expectancy approximately seventeen years lower than that of the total population (AIHW 2007b).

Literature and statistics in relation to gay and lesbian older people are sparse, as much of the research focuses on younger people, and much of the research on older people fails to acknowledge sexuality, either hetero or homo (Thorson 2000). Gay and lesbian older people are often regarded as a subculture, and subject to prejudice and discrimination (Thorson 2000). Fullmer (1995, in Powell 2006: 59) notes that 'older gays and lesbians have learned through a lifetime of experience that they will likely be discriminated against if it is known that they are homosexual'. Older gay men and lesbians have few, if any, positive role models for forming relationships, ageing or creating alternative family structures (Powell 2006). Social structures and institutions may discriminate against homosexual older people—for example, aged care services may structure activities and policy around the assumption that their clients are heterosexual.

Elder abuse crosses national, class and cultural boundaries. Both men and women are abused, and older people who are physically and mentally f t are subject to abuse as well as the frail and dependent (Valsler 1996). People from what are perceived as disadvantaged or vulnerable groups are over-represented in elder abuse statistics. Research has found that people with some form of decision-making disability (such as dementia) are more likely to be subject to abuse (Boldy et al. 2002). Females are also more likely to experience elder abuse than males, although a substantial proportion of men are also abused (Boldy et al. 2002; Faye & Sellick 2003; Sadler 2006). Older aged (aged 75 years or older) have also been found to be more likely to experience abuse (Boldy et al. 2002). In the case of residential aged care, studies have shown that abuse is more likely to occur in institutions where the approach by staff has become depersonalised and dehumanised to the extent that the older person is viewed as an object rather than a human being (Valsler 1996).

Rights-focused advocacy and empowerment

Elder abuse responses have been linked to human rights through the use of a rights-based advocacy approach to intervention. Current Australian interventions into elder abuse tend to follow an advocacy model with strong foundations in empowerment and human rights (Black 2008). The rights-based advocacy model involves providing information and support to an older person in order to empower them to address their situation of abuse (Faye & Sellick 2003). The advocacy model works with the individual and their concerns, while seeking to redress macro level disadvantage—for example, disadvantage in relation to age or frailty, which may have contributed to the abuse (Cripps 2001). The focus is on empowering and supporting the older person to assert themselves in order to redress the abuse being experienced and to uphold their own rights and best interests, where possible.

Recognition of the need for advocacy has grown out of the human rights push for equality in Western societies and an acknowledgement that not all people are equal and some groups are at more risk of having their rights abused than others (Sorensen & Black 2001). Sometimes legislative protection is inadequate, as wrongs may be hidden because the vulnerable person may not have the means to complain (Rayner 1993, in Parsons 1994: ix). People who are marginalised, excluded or unable to participate in mainstream society are very dependent on the people who care for them, be they family, friends or care workers, to look after them appropriately and support their best interests. This dependent relationship unfortunately holds the potential for abuse and exploitation, given the unequal distribution of power between the parties (Black 2004). Advocates work to empower people, assisting them to self-advocate where possible and advocating on their behalf if necessary. An advocate may provide information and advice in order to assist a person to take action to resolve their own concerns or may take a more active role in representing the person's rights to another person or organisation which has the power to make life-affecting decisions for the individual. It must be remembered that advocacy is far from easy and unproblematic. It may involve being immersed in situations that are very distressing for the people involved, and a range of conf icts and dilemmas can arise. Advocates bring their own sets of values and beliefs to the situation, and these may conf ict with those of the person they are advocating for. It is important to remember that the advocate's role is to help people get justice, not to judge them, try to change their values or inf uence their wishes.

Case study 13.1 has been included to illustrate the way in which rights-based advocacy and empowerment may be used in situations of elder abuse.

There are many advocacy agencies in Australia that work to advance and maintain the rights of vulnerable groups, such as older people, people with disabilities, women, children, and people from culturally and linguistically diverse and Indigenous backgrounds. Advocacy agencies are involved in conducting community education as well as providing individual and systemic advocacy. This is undertaken with a view to promoting positive attitudes towards older people and raising awareness of their rights and the potential for abuse that exists. Community education targets the level of social structures and is a proactive form of systemic advocacy which empowers older people by reinforcing the fact that they have rights and there is assistance available to support their rights, should they require it.

Conclusion

It has been proposed that critical theory has been important for social workers in providing a link between theory and practice in its insistence that theory be grounded in practice and vice versa (Ife 1999). This chapter has explored a number

Case study 13.1

Mr Jeffries is a 73-year-old man who has recently moved into residential aged care. His friends contact a social worker to report concerns that he has been forced into residential care against his will and that his daughter, Sarah, is selling off his house against his wishes. The friends report that the aged care facility is not allowing them to visit Mr Jeffries, under instructions from his daughter, who has told the facility that they are undesirable characters who frequently borrow money from Mr Jeffries without paying it back.

The social worker visits Mr Jeffries at the facility and he asserts that he did not want to leave home, but was convinced by Sarah that he was here for 'respite', as a temporary measure. The social worker discovers that Mr Jeffries has signed over an enduring power of attorney to his daughter, as she has told him frequently over the last couple of years that he is 'losing his mind' and is not capable of looking after his finances any more. Mr Jeffries tells the social worker that his friends have borrowed money from him in the past but have always paid it back, and says he would like them to be able to visit him.

The social worker and Mr Jeffries meet with the facility manager and explain that Mr Jeffries would like his friends to be able to visit. The social worker reminds the manager that it is Mr Jeffries' right to decide who visits him, and not his daughter's. With assistance from the social worker, the facility manager organises an appointment with a psychogeriatrician, who tests Mr Jeffries' mental capacity and reports that he shows no signs of mental impairment. The psychogeriatrician says that Mr Jeffries has decision-making ability and is perfectly capable of managing his own affairs if he wishes to.

The social worker informs Mr Jeffries of his rights, and says that he does not have to live at the facility if he does not want to, and tells him about a range of community care services that are available to support him to live at home independently. She tells him that, as he still has decision-making capacity, he is able to revoke the enduring power of attorney that Sarah holds, and she assists him in doing so. The social worker encourages him to get in contact with other family members to provide support and assistance. Mr Jeffries calls his son James, who lives interstate, and tells him what has occurred. James is concerned and horrified, and flies over immediately to assist his father to sort out his affairs. Mr Jeffries, supported by James, contacts the real estate agent who has been advertising his home and stops the sale going through. Mr Jeffries then draws up a new enduring power of attorney naming James as his attorney, but only in the event that Mr Jeffries loses decision-making capacity. »

The social worker explains to Mr Jeffries that he can report what his daughter has done to the police and press charges if he wishes. Mr Jeffries decides he does not want to pursue legal action as the sale of the house was able to be stopped and he still would like to be able to patch up his relationship with his daughter in the future in order to maintain contact with his grandchildren.

of theoretical perspectives which may be applied to the area of abuse and mistreatment of older people, as well as addressing the systemic discrimination and exclusion that pervades. Utilising a critical social work approach in elder abuse work permits us to focus on both macro and micro issues. Critical social work allows analysis of the relations of power within the social context as well as the individual situation, serving to highlight them and indicate sites for action.

14

disabling discourses and enabling practices in disability politics

Kelley Johnson

> We are in the society of the teacher-judge, the doctor-judge, the educator-judge, the social worker-judge; it is on them that the universal reign of the normative is based; and each individual, wherever he [*sic*] may f nd himself, subjects to it, his body, his gestures, his behaviour, his achievements (Foucault 1979: 304).

I f rst read these words when I was undertaking a PhD which focused on the deinstitutionalisation of a group of women with intellectual disabilities (Johnson 1997). As a person who had worked with disabled people for an extended period of time and had traversed at least three of the professions Foucault pinpoints, they were uncomfortable reading. I had not seen myself as wielding power over others, as a frontierswoman patrolling the boundaries of 'the normative', nor had I seen myself as a judge, someone who wielded power over others—not only in terms of their external lives, but over the way their very subjectivity was framed and constituted. Yet while the words challenged, they also opened up new ways of thinking about myself, about work and about the world in which I lived. The words still have force and serve as a useful jolt which leads me into a ref ective and critical stance in relation to my work. In this chapter, I therefore take them as a key theme and develop a discursive approach to disability.

Although discourses have been def ned in many diverse ways depending on the particular theoretical and disciplinary orientation of the writer (Fairclough 1992), in this chapter they are def ned as:

> ways of constituting knowledge, together with the social practices, forms of subjectivity and power relations which inhere in such knowledges and the power relations between them. Discourses are more than ways of thinking and producing meaning. They constitute the 'nature of the body,' unconscious and conscious mind and emotional life of the subjects which they seek to govern (Weedon 1987: 108).

From Weedon's perspective, discourses allow us to speak of some things and they exclude others from our thoughts and our consciousness. They set the boundaries of what can and cannot be said at a particular time and in a particular culture. They establish through disciplinary knowledge and professional work the boundaries of the normative and that which is seen as lying outside such boundaries. They are formed through knowledge and power, and as a consequence they shape not only the way people live their lives but how their very subjectivity is constituted. Discourses shape the way we see ourselves.

In adopting this approach to the chapter, I am advocating a postmodern and critical approach to the way in which social workers work with disabled people (see the following section for a discussion of the language used to 'label' this group of people).

A postmodern and critical approach to social work practice is primarily concerned with practising in ways which further a society without domination, exploitation and oppression. It focuses not only on how structures dominate but also on how people construct and are constructed by changing social structures and relations, recognising that there may be multiple and diverse constructions of ostensibly similar situations. Such an understanding of social relations and structures can be used to disrupt dominant understandings and structures and as a basis for changing these so that they are more inclusive of different interest groups (Fook 2002a: 18).

The implications of this approach in social work with disabled people involve a commitment to understanding the way in which social structures and processes currently affect the lives of this group and to working to change those structures which are oppressive. However, such an approach also recognises the importance of the agency of disabled people in relation to their own lives.

Therefore, in this chapter I want to explore some of the issues raised by Foucault's statement in relation to working with disabled people. My main aim is to challenge the view that disability is a f xed medical condition of an individual and that assisting individuals to 'deal with' their disability is a primary function of social workers. Rather, I want to share the complexity of the issues confronting disabled people and to explore some of the ways in which *they* have positioned professionals such as social workers. Using some of the research and the work I have undertaken with disabled people (particularly people with intellectual disabilities), I want to explore three issues:

- the need to see disability as discursive and socially constructed
- the position of social workers in relation to disabled people
- learning from different discourses in relation to disability.

However, before addressing these issues, it is important to ref ect on the language which is used to describe disabled people, for words are fundamental to the knowledge that we acquire, to the theories we develop about others and the way we behave in relation to them. This becomes particularly apparent when we look at the ways in which language about disability is considered over time.

The importance of words

How we use words in reference to others is important and highly politicised. Labels (particularly those which are perceived to be 'negative' by others in the community) are always problematic. Disabled people object strongly to the term 'the disabled', which identif es individuals and groups solely in terms of their disability and which objectif es them as people. But the issue of how to describe disability remains highly contested, and social workers and other professionals should be careful. Some groups of disabled people prefer the term 'people with disabilities', arguing that their identity as people is more important than their ascribed disability. Others argue strongly for the term 'disabled people' on the grounds that the focus should be on how social structures disable them. In relation to 'intellectual disability', the term 'people with intellectual disabilities' is widely used by self-advocates in Australia. However, in the United Kingdom the term used by self-advocacy organisations is generally 'people with learning diff culties'.

In this chapter, I have used the term 'disabled people' in general references but when I am discussing 'intellectual disability' I use 'people with intellectual disabilities', as this is the preferred term of self-advocates. If you are going to have to live with a label, it is important that those who work with you use the one that you prefer.

Thinking about discourses

Foucault was clear in his discussion of discourses when he said they were not necessarily oppressive or for that matter freeing. However, by their very nature they both open up ways to see others and simultaneously limit them. In this section, I brief y describe three of the discourses to which disabled people have been subject.

The medical, individual or tragedy discourse

Much of the knowledge gained in the twentieth century about 'disability' developed from disciplines such as medicine. It led to some ways of preventing particular forms of impairment. For example, phenylketonuria—which causes severe intellectual disabilities—was found to be preventable by the use of a strict diet for babies. This form of knowledge also led to the categorisation of groups of people as having particular syndromes or forms of 'disability', and it def ned disability in terms of an individual's lack of capacity:

> disability refers to 'limited activity'—not being able 'to do things', and a 'disabled person' is someone who has a medically certif able 'condition' that prevents him or her carrying out the full range of age-related activities considered normal (Thomas 2007: 12).

This def nition places the 'disability' f rmly within the individual. It is seen as a characteristic which places them outside the boundaries of the 'normal', and positions them as someone who is unable to live independently or without support. In this def nition, there is an assumption that there is something that can be called 'normal', although it is not def ned. It suggests that disability is unchanging and static, and it positions the person f rmly as a 'patient' or as someone with a medical condition. The role of professionals in relation to people with disabilities within this framework involves caring for them, supporting them, f xing them or f nding ways to 'cure' them. The def nition does not specify particular kinds of disability, but usually such an approach encompasses people with intellectual, psychiatric, physical or sensory impairments. This way of thinking about disability has been labelled as the medical or individual tragedy model by some disabled activists (Oliver 1996; Thomas 2007).

However, not even the 'medical discourse' is unitary in its approach. In relation to people with intellectual disabilities, for example, the medical view is intertwined with the development of social science disciplines such as psychology in the early twentieth century and with the then widely accepted theory of eugenics. The latter theory positioned people with intellectual disabilities as a genetic threat to the general population because they were believed to transmit their 'disability' to their children and to be promiscuous, hence leading potentially to the birth of large numbers of children with disabilities. Early IQ tests were developed in part to identify children with intellectual disabilities whose 'disability' may not otherwise have been detectable and then to separate them from the community (Rose 1979). This perceived threat that these people were believed to pose was one of the factors (though not the only one)[1] leading to institutionalisation of many people with intellectual disabilities (and is illustrated in Case study 14.1). In some countries until the 1970s, women with intellectual disabilities were forced to undergo sterilisation if they were leaving an institution to live in the community (Sigurjonsdottir and Traustadottir 2000).

Case study 14.1: Jane's experience

Jane was one of 21 women with whom I worked in an ethnographic study on deinstitutionalisation in the 1990s. She lived in a locked unit in a large institution in Australia. She was 28. She was 'diagnosed' as having moderate intellectual disabilities and challenging behaviour, and was perceived by the nurses at the institution as being a danger to herself and to others. Jane had lived in the wider community in hostels and supported housing. She enjoyed partying and sex, and her advocate reported that one of the reasons for her admission to the institution was the 'trouble' her presence caused among men living in the hostel with her. Jane was sometimes aggressive and attacked some members of staff. Her psychiatric report stated that Jane's behaviour was due to her intellectual disability. She attended anger-management classes.

However, Jane had been sexually abused by the men in her family from childhood. While this was known to the people at the institution, her history was not taken into account in either the psychiatric reports or in the support that she was given. Rather, her behaviour was interpreted in terms of her 'disability'. She was not offered counselling for her experience of abuse. The medical report was important because it recommended her continued exclusion from the community.

As a social worker, what would you want to take into account in thinking about Jane's future?

A new discourse: the social model of disability

The social model was developed by disabled people and strongly counters the individualistic medical discourse described in the previous section. It repositions disabled people from being sick or in need of care and individual support to an oppressed group within society:

> Disabled people are an oppressed group in society. To understand this it is necessary to grasp the distinction between the physical impairment and the social situation called 'disability' of people with such impairment. Thus we def ne impairment as lacking part of or all of a limb, or having a defective limb, organ or mechanism of the body; and disability as the disadvantage or restriction of activity caused by a contemporary social organisation which takes no or little account of the people who have physical impairments and thus excludes them from participation in the mainstream of social activities (Oliver 1996: 22).

This model is important because it redef nes disability as something that affects an individual from the outside. While someone may have an impairment, the disability they experience comes from the failure of the society to provide the supports and to remove the barriers which prevent them from leading full lives. The social model is described by one of its originators, as follows:

> The social model provides a view of disability which argues strongly that social change and particularly structural change are fundamental to removing the idea of disability. For example if our society was able to provide physical access to all spaces then the 'disability' of lack of access to buildings would disappear for those who use wheel chairs (Oliver 2004: 21).

The social model shifts the focus of working with people from individualising their situation and providing support to working for social change and removing the barriers which prevent people from living fulf lling lives. Among the barriers are 'inaccessible education systems, working environments, inadequate disability benef ts, discriminatory health and social support services, inaccessible transport, houses and public buildings and amenities and the devaluing of disabled people through negative images in the media' (Oliver 2004: 21). Case study 14.2 illustrates such barriers. An impairment is only seen as limiting because of the failure of society to provide for equality for all its citizens. The social model provides a basis for disabled people and their supporters to take action on inequality and injustice. In the United Kingdom, and to a lesser extent in Australia, it has inf uenced government policies and practices. Further, it has led to changes which promote the inclusion of disabled people in areas such as education and employment, as well as to a movement towards individualised budgeting where disabled people manage their own money and are able to purchase support, and to have more choice and control over their own lives. While the social model has provided a different way of viewing the issues affecting the lives of disabled people from that offered by the medical model, it too has limitations. It has been criticised for focusing primarily on the political issues affecting the lives of physically disabled people and not suff ciently taking into account the needs of people with an intellectual disability (Chappell 1998), for distorting the psychic realities of disabled people (Watermeyer & Swartz 2008) and for a failure to take the signif cance of 'impairment' suff ciently into account (Shakespeare 2006).

Case study 14.2: barriers to health care

In 2003, a study was undertaken at La Trobe University to explore the barriers women experienced in accessing cervical screening. Fifty disabled women talked about their experiences of attempting to access services in either individual interviews or in focus groups, and an audit by a disabled researcher was undertaken in three services. While not all women were negative, the majority commented on difficulties of access, which were both physical and attitudinal. Among the barriers documented in the study were:

- the lack of adjustable tables for examination
- a stated belief by some medical practitioners that cervical screening was not important for the individual because she was disabled
- a refusal by funding bodies to provide support for personal assistants to support a woman going to an examination
- failure by services to provide accessible information to women who found printed material difficult to access
- failure to use existing hearing loops in services because staff did not know how to use them
- inaccessible buildings
- failure by some services to take into account women's needs for a longer examination time (Johnson et al. 2003).

As a social worker, if you are not disabled how do you go about identifying the barriers which might be important in someone's life? Can you? Should you? How do you balance 'impairment' and 'disability'? Where should your focus be as a social worker?

The rights discourse

Discourses are constantly changing as knowledge develops and wanes in particular areas, and as we are informed by particular world or national events. The focus on rights for disabled people was part of a wider emphasis on this issue following the Second World War, when there was an increasing emphasis on rights for marginalised groups, including women, African Americans and Indigenous people. By the latter part of the twentieth century, rights were becoming an important discourse in thinking and talking about disability (Whitehead 1992). Such a discourse focused on the need for disabled people to be able to live 'as normal a life' as possible, to move from the segregated systems of care in which many had lived and to have clearly stated rights as citizens which could be protected. A strong example of the application of a rights discourse can be found in the class actions undertaken in the United States to close large institutions. These cases were based on the constitutional rights of people with intellectual disabilities as American citizens and on their right to adequate care and treatment (Johnson & Tait 2003). The rights movement found its expression in anti-discrimination and disability legislation, with a strong focus on asserting and protecting people's rights. At an international level, the importance of rights for persons with disabilities has recently been aff rmed in the UN Convention on the Rights of Persons with Disabilities (United Nations 2006) which, when ratif ed, has the force of an international treaty, binding the government of each country to working towards its goals of inclusion by people with disabilities in their communities, in education, in work and in the development of relationships.

The rights discourse has underpinned much of the movement towards the inclusion of disabled people in their community rather than excluding them from it. However, it is not unproblematic, partly because of the very meaning of rights:

> First rights should be distinguished from the interests which they seek to secure; the legitimate interests of young people, or the disabled [*sic*], in obtaining f nancial security and a reasonable standard of living do not necessarily found a right to the realisation of these ends. Secondly expression of rights must be reasonably precise, they must rise above the rhetorical statements of hopes or expectations. Vague platitudes are not rights. Thirdly rights should carry a capacity for engendering . . . compliance. A right which cannot ever compel (or persuade) compliance does not qualify (Carney 1991: 60).

This def nition raises a number of issues about rights, and perhaps partly explains why stated rights have sometimes been diff cult to put into practice. Case study 14.3 shows the diff culties that can arise in asserting rights. Disabled people and their supporters can use rights which are part of legislation or international conventions or found in policy statements but they need power to enforce such rights. This can be diff cult for some disabled people, particularly if they are alone (see, for example, Millear with Johnson 2000). Rights are also relative across different groups so, for example, parents' rights in practice are often balanced against the rights of people with disabilities. Further, one right may be privileged over another. For example, in the Republic of Ireland the *Crimes Act (Sexual Offences Act)* 1993 effectively prevents people with intellectual disabilities from

Case study 14.3: claiming rights

> Under the old *Equal Opportunity Act* I fought a number of areas of discrimination and one of those was on sexual harassment and the other one was against a record shop and a third one was against a stupid workshop that didn't believe in having married people in it. In the record shop they asked me for my driver's licence (as a guarantee for a cheque). I said, 'Excuse me visually impaired people don't have a driver's licence' and I thought that was discriminatory and I went through an outside conciliatory meeting with the person and they hopefully improved their things with people like me. Later they developed a simple system that I could use (Millear with Johnson 2000: 245).

Amanda is a strong self-advocate who has been labelled as having an intellectual disability and a visual impairment. She has a good knowledge of the law and her rights. Under the *Disability Discrimination Act* she took the Scouts to the Australian Human Rights and Equal Opportunity Commission because they refused to allow her to be a warranted leader on the basis of her disability. Amanda sought legal assistance but the case took 39 months and she found it difficult and at times traumatic. She won the case, but did not ever become a warranted leader.

Amanda's account raises the issues of how difficult it can be for people to assert their rights. It demands constant vigilance, knowledge and also a degree of support from others.

What would it mean for you as a social worker to work from within a rights discourse? As a social worker, how would you support someone through a discrimination issue? What would you need to know about rights and disability to do this?

having sexual relations unless they are married. This act was instituted to protect people's rights against sexual abuse but its unintended consequence was to transgress rights stated in both the Irish Constitution and international charters to which Ireland is a signatory. Once enacted, legislation such as this is very diff cult to change.

In spite of these diff culties of translating rights into realities, a rights discourse offers opportunities for constructive social change. It moves from social efforts to compensate through services and interventions for a 'natural disadvantage' seen to be inherent in the individual, to action to 'determine how society can accommodate a range of differences that, from a justice- or rights-based approach, are neutral, (Stainton 2007: 92).

Some reflections on discourses

In this chapter, I have only been able to give a brief description of three of the multiple discourses which frame and shape the lives of disabled people. What can be learned from this account?

The f rst point to make is that disabled people are not one group. The attribution of the label 'disability' can be a veil that covers difference with a semblance of sameness. Multiple groups of people are included within the label and often treated as if their needs were the same. Issues of gender, age, culture, identity, different needs for support or particular lifestyle preferences can be covered over by the label. For example, government policies and professional practice currently stress independence, choice and employment as desirable life opportunities for people with intellectual disabilities. They are. But there are some people within this group for whom these particular values may not be central. For example, people with very high support needs may not be able to take up employment and may not be able to live independently in the community. Questions then remain about how these people can live fulf lling lives and how they f t within existing discourses.

Second, some people who may be given the label 'disabled' by professionals completely reject it, however it is used. For example, 'deafness' is seen by many deaf people as a cultural difference, not a disability. Deaf people have their own language, arts and culture. The diff culties they encounter are seen as the failure of hearing people to acknowledge or to come to know this culture (Goggin & Newell 2005; Ladd 2003).

The discourses which I have brief y described draw on issues, values and knowledge which often lie outside of 'disability', and they have changed with time and with different emphases within the wider society. The institutionalisation of disabled people in earlier times, for example, has been attributed to 'the rise of capitalism . . . the expansion of state activity into new areas of economic and social life and the emergence of professionals [and] the growing inf uence of eugenicist ideas about the quality of the population' (Chappell 1998: 212). Similarly, it could be argued that the current focus on independence, individualism and choice ref ects the values of a late capitalist society.

Discourses are not f xed, and neither is our view of disability. They change over time and often in response to resistance by the people who are subject to them. The social model is a direct reaction by disabled activists to the oppression they perceived in society and which they saw as being in part due to the medical or individual discourse of disability.

As the above brief account reveals, coming to terms with disability is complex and is linked to wider social issues, to social pressures and to particular disciplinary frameworks. Clearly, how we think about disability will shape the way we work with people who have been given the label.

Finally, it would be easy in this chapter to see discourses as rising and falling in a linear fashion, so the medical or individualised discourse of disability gives way to the social model and a more rights-oriented approach. However, it is probably also clear that these discourses exist simultaneously with a greater or lesser focus in the society. Even the eugenicist theory, which is now discounted, lingers on in the negative views about sexuality and people with intellectual disabilities.

The position of social workers in relation to disabled people

> The dominant discourse on disability in social work has been that of an individual/ medical model, which largely relegates the 'problem' of disability within the individual (Hiranandani 2005: 1).

Given the complexity of dis(abling) discourses encountered in this chapter, it is hardly surprising that the social worker's position may be a contested and often ambiguous one when they are working with disabled people. The nature of their role and how they are perceived depend greatly on the discourse within which they are operating. They were, and sometimes still are, boundary workers establishing the normative and identifying and managing those who lie beyond its borders. Social workers were part of the institutionalisation processes which led to many disabled people living in segregated settings. Their role within the institutions and in services was very much focused on the support and management of individuals (Judge & van Blumelen 2002). However, they were also part of the movement towards people leaving such institutions (West 2000).

So, with changing discourses have also come changing roles. An increasing focus on the importance of disabled people being involved in decision-making about their own needs and lives with an accompanying focus on individualised planning and budgeting has led to a focus on case management for some social workers. This new role has been conceptualised as:

> The overarching set of functions in a service system that seeks to organise comprehensive individually tailored packages of support for people with intellectual disabilities. These functions are:
> - information collection, assessment, planning and prioritisation of needs
> - allocation, development and negotiation of resources
> - implementation, monitoring and review of support plans (Bigby et al. 2007: 17).

While this role offers opportunities for working with disabled people in taking more power in their lives and in asserting and protecting their rights as citizens (Stainton 2007), some case managers have reported that it can involve working with individuals to adapt their needs to scarce resources with little time to become familiar with the individual or to work for structural change (Gough 2007).

As the discourses have shifted and changed, the views of disabled people have become much stronger and, with the rise of the social model in particular, there has been an increasing critique of the role of professionals, including social workers. Non-disabled professionals are identif ed by some disabled groups, organisations and individuals as being part of an oppressive society which has positioned them as 'dependent' and as groups to be controlled. Writing from a social model perspective, Oliver sees professionals as sited within the medical discourse:

> the medical profession, because of its power and dominance, has spawned a whole range of pseudo-professions in its own image—physiotherapy, occupational therapy, speech therapy, clinical psychology—each one geared to the same aim: the restoration of normality. And each one of these pseudo-professions develops its own knowledge base and set of skills to facilitate this. They organise their interventions and intrusions into disabled people's lives on the basis of discrete and limited knowledge and skills (Oliver 1994: 37).

It is not diff cult to see how social workers would f t into this professional prof le. However, for social workers who see their roles as standing in solidarity with groups who are oppressed and advocating with them, the rift that exists between some disabled people and 'professionals' can be a diff cult issue with which to work. This takes us back to a consideration of a critical approach to social work theory and practice. It is probably apparent from this chapter that social workers need to be committed to social change which will positively affect the people with whom they work. This necessitates not only an understanding of the shifting nature of discourses specif c to a particular group, but a wider knowledge of how the society itself is changing and how this impacts on social work practice. It also means being able to stand by the individual, to see not only the person's impairment but also how gender, class and culture may affect the way they see the world. These skills mean that critical ref ection on theory and practice are integral to the social worker's role.

Conclusion: learning from different discourses in relation to disability

Socrates stated that an unexamined life is a life not worth living, and this is as true of our professional lives as it is of our personal ones. The failure to ref ect critically on the discourses within which we operate as professionals can lead us into oppressive stances in relation to those with whom we believe we are advocating. Social workers who were involved in institutionalisation did not see their roles as increasing the segregation of disabled people, but rather believed that they were serving the needs of the community and disabled people. For social workers to work effectively with disabled people, they need to turn a critical gaze on both the knowledge that they receive and on the ways in which they exercise it in practice, for with knowledge comes power.

In describing the role of an intellectual, Foucault commented:

> The work of an intellectual is not to shape others' political will; it is through the analyses that he [*sic*] carries out in his own f eld, to question over and over again what is postulated as self evident, to disturb people's mental habits, the way they do and think things, to dissipate what is familiar and accepted, to reexamine rules and institutions and on the basis of this reproblematisation . . . to participate in the formation of a political will (in which he has his role as a citizen to play) (Foucault 1988: 265).

If we substitute the word 'professional' for 'intellectual' in this quotation, we come close to understanding how social workers can work with others in creating change.

15

opening spaces for alternative understandings in mental health practice

Selma Macfarlane

This chapter aims to open spaces for alternative understandings of mental health and illness. I take a broad view that mental health practice occurs not only in designated mental health services but across many settings where social workers work. I use a range of critical approaches to problematise dominant medical model/psychiatric discourse and consider other perspectives. Some of the questions I explore are: How is it that we value certain types and sources of knowledge and expertise around mental health and illness above others? How might racism, patriarchy, violence and/or poverty shape the anxiety or depression experienced by growing numbers of people? Is there anything about our (post)modern society of consumption and technological development that fosters alienation or despair? And what might a consideration of such questions offer to social work practice and the wellbeing of individuals and communities? I draw on postmodern, feminist, anti-racist, ecological and consumer-led recovery discourses to go beyond the individually pathologising nature of medical model/psychiatric discourse. Given that, after twelve years of mental health reform in Australia, 'any person seeking mental health care runs the serious risk that his or her basic needs will be ignored, trivialised or neglected' (Mental Health Council of Australia 2005: 1), critical perspectives may be more important than ever.

The terms 'mental health' and 'mental illness', as well as 'consumer', 'client', 'service-user' and 'worker', are fraught with problems and, from a critical perspective, in need of serious de- and reconstruction. I am, however, guilty of using them throughout this chapter, for convenience's sake. Critical perspectives draw attention to the fluid and complex nature of identity and the oppressive implications of binary oppositional thinking such as that expressed by the categories above. The lines between these categories are often blurred: we all consume services; clients can and do become workers and vice versa; and psychological wellbeing fluctuates across each individual's life experience.

While the language used to construct mental illness is both powerful and problematic, I agree with Rogers and Pilgrim (2003: 16) that 'madness and distress are real . . . [and] ref ect real phenomena of fear, sadness and alienation . . . [however] we do question . . . whether professional codif cations of madness and misery are superior to lay views and understandings'. It is to this issue—the professional codif cations of psychiatry, as expressed largely through the DSM (*Diagnostic and Statistical Manual of Mental Disorders*) and its revisions—that I now turn, problematising modernist grand narratives that categorise, universalise and decontextualise human experience.

Challenging grand narratives of mental health and illness

Critical approaches acknowledge that the organisation of society is not so much 'natural' as created through social practices, discourses and institutions (Pozzuto et al. 2005: 33). We are embedded in layers of culturally, historically and socially produced 'truths' that become 'normal' given their dominance at particular times. These 'grand narratives'—around, for example, mental illness—naturalise certain explanations and marginalise others. It is argued from a critical perspective, however, that totalising discourses such as the DSM cannot adequately describe complex human experiences that are shaped by social and contextual factors.

Postmodern critical perspectives highlight the power of grand narratives, controlled by dominant groups—often in their own interests—to construct others in relation to their truth. As Duffy et al. (2002: 364) observe: 'the DSM represents the dominant cultural narrative about emotional, behavioural, and psychological problems . . . [shaping] the thinking and practice of most clinicians'. Biomedical constructions are supported by and intertwined with social policy and legal systems, further legitimising medical treatment and management of psychological distress, and delegitimising alternative perspectives (Morley 2003: 66).

Psychiatry has power to be both oppressive and enabling; however, its *position* in patrolling 'the boundaries between reason and unreason, between sanity and madness' creates a 'monologue of reason about unreason' capable of excluding other voices (Thomas & Bracken, 2004: 366). Using language of democracy, rights and accountability—central concepts in critical practice—Thomas and Bracken (2004: 361) say that service users, while a diverse group, share a belief in the right to 'interpret their experiences in their own way, and to receive help accordingly'. From a critical perspective, it is startling and disturbing to note, for example, that research exploring consumers' perspectives towards the impact of pharmacotherapy in the recovery process remains almost non-existent (IPP-SHR 2008: 1).

Mental health research has consistently privileged some truths over others. Service user-controlled research challenges the disempowering nature of traditional research, and is explicitly political and change oriented (Turner & Beresford 2005). Service user-controlled research highlights the distortion—rather than the neutrality—of research conducted from a supposedly objective distance. This distortion includes misunderstandings resulting from power imbalances between expert/client and researcher/researched; inadequate awareness by distanced interpreters of their own standpoint; discrimination relating to structural inequalities; commitments to agendas and values that limit empathy; and socialisation into understandings that inferiorise others (Glasby & Beresford 2006; Turner & Beresford 2005). Glasby and Beresford (2006) argue that medical research and systematic reviews have merit, but are only part of a range of ways of understanding human experience. Mary Boyle—a professor of psychology in the United Kingdom—observes that the divisions created between 'normal' and 'abnormal' by the psychiatric diagnostic system have hindered effective responses. She suggests abandoning diagnosis entirely if we want to understand and meet people's needs (Boyle 2007: 291).

Consumer/recovery movements

Critical approaches to mental health and illness include and privilege consumer literature, action, leadership and involvement. The roles of consumer groups and users/survivors of the mental health system have been pivotal in consciousness-raising around mental and psychological distress and the development of recovery orientations in services.

The recovery movement promotes service user involvement in the development of mental health policy and practice; this has become politically mandatory in countries like Australia, New Zealand and the United Kingdom, where the term 'recovery' now features in policy documents. While increasingly acknowledging structural factors shaping mental (ill)health and the importance of consumer participation, in many respects policy rhetoric remains aspirational (O'Hagan 2004). Some suggest that contemporary models of service user involvement are tokenistic. Stickley (2006) argues that, rather than 'kowtow' to dominant discourse, service users need to 'call the tune' and 'establish power positions outside the traditional hierarchy'—for example, by securing funding for independent service user-led projects (2006: 570).

While service user involvement or leadership is an important step forward for critical mental health practice, here again we must acknowledge diversity and context, and be open to challenging our assumptions around what may be experienced as empowering or emancipatory. 'Giving voice to rarely spoken stories is not guaranteed to be a rewarding experience' (Gray 2007: 426): speaking out does not guarantee being heard, and lack of speech may not mean absence of agency. Referring to Foucault (1978), Gray (2007: 427) suggests that being quiet 'can tell of an agentic subject resisting "technologies of domination" that operate to compel confessions'. In her work with women taking an activist stance to inspire change in the mental health system, Gray observed that personal agency was demonstrated by the women through their decisions, and at times refusals, to speak about personal details.

Power, empowerment and emancipation

Issues of power, according to Manning, are f rmly 'embedded in the nature of mental illness and the history of psychiatry' from the presentation of mental illness as a disease through to the professional's position as expert (Manning 1998: 90). Power differentials are exacerbated by labelling processes which distance service providers and override def nitions of problems and needs by those directly experiencing psychological distress. While promotion of an illness model aims to decrease public prejudice towards people with a psychiatric diagnosis, Read (2007) found that diagnostic labelling *increased* the perceived seriousness and intractability of a person's problems, exacerbating social distancing and rejection. Mental health practitioners are not immune to these dominant perceptions.

Critical practice involves a shift in position from expert to co-collaborator; postmodern perspectives on power are useful in understanding that sharing power does not imply a 'loss' of power or devaluing of one's own expertise. Bishop (2002) uses the evocative term 'becoming an ally' to describe practice based on an understanding of oppression, support for people in empowerment processes and working with others to challenge oppression. Empowerment requires knowledge-sharing, building dialogical relationships, linking the personal and the political, and challenging oppressive structures and discourses (Manning 1998; Healy 2005d; Ife 2005a). Critical practice, Healy (2005d) reminds us, manifests in large and small ways—at micro and macro levels—from interpersonal relationships to advocacy for policy change.

Issues of power and inequality are seldom acknowledged within the dominant medical model/psychiatric discourse; however, from a critical perspective power and inequality are considered central to experiences of psychological or mental distress. Tew (2005) observes that 'factors such as oppression, injustice, social exclusion or abuse at the hands of powerful others may be implicated in the sequences of events that lead up to many people's experiences of mental or emotional breakdown' (2005: 71). The development of critical psychiatry has been described by some as the profession's renewal, creating spaces for alternative voices to be heard, and taking a political stand that acknowledges how poverty and social exclusion have traditionally been overlooked in understanding psychosis and mental ill-health (Double 2006).

Structural inequality

Critical theory is based on acknowledging and taking action to challenge oppression and inequality. That oppression and inequality are linked to mental health is clear: 'mental health problems are socially patterned . . . and ref ect [and contribute to] social divisions' (Rogers & Pilgrim 2003: 16). While there are many forms of social inequality, my focus here is primarily on race and racism, gender and patriarchy, and their impact on mental (ill)health.

Sociological literature indicates that racial discrimination is both an acute and chronic stressor linked to mental and physical health problems (Mossakowski 2003: 318). Critical race theory examines the inf uence of race and racism on individual and group experiences, drawing attention to social contexts of structured inequality and the harm this causes, radically challenging the individualised nature of psychiatric pathology and research. Brown (2003, 2008), for example, points to the consequences of race-related hopelessness among black men in the United States—manifested in suicide, substance abuse and criminality—and the 'anti-self issues' that occur as racial minorities try to maintain a positive identity in a society that consistently constructs 'the other' as defective (Brown 2003: 296).

Critical practice involves awareness of cultural and historical factors that shape experience and meaning systems. Yip (2006b) points to variations in cultural conceptions of mental health and mental illness regarding, for example, self-actualisation, individual rights and emotional assertiveness, and how Western constructions may be inadequate and/or damaging. Workers may be so embedded in their own cultural location that others are ignored or invalidated.

Miller et al. (2006) explore the usefulness of Western biomedical models in treating psychological distress of war-affected communities, suggesting that organisations seeking to work with these groups need to understand the 'local idioms of distress—the particular ways in which psychological distress is experienced, expressed and understood in specif c cultural contexts' and help-seeking behaviours in those contexts (Miller et al. 2006: 409). Timimi (2007) also points to institutionalised racism implicit in Western psychiatric conceptual systems, and the meaninglessness of concepts such as depressive guilt and hopelessness to some non-Anglo cultural understandings.

Understanding the mental health implications of patriarchy and sexism is also crucial to critical mental health practice (as is heterosexism, which is not addressed here). While acknowledging that other social inequalities are important, Williams (2005) suggests that gender is particularly salient to personal psychological wellbeing; her focus is on damage to women, although she acknowledges men are also harmed by oppressive practices towards women. Williams maps social inequalities that impact on women's mental health in terms of access to resources that promote mental health (money, work, status), exposure to mental health risks (devalued or unpaid work, relations with men, and abuse and violence), and processes that maintain the status quo (being a 'good woman', devaluing emotions). She suggests that workers cannot adequately support women unless they have an awareness of structural disadvantage and how psychiatric discourse masks social determinants of mental distress. A striking example, provided by Morley (2003: 76), is applying a medical label to the responses of women who have been sexually assaulted, medicating their pain and outrage, and individualising the causes of and solutions to 'her problem'.

Hart's (2006) examination of the construction of women's depression in mainstream Western magazines highlights the disciplinary mechanisms inherent in locating 'the problem' within the individual woman's body, while minimising the complexity of cultural, social and political factors at work in that experience. Women are encouraged to engage in self-monitoring and disciplining, and expected to pursue whatever self-improvement and self-transformation is necessary to control problematic experiences. This creates a reliable scapegoat for social inequalities while simultaneously creating unattainable ideals of femininity and mental health. Existential questions 'about the meaningfulness of one's life and sociopolitical questions about happiness (e.g. should I stay married, have children and leave work, try to look younger, slimmer etc.) [are transformed] into technical questions about the most effective ways of coping or managing one's emotional life and malfunction' (Rose 1996, cited in Fullagar & Gattuso 2006: 10).

Critical practice requires mindfulness of multiple identities and how they intersect in specif c contexts (see, for example, Mullings & Schulz 2006). Sharma and Rees (2007) examined mental health problems experienced by women in remote Australian mining towns and found that, as well as geographical remoteness, isolation and extreme climate, additional social factors impacted signif cantly on the women. Most prominent was the patriarchal nature of the towns, where female partners were bound largely to the private sphere of the household. This was compounded by the unsociable work hours of their mining partners and considerable time spent by their partners with male coworkers during leisure time. Mining towns, the authors suggest, 'epitomise the heart of Australia's "blokeland"' (Sharma & Rees 2007: 4), where limited resources, support and opportunities for women affect their mental health. Recently arrived families, in particular, experience a lack of community connectedness, which further hides violence or abuse that may be occurring in the home (Sharma & Rees 2007: 5). The intersecting social factors of rurality/remoteness, patriarchy and work culture, in this context, combine to create particular experiences of psychological and mental distress that cannot be understood in terms of individual pathology alone.

Work itself has been strongly linked to mental health in recent years. It is easy to see how unemployment and poverty place severe stress on individuals, families and entire communities. Overemployment, underemployment and unhealthy jobs have also been identif ed as contributors to mental ill-health (Morrow et al. 2002; Rogers & Pilgrim 2003). Exclusion from meaningful work is recognised as a contributor to mental and psychological distress, and the workplace is both a potential contributor and threat to wellbeing. Women and others who combine caring with low-paid employment, persons experiencing racism, ableism or other forms of discrimination, bullying and pressure to consistently raise production eff ciency, youth unemployment or underemployment, lack of job satisfaction, inequality that transfers from educational to employment opportunities, work in high burnout environments, and poor work/life balance are all factors requiring critical attention. In a society dominated by consumerism and neo-liberal agendas, the impact of work on material, mental and emotional experience remains profoundly underestimated.

Indeed, what does the psychological (ill)health of a society imply about the character of that society? Rogers and Pilgrim (2003) suggest that levels of psychological/mental distress are markers of 'social progress, levels of current alienation and the success, or otherwise, of social policies designed to improve the quality of life of . . . citizens' (2003: 43). One must wonder why it is that, as stated at a recent mental health conference in Australia, most mental health problems are identifable before the age of 25. What is it about young people's lives that creates such distress? The more individualised and medicalised our responses to the problems of mental and emotional distress, the easier it is to ignore social injustice and other aspects of the larger social picture that shape personal experience.

Ecopsychology and consumerism

Critical approaches, with their emphasis on challenging taken-for-granted assumptions and the impact of the social on the personal, encourage us to question the 'givens' of any society. As new human problems gain prominence due to changing cultural, environmental and social circumstances, new ways of understanding and responding become necessary (Mack 1995). Kovel, for example, argues that contemporary Western societies suffer from 'anthropocentric delusions' that the current rate of destruction of natural environments is unimportant, resulting in an 'ecodestructive complex' reaching or surpassing crisis dimensions (2007: 122). Kovel observes that human beings are unavoidably part of nature, and the larger ecological crisis is not only generated by humans, but extends deeply into 'an ecologically pathological society' (2007: xii). Ecopsychologists are convinced that, in order to heal the mind, the earth—and our connections to it—must be restored. The restoration of these connections occurs in many ways; in my own interviews with people who had used mental health services, connection with the natural world featured in varying ways in their recovery processes, whether it was planting a tree, walking along a beach or simply having the opportunity to go for a drive in the countryside.

Distancing from the natural world is accompanied by our addiction to technology—'techno-addiction'—which, like other addictions, engenders total immersion and daily dependence, and can result in 'denial, dishonesty, control issues, thinking disorders, grandiosity, and disconnection from one's feelings' (Glendinning 1995: 46). Glendinning (1995: 79) proposes that technological society's dislocation from nature creates traumatic stress that begins in childhood—not as a rare event, but as a societal malaise, whereby our psyches *restructure themselves to survive* by fnding temporary nurturance in substances, violence, sex, material possessions and machines. Kanner and Gomes (1995: 79) propose that consumer culture produces 'fantasies of endless comfort and convenience, of every wish instantly becoming the world's command'. This narcissistic position, they say, is characterised by 'an infated, grandiose, entitled and masterful self-image or "false self" that masks deep-seated but unacknowledged feelings of worthlessness and emptiness' (1995: 79).

Constant exposure to advertisements encourages (over)consumption from an early age, suggesting that products can solve life's problems, while reminding those who cannot afford such products that they are doomed to insignif cance, unhappiness and failure (Durning 1995; Kanner & Gomes 1995). Hooks (1994, cited in Kanner & Gomes 1995: 87–8) ref ects on how 'systems of representation' such as advertising impact on poor people, observing that poverty and inability to consume and benef t from the trappings of aff uence (read 'normalcy') become synonymous with 'depravity, lack and worthlessness'. The psychological consequences of internalised oppression (and dominance), while highly relevant to a critical perspective, are rarely acknowledged by discourses that promote views of individual inadequacy, illness and pathology.

The range of critical perspectives explored brief y in the preceding paragraphs, from consumer and recovery perspectives to critical race theory and feminism to aspects of contemporary Western society, open up some alternatives to dominant bio-medical constructions of mental health and illness. Some of these ideas may capture your interest or resonate with your own observations, feelings or experiences. In the next section, I look more closely at some of the potential implications and challenges for social work, in drawing on critical perspectives to inform practice. I begin by discussing some possibilities as to why social work seems to have shied away from critical approaches to mental health.

Why has social work shied away from critical approaches to mental health?

Although social work's uniqueness—both traditionally and more critically—is often considered to be its emphasis on the person in environment, in relation to mental (ill)health, social work has been problematical in drawing fully on this orientation, despite indicators even in mainstream policy documents of its relevance. For example, the recent VicHealth Mental Health Promotion Framework identif es social factors, 'such as the larger structures of society (the distribution of wealth, the nature of hierarchies), the circumstances of the immediate setting and the support available', as crucial determinants of mental health. It identif es social connectedness, discrimination, conf ict and violence, and economic participation as key mental health determinants (Victorian Health Promotion Foundation 2005). So why does a critical approach still appear to be lacking in social work's positioning and response?

One suggestion is that social work's quest for professional recognition, with specif c technical expertise, has generated uncritical alignments with medical, psychiatric or scientif cally based disciplines, albeit with social workers accepting supportive or supplemental roles (Bainbridge 1999; Kirk 2005; Ferguson 2008). As the range of diagnosable 'disorders' has extended and broadened in the past few decades, so too has the diversity of professions and services involved with their treatment, allowing more social workers to engage in mental health practice. Kirk suggests that while these factors seem to open the way for social work to assert itself and (re)claim a critical perspective, the profession has, surprisingly, not responded. He suggests that one reason for social workers' silence may be a perceived (and perhaps real) lack of authority and autonomy, which has conditioned social workers to adapt to the priorities of other professions to survive: i.e. social work has been 'co-opted by the establishment' (Kirk 2005: 10). According to Bainbridge (1999: 186), the seduction of the medical model and the search for professional legitimacy (Dietz 2000) have meant that social work has embraced dominant knowledge systems in ways that have maintained the subjugation of alternative voices and local/experiential knowledge of clients, and reinforced oppressive relationships.

Morley (2003: 68–9) suggests that social work models commonly employed in mental health practice, such as strengths-based perspectives, advocacy and empowerment models, and consumer participation models, do not go far enough in challenging the medical 'truth' on which they are based. She observes that these approaches retain an emphasis on presenting symptoms divorced from social context, and continue to frame work with people experiencing psychological or emotional distress in medical terms. Reluctance within mental health systems and services to take social inequalities seriously may be both professionally functional (preserving the status quo) and less personally challenging for workers than questioning the benef ts gained from existing social relationships and listening closely to what people with mental health needs actually say about their lives (Williams 2005: 163).

Implications and challenges of a critical approach to mental health for social workers

The radical potential for social work to act as a force for emancipatory social change has always sat uneasily beside expectations that social work should engage in practices of social control, resource rationing and surveillance (Ferguson 2008: 15). Yet, according to Ferguson, it is the 'radical kernel' of social work, 'the inherent tension between its controlling role on the one hand and its potential to be a force for . . . social justice on the other, that make social work different' and worth preserving (Ferguson 2008: 21). Pozzuto et al. (2005: 25) observe that social work can consider itself 'nestled within mainstream society, accepting directives for the maintenance and functioning of that society' and viewing its 'proper place' as solving individual problems within the 'mechanisms of the current social order'. Or social work as a profession can acknowledge, more critically, that the function of 'helping' the individual necessarily includes a critique of the social (Pozzuto et al. 2005: 34).

Dietz (2000) suggests that clinical practice must address the dialectical relationship between private troubles and public issues, and aim at transforming professional relationships that disempower clients (2000: 503). This view contrasts with those of others, who suggest that clinical practice and critical practice are at odds (see, for example, Renouf & Bland 2005: 423). According to Dietz (2002), clinical practice *must* be political, and involves helping individuals to understand their experience in its social and political contexts, questioning pathologising discourses, and joining others in naming inequality and transforming relationships of domination (2000: 504). Practice skills then include asking questions such as 'What happened to you?' rather than 'What is wrong with you?' and listening for clients' experiences of oppression and/or abuse. Narrative therapy, for example, is a practice approach that acknowledges and works with both individual and cultural-social narratives (Pozzuto et al. 2005). Critical practice can also include workers acting as allies in helping to create 'democratically run spaces [such as self-help groups] . . . to exchange support, relate experiences' and learn from others (May 2007: 2).

Kirk (2005: 12) states that 'social workers need to be more sceptical of psychiatric claims and more critical minded about mental health practice'. This is not always easy: deconstruction takes time, and reconstruction is challenging, 'given all [the] vested interests' (Bainbridge 1999: 189)—particularly in systems such as mental health, which are hierarchically organised and resistant to change (Swift & Levin 1987, cited in Manning 1998: 103). Programs or services, even when theoretically based on empowerment principles, can become compliant with prevailing systems, and come to 'look more like the traditional system in order to survive' (Manning, 1998: 104).

Critical practice may include consciousness-raising with multidisciplinary team members around—for example, consumer self-determination (Bailey 2002)—as well as clients' expertise in their own lives (Leibrich 1998), and the impact of wider structural factors on personal experience. Alberti (2000) attests to the usefulness of constructing organisations and multidisciplinary teams, as well as service networks, as 'clients' in their own right, requiring relationship-building and thoughtful intervention. If knowledge is developed and expanded through interpersonal connections, critical practitioners may need to consider fuller involvement with those aspects of systems and/or services that are most challenging to critical values, rather than distancing (Alberti 2000).

Tew (2005) aff rms that establishing dialogue across professional and consumer groups, and developing 'co-operative power across . . . previously entrenched "us" and "them" divisions' is important in de/reconstructing unhelpful binary oppositional positioning (2005: 79). Cross-cultural analysts Antal & Friedman (2003) propose that effective and respectful cross-cultural (or, I suggest, cross-disciplinary) practice combines high advocacy—expressing one's position clearly—with high inquiry—exploring and questioning one's own beliefs or reasoning, as well as those of others. This suggests critical practitioners engage with others to explore assumptions and belief systems (skills in 'negotiating reality') and use 'cultural differences' as resources for learning and generating holistic and empowering responses in specif c contexts.

Postmodern views of power suggest that power relations are continually shifting as oppression is contested at the macro and micro levels (Tew 2005). Power, according to Tew, is always present in the everyday discourses and interactions that take place between people. Encouragingly, he suggests that the aggregation of critically informed micro-level responses can contribute to wider social change (2005: 77–8). This is important for workers who doubt their capacity to practise critically in traditional or hierarchical environments. Mathieson's concept of the unf nished (cited in Fook 1993, cited in Alberti 2000: 47) is useful to critical mental health practice, as it is 'an approach which views small achievements as legitimate as long as they are kept open to change' and are continually viewed as being part of larger scales of social change. Case study 15.1 illustrates one social worker's attempt to work critically in a specif c context.

Critical practitioners can also be involved outside traditional social work settings—for example, in programs that draw public attention to the psychological damage done by corporate advertising, particularly to children, or involvement in critical analysis of the dependencies and alienations created by new technologies (Kanner & Gomes 1995: 89). Social workers who are concerned with 'reanimating our connection with the Earth' can challenge powerful institutions and structures that engender environmental destruction and extreme consumerism, by working with policy-makers, corporate leaders, economists and others to create social change (Mack 1995: 285).

At a micro level of practice, recovery-based perspectives construct persons experiencing psychological distress as heroes who have survived against great odds and ask workers to remain hopeful despite consistent rejections from distressed persons to engage in opportunities or to exercise agency (Deegan 1996). 'There is more to the recovery process than simply recovering from mental illness': the effects of poverty, stigma and traumatic experiences of being subjected to some of the damaging

Case study 15.1

Kim works in a support service for women who have experienced psychological distress/upheaval. She is a social work graduate, keen to enact her commitment to critical practice. Her practice includes:

- taking seriously her clients' past experiences of sexual assault/violence, and making referrals to specialist feminist-based counsellors and creating spaces for women to share experiences in a supportive group
- ensuring that when issues such as body image or the devalued work of women arise, they are explored critically and sensitively, linking the personal and the political
- facilitating opportunities for gardening, bushwalking and shiatsu
- critically reflecting on her reluctance (even fear) to share consumer literature with service users, then beginning the establishment of a library of consumer/survivor literature at the service, together with the women
- initiating knowledge-sharing workshops with the local mental health service network
- raising structural factors, such as the impact of poverty, domestic violence, heterosexism or racism on mental health, in wider policy forums.

aspects of mental health treatment also need to be recovered from (Deegan 1996: 96). Workers' ability to remain connected, to 'refuse to be dehumanised . . . to be bold and brave and daring enough to remain human hearted while working in the human services' (Deegan 1996: 97), is a critical challenge. The gaining of wisdom implies moving beyond 'mere recognition of illness' to holistically 'encounter[ing] the human being who comes for help' (Deegan 1996: 92).

Finally, ref exivity and honest examination of our own assumptions are vital to critical approaches. What shapes 'our own individual ontology of sanity and madness'? (Bainbridge 1999: 191). How do our views and beliefs shape and rationalise our practice and how does this impact on our emancipatory intent? As social workers, commitment to critical practice enables the opening out of spaces for a wider range of understandings and responses to mental and psychological distress; as a profession committed to the wellbeing of individuals and emancipatory social change, we should expect no less of ourselves and our profession. If social workers don't engage in critical mental health practice, who will?

16
weaving together the personal and the political in loss and grief

June Allan

Loss and grief are part of the life experience of each of us. Anecdotal evidence from practitioners suggests that the circumstances of people who see a social worker are frequently complicated by losses that have had a profound and enduring impact on their own and others' lives. Critical social work has previously paid little attention to practice issues concerning loss and grief, which have been dominated by psychological theories such as psychoanalytic, stress, attachment and psycho-social transition theories (Stroebe & Schut 2001, 2008). However, increasing recognition of ways in which people are linked to and inf uenced by their social world, and new theories for understanding grief shaped by sociological and social constructionist perspectives (e.g. Klass et al. 1996; Walter 1999; Neimeyer 2001; Small 2001; Currer 2007; Howarth 2007; Stroebe & Schut 2008), are resulting in richer understandings of loss and grief at the personal and social levels.

In this chapter, I invite readers to ref ect on the assumptions made in relation to loss and grief in our society, and to question taken-for-granted ideas and practices in this aspect of work in the human services. Modern Western literature typically depicts only isolated individuals and families dealing with their own private grief, yet these experiences are social, as Howarth's (2007) recent work shows. This can be seen in events such as the tragic loss of life in the Indian Ocean tsunami and the Bali bombings; the catastrophic daily loss of life in parts of Africa as a result of the AIDS pandemic; the disastrous loss of life that has occurred in places like the Balkans and the Middle East as a result of wars and civil conf ict; the mass movement of environmental refugees across the globe, displaced and homeless; and, much less 'dramatic', the huge numbers of people who visit cemeteries each year in Australia;[1] the women and men struggling with the breakdown of an intimate relationship; the distraught widow with whom I worked to assist her to make meaning of her life following the sudden death of her life partner. Loss and grief are experiences of everyday life, arising from a multitude of events, both ordinary and extraordinary.

Frameworks upon which social workers have tended to draw in understanding and responding to loss and grief have traditionally focused on individualistic, pathologising approaches. Ways of working that integrate individual experience with the broader context are needed, incorporating social, cultural and political understanding and educative, empowering and collective ways of working that respectfully work with the meanings those who are grieving give to their experiences. I explore contemporary understandings of grief in the context of social, political and cultural inf uences and the inf uences of dominant discourses regarding grieving processes. Themes and contradictions are teased out, and implications for practice discussed. Grief, and working with people to live constructively with their grief, can only be understood through the knowledge that the personal, social, political and cultural are intimately bound together.

The language of loss and grief

'Loss', a term that is frequently viewed negatively and often used interchangeably with 'death', takes many different forms. The notion of loss can be thought of simply as no longer having something or someone that we used to have (Miller & Omarzu 1998: 4). Unlike 'change', which is a neutral term, loss is about absence and refers to detrimental aspects of some sort of change (Currer 2007: 15). The types of loss people experience can be understood in two general ways. The f rst is physical, 'where something tangible has been made unavailable' (Miller & Omarzu 1998: 6), such as the death of a loved one, or loss of a body part such as a breast or limb. The second, symbolic losses, occur 'where there are abstract changes in one's psychological experiences of social interactions' (Miller & Omarzu 1998: 6). This includes circumstances such as the loss of a sense of self-worth experienced through retrenchment, loss of a sense of peace through wartime trauma or victimisation in family violence, or loss of dreams and ideals. Secondary losses, those losses that result from a primary loss, can have signif cant implications for individuals. A primary loss—for example, the loss of a limb—can lead to secondary losses, such as loss of employment. Factors such as f nancial security and social support can also help avoid secondary losses, indicating that socio-economic and other social factors are important considerations in the experience of grief (Currer 2007: 6–8). 'Bereavement' is a term specif cally associated with loss through death, signifying 'the situation of an individual who has recently experienced the loss of someone signif cant through that person's death' (Stroebe et al. 1998: 83).

'Grief', the response to loss, is customarily deemed to be natural, universal, psychological and physiological (Marris 1996; Walter 1999) and is now interpreted as both an emotional and cognitive process (Currer 2007: 16). Typically linked to sadness, grief covers a broad range of emotional, physical and behavioural responses, including anger, regret and a sense of betrayal and injustice. 'Mourning' is commonly associated with the process of grief (e.g. Walter 1999; Harvey 2000; Hagman 2001). It usually refers to the customary social responses associated with death-related losses (Currer 2007: 17). Cultural norms about how people should behave and feel, such as customs and rituals that are ordinarily part of mourning processes (e.g. Walter 1999; Marris 1996), serve as a mechanism for the regulation of emotion and grief within societies. This regulation is further discussed under the 'rules' of grieving.

Loss and grief as social, political and cultural experiences: themes and contradictions

A number of signif cant factors in Australia's past and present have inf uenced attitudes to loss and death, and shaped professional responses to people who are grieving. Kellehear (2000a), Damousi (2001) and Jalland (2006) have made major contributions to our understanding of these factors. Those discussed here are Australia's race relations, multiculturalism, medicalisation, secularisation and gentrif cation, and the development of 'grief and bereavement care', a term used to cover the counselling services and mutual help groups tailored to loss and grief.

Australia's race relations history and institutional racism are important factors in understanding the pattern of public grieving and remembrance of loss and death. In honour of the tragic loss of life and injuries sustained in the First World War, white communities across Australia established memorials (Damousi 2001). The Australian War Memorial was built as a sacred and spiritual symbol of the sacrif ce of Australians in war. However, only recently has the impact on Indigenous Australians of policies of the colonial government, and later the federal and state governments, been recognised. Acknowledged are the cumulative and adverse effects of the experience of massive and continuing losses of land, culture, identity, family and children (Kellehear 2000b; Raphael 2000; Damousi 2001), as documented in the *Bringing Them Home* report on the forcible removal of Indigenous children from their families (Human Rights and Equal Opportunity Commission 1997).

The growing movement for reconciliation and response is now resulting in the development of programs of support for reunion of families, and counselling and healing programs for the trauma and grief Indigenous people have experienced (Raphael 2000), although some of these positive developments are challenged by policy initiatives such as the current federal government intervention in the Northern Territory, discussed in Chapter 8. A momentous step towards reconciliation is the National Apology to the Stolen Generations made by Prime Minister Kevin Rudd in 2008, a step that Kellehear (2005) exhorts communities to undertake at local levels. An Indigenous people-centred approach to decolonisation that includes the healing needs of individuals, families and communities is developing (Atkinson & Ober 1995; Fredericks 1995; Brown 2001; Wingard 2001a, 2001b; Atkinson 2002) alongside the belief that, to address the abuses and losses that have occurred and work towards social justice and equal human rights, it is necessary to also address the systems and structures of oppression and the cultural awareness of white people (McKendrick & Thorpe 1998; Nelson 2007). Raphael (2000) asserts the value of the development of a culturally appropriate model of narrative therapy for its focus on storytelling and oral tradition, and its orientation to families and social groups. Such a development is seen in Galloway and Moylan's (2005) account of the healing camp for Indigenous women in Cairns using narrative ideas in a community gathering. Towney (2005), a Wiradjuri man, describes an approach to conversations with Indigenous Australian men that involves the use of narrative practices in culturally appropriate ways.

Australia's increasing cultural diversity has also been a most important inf uence on attitudes and responses to major losses. Postwar European immigration and further waves of immigrants from many different cultural and racial backgrounds[2] have contributed to a growing recognition and acceptance of difference and diversity in human behaviour and social responses. People from some of these cultures have brought with them values and norms requiring openness and outward expression of grief as respect for the dead. Over the years, this—along with other factors favouring the expression of feelings—has changed the nature of Australian society and the ways it has dealt with loss (Raphael 2000; Damousi 2001; Jalland 2006).

Noting the wide range of cultural and religious patterns and behaviours now seen in contemporary Australia, Campbell et al. (2000: 69) draw on Kagawa-Singer's (1998) metaphor of weaving cloth to describe 'how many cultures may use looms and threads (universal aspects of behaviour)' to create a 'great diversity of recognisable patterns or styles (culture-specif c behaviours)'. Campbell et al.

(2000) warn that workers may fall into the trap of superimposing parts of their own tapestry on to those with whom they work, unless they have sound transcultural understanding. Numerous writers point to the necessity of understanding the diversity of spiritual and cultural meanings in different settings (e.g. Fukuyama & Sevig 1999; Arulampalam et al. 2005; Chan et al. 2006; Currer 2007; Rosenblatt 2008). Desai and Bevan (2002) also highlight how traditional approaches to loss can ignore people's experiences of racism.

The British-inf uenced middle-class values that dominated the colonial Australian way of grieving—stoicism, privacy, reserve and avoidance of discussion of taboo topics such as sexuality and death—persisted after the overwhelming loss of Australian lives in the First World War, becoming eroded somewhat f rst by the impact of a strong Irish inf uence and later by the post-Second World War immigration (Griff n 2000; Raphael 2000). More recently, however, there has been a strong inf uence from the United States in relation to matters of loss, death and grieving. Two ways in which this has occurred are seen in the prominence of a dominant model of grief, and the corporatisation of the funeral industry.

First is the profound inf uence of the 'stage theory' of dying and loss, brought to prominence by the Swiss-American psychiatrist Elisabeth Kübler-Ross (1970; Kübler-Ross & Kessler 2005). Kübler-Ross popularised psychological ideas about death and dying, encouraging greater openness about dying. Second, American business practices have signif cantly inf uenced the funeral industry in Australia. In the early 1990s, small Australian funeral businesses were taken over by larger companies and international corporations, in particular the United States-owned Service Corporation International (SCI). A decade later, these American companies withdrew, but the Australian f rm InvoCare, which took over SCI, now directs the funerals of one in f ve Australians. This increased concentration of ownership with its corporatised practices has led to costlier and 'supersize' funerals, part of the American legacy (Jalland 2006; Larkins 2007).

The processes of medicalisation, secularisation and gentrif cation have all contributed, among other things, to the emergence of professionals whose focus is grief and death. The rise of modern medicine saw the health and disease issues of people ('patients'), and hence dying and death, become the province of medical experts (Jalland 2006; Howarth 2007). This paved the way for professionals with expertise in helping people deal with these matters, typically focusing on individuals. During the 1980s, a more participatory style of health-care culture developed, with healers, patients and their communities working together on health outcomes. Through these developments, death came to be seen as a health matter, to be aided through palliative care or medically assisted suicide in the pursuit of the 'good death' (Kellehear 2000b: 6–7), one in which some control could be exercised (Currer 2007).

The gentrif cation of Australian society (Kellehear 2000b) through the growth of the middle class contributed to the development of professionals as a group. Smaller social networks, medicalisation and a rising life expectancy all contributed to the fact that families experience death less frequently in contemporary Australia. With the development of the isolated nuclear family, individuals know less about what to expect regarding loss and death, and increasingly academic and professional information has outweighed personal and community experience in the provision of advice and direction (Kellehear 2005).

At the same time, the secularisation of Australian society through the separation of church and state (Griff n 2000; Kellehear 2000b; Freeman 2005) has resulted in understanding, processing and managing death commonly becoming matters for medicine and law rather than for religion. Deaths are typically explained in medical rather than religious terms, and disasters are commonly regarded as occupational health and safety issues rather than as 'acts of God'. Volunteer rescuers, police and f remen become the 'angels' and 'saints'. Death and the funeral moved out of the family home during the twentieth century (Griff n 2000; Larkins 2007). Materialist ideas in which death is 'a product of physical processes' (Kellehear 2000b: 5) have become popular, although religious ideas about death remain popular—albeit in different forms, such as New Age concepts, or spiritual notions emerging from a combination of Eastern religions and Western mystical traditions. Secularisation, along with the growth of professionals and the process of medicalisation, increasing aff uence and women's growing independence, has fostered an individualistic counselling approach.

Thus 'grief and bereavement care' has taken the place of social mourning as an accepted way for people to grieve in contemporary Western life, with modern-day therapy substituting in many situations for functions once played by religion (Walter 1999).[3] But the culture of professional experts and counselling is a contentious issue. Some authorities regard counselling as a useful resource to assist people to grieve, as attested to by the vast array of literature on grief counselling (e.g. Rando 1993; Gunzburg & Stewart 1994; Attig 1996; Neimeyer 2001; 2006; Chandler 2005; Freeman 2005; O'Shea 2005). Others question it, however. Little (1999), for example, describes what he considers to be the inappropriateness of professional support in the immediate aftermath of the Thredbo landslide in 1997 in which a number of people were killed, commenting that 'at the start the handling of the disaster looked like a disaster itself'. Grief and mourning became a fashionable topic in the media, and public and professional expectations inappropriately managed and rushed the grieving process. All of this, argues Little, may have 'inhibited genuine grieving, which takes its own time and proceeds in its own way' (1999: 88). Bereavement care can be quite prescriptive, and may or may not suit individuals, depending on how much freedom they seek for themselves. However, it may also offer a refuge from a society that many grieving people feel has policed them too harshly, having had 'bad experiences with families and professionals who they feel do not and cannot understand' (Walter 1999: 202–3).

These differences and contradictions become more complex because of the rules and norms on how we are 'allowed' to grieve, who is 'allowed' to grieve, and who we are 'allowed' to grieve for.

The 'rules' of grieving

The emotions of grief are often raw, disturbing, volatile and unexpected. People who are grieving are prone to feelings of anger. These emotions are therefore to be regulated, a phenomenon thought to occur in all societies (Rosenblatt 1997, cited in Walter 1999: 119; Currer 2007). How and why regulation should occur, however, are matters of considerable debate, and opinions are divided on whether the emotions of grief should be contained or expressed. The position often aff rmed by popular Western culture is that the emotions of grief should be contained, at least in public (Walter 1999). Further, Holst-Warhaft (2000) suggests that grief not contained can become political outrage and translate into violence, noting that revolutions and riots have often begun with funerals in different parts of the world. Mourning rituals and memorials attempt to 'bring order to the emotional chaos of grief' (Holst-Warhaft 2000: 18).

Yet, at the same time, the view persists that grief should be allowed to express itself naturally and that its expression may be appropriate and healing (Walter 1999; Raphael 2000). It must be talked through if the person is to 'recover', a position reinforced in the cultural shift from denial to the growing expression and public recognition of grief fostered by a more permissive climate and greater freedom of self-expression emanating from the United States (Jalland 2006). Now both governments and activist groups use disasters, public mourning and rituals as political tools to capture world opinion, draw attention to issues, or hasten progress and legislative change. Grief, an empowering and enabling force, can effectively be mobilised for political purposes to give the bereaved a political voice and to enact change (Damousi 2000; Walter 2006). A clear example of this is the hastening of gun law reforms in Australia following the tragedy at Port Arthur in 1996 in which 35 people were murdered (Altmann 2006).

There is debate in the literature as to whether males and females grieve differently (e.g. Golden 1997; Walter 1999; Martin & Doka 2000; Reynolds 2002). Walter (1999) maintains that there is a considerable body of evidence to suggest that males have a more contained way of grieving and that females prefer to express their grief, still stereotypically portrayed (Filak & Abel 2004). However, while strands of that remain true in the Australian community, particularly among Anglo-Saxons (Howarth 2007), there is now recognition that ways of grieving are not necessarily tied to the gender of the grieving person, associated with the knowledge that some women may seek action-oriented healing, and some men may use relational skills to heal their grief (for example, Golden 1999; Martin & Doka 2000; Doka & Martin 2002). A so-called 'feminine' style centres on the open expression of feelings, is social and support-seeking and relational-oriented. A 'masculine' style is more instrumental, demonstrating an action-oriented, cognitive and solitary style of grieving (Golden 1997; Martin & Doka 2000). It is inappropriate to perpetuate these stereotypes, and terms such as 'intuitive'/'expressive', 'instrumental' or 'blended' (a mix of these with an emphasis on one) are more appropriate to describe the styles of grieving adopted by individuals (Martin & Doka 2000). Clearly, the issue of gendered grief will continue to be the focus of continuing research and debate, but while it is important that practitioners understand and respect people's individual styles of grieving, they nevertheless should also approach their work with a gendered understanding of styles of grief.

If an event is not perceived to be a socially signif cant loss, it can cast people into disenfranchised grief—that is, 'grief experienced when a loss is not or cannot be openly acknowledged, publicly mourned, or socially supported' (Rando 1993: 498). This arises because societies have sets of norms about and for whom people should grieve. These norms or grieving rules may not correspond to the nature of relationships, the sense of loss or the feelings of the grieving person (Doka 2002). Grief is disenfranchised for f ve main reasons. First, it may occur where the relationship is not recognised by society, especially if it is not based on familial ties, such as a lover (including homosexual—for example, Whipple 2007—or extra-marital relationships), friend, colleague, caregiver or step-parent, ref ecting in part the legal status accorded to these relationships. Second, the loss itself may not be recognised because it is not regarded as socially signif cant (such as abortion, relinquishing a child for adoption or foster care—for example, Robinson 2007—or loss of a pet). Third, grievers themselves may not be acknowledged as they may be considered to be socially incapable of grief, such as the very old—for example, Moss and Moss (2003)—or the very young, or people with intellectual impairment. Fourth, the death itself may be disenfranchising where its circumstances create shame and embarrassment, such as death from a disease like AIDS, or from self-destructive causes like suicide. Finally, the ways individuals grieve can contribute to disenfranchisement where grieving rules in a given society are not followed (Doka 2002). Practitioners and communities therefore need to be sensitive to the needs of those whose grief is not acknowledged by society.

It is clear that the discourses on loss and grief contain many contradictions for grieving people to negotiate—at a time when they are likely to be at their most vulnerable. I now consider more closely actual grieving processes and the practice implications of dominant and changing theoretical discourses.

Grieving processes: theories and practices

Three sets of competing discourses, considered in the preceding discussion, are evident in the conceptualisation of grieving processes. These concern, first, the notion of grief as a series of stages, following a linear trajectory to completion or resolution, as popularised by the 'stage theory' developed by Kübler-Ross (1970) and later by others such as Worden (1991), Parkes (1996) and Kübler-Ross and Kessler (2005). The second discourse involves the culture of containment and control compared with the culture that supports the expression of grief. Finally, there are competing discourses concerning the social integration of the dead in society: whether the living should leave behind their relationship with the dead, or maintain continuing bonds.

The notion of continuing bonds has been supported by a range of research studies and evidence from bereaved people themselves, suggesting that, rather than detaching themselves and moving on from deceased persons, individuals instead need to develop meaningful symbolic ways of holding on to the dead (White 1988; Klass et al. 1996; Walter 1996, 1999; Foote & Frank 2000; Neimeyer 2000; Klass & Walter 2001; Howarth 2007). The notion of grief or bereavement as something that 'ends' no longer fits, and is being replaced by the idea of negotiation and renegotiation of the meaning of the loss over time. There is recognition that major losses impact on people for the rest of their lives, and that as they change they experience an altered but continuing relationship with the deceased person (Silverman & Klass 1996). New connections with the deceased are constructed and reconstructed as the meaning of the loss is negotiated and renegotiated.

The modernist view of grief that dominated among health professionals in the twentieth century provides people with some idea of what to expect when they are grieving, but that is now being challenged. More recent views claim that everyone grieves differently, and there is no single way to deal with grief reactions (Walter

1999; Kellehear 2000b; Howarth 2007). What are the implications of these different perspectives for work with individuals and communities?

Individual counselling

There are numerous critiques of the dominant modernist discourse of the grieving process in which time is expected to heal and the bereaved are expected to restrain their displays of grieving to appropriate times and places (e.g. White 1988; Walter 1996; Foote & Frank 2000; Neimeyer 2001; Goldsworthy 2005; Howarth 2007). If the expression of grief is too short, too long, delayed, too demonstrable or not demonstrable enough, then the mourning is judged to be 'complicated' and is pathologised (Foote & Frank 2000).

Key researchers in the f eld agree that complications of grief do exist (Kristjanson et al. 2006; Lobb et al. 2006). There is a move, driven by Prigerson and her colleagues (2008) in the United States, for complicated grief, or what they refer to as 'prolonged grief disorder', to be included in the *Diagnostic and Statistical Manual of Mental Disorders*. Currer (2007) recognises that we might not like classif cations because they risk missing people's unique experiences of grief. But she reminds us that some grieving people, who themselves want to change their responses and f nd relief, may welcome such a classif cation. In a risk-management society, it may also afford people access to counselling support through health insurance to which they may otherwise not be entitled.

However, with these developments come concerns that the term may be misused and be culturally bound unless def ned in a way that recognises, for example, Indigenous people's experiences of 'broad-based cultural losses' (Walle 2004: 52 in Lobb et al. 2006: 31). It also raises questions about distinctions between normal and complicated grief (Lobb et al. 2006). Walter (2006) regards these developments as again pathologising grief, a ref ection perhaps of society attempting to create order amongst the chaos of ongoing suffering. He questions the appropriateness of this.

An alternative narrative proposes that the story of the person who is seen to have problems such as complicated grief should be reinterpreted as the dominant discourse exercising power over the person's life. The 'problem' story is reinterpreted as a form of resistance to the power of the dominant discourse, and counselling is then seen as nurturing resistance to the dominant discourse (White & Epston 1990; White 1993, cited in Foote & Frank 2000: 177–9). As most people's stories draw on the dominant discourse, the personal problems they bring to counselling can be seen to emanate from the 'lack of f t' between their lived experience and the dominant socio-cultural story being imposed on them. Discussing family bereavement in the context of immigration and inter-ethnic marriage in America, Shapiro (1994, 1996, cited in Walter 1999: 152) recognises that the way in which a person feels most comfortable grieving may not f t with the dominant cultural expectations of the community in which he or she lives. She suggests that the aim for practitioners is therefore to focus with the person on the best f t between their own style and the cultural expectation. The main learning for critical social workers is to be open and f exible, holistically considering the person's experience within their social, political and cultural contexts.

The aim of narrative work is to assist clients to critique the imposed story, freeing them to develop their own story to give meaning to their experiences, and recognising how the dominant discourse works to deny this story (Foote & Frank 2000). Neimeyer (2006) suggests that meaning-making or meaning-reconstruction in response to a loss is the central process of grieving. I have provided an example of this elsewhere (Allan 2005).

Groups, communities and activism

While individual counselling has its place in supporting individuals and countering dominant but unhelpful messages received from the community, family or professionals, a sense of community is important for those who grieve (Klass & Walter 2001; Kellehear 2005). As Little (1999) asserts, a robust social fabric is fundamental to people's wellbeing. Social workers can contribute much by helping to build stronger communities and social infrastructure that help when grief strikes, and by linking those who grieve with existing communities of support. Self-help groups for loss and bereavement such as Solace and The Compassionate Friends can provide such communities of support for many, and have become popular in Australia. These groups are valued for their reliance on experiential rather than professional knowledge, forming communities of experience not shared by mass society, professionals or families. They have their own subculture in which continuing bonds are aff rmed, providing an alternative to dominant discourses in mainstream culture. Some may have activist aims, channelling emotions such as anger into political activity (for example, strengthening sentencing laws).

Much can be learnt from other alternatives to Western individualistic approaches. The Memory Box Project (Morgan 2000) is one example. This project with HIV-positive women in Uganda encourages the women to create memory boxes to leave for their children. The memory box of Maki Lufhugu, for example, contains, among other things, her skaf-tin (lunch box), her favourite hat, a memory book of photos and press clippings, and her life story written in her own handwriting.

Detailed information about the women and their origins decreases the risk of fear, confusion and loss of identity for their children, thereby lessening the distress of their grief (Morgan 2000). The personal story book of the Bambanani Women's Group in Cape Town (Morgan & the Bambanani Women's Group 2003) is another wonderful example of creative and communal approaches.

Grief can be a powerful motivator for bringing about change and striving for a more socially just society. Not only can the power of disabling discourses be challenged through individual counselling and groups, as already discussed, but social workers can also work with or advocate for people who grieve to work towards change. Activism has several functions: healing, education, awareness-raising, and attitudinal and social change. It can occur through lobbying and campaigning for legal and other reform, public rituals, speaking out on issues, public storytelling, setting up new support or action groups, and publishing (e.g. Ryan 2000; Kellehear 2001; Wingard & Lester 2001; Morgan & the Bambanani Women's Group 2003; Prieto with de Ungria 2006).

There are numerous other examples of effective activism. Some individuals decide to care for others or do volunteer work, all of which serves in some way to develop a sense of community. Others, through their own experience and disaffection with existing services, establish new support groups. Following the death of her father in a construction incident, Liz Moyabad founded the Industrial Death Support and Advocacy (IDSA) in 1995 in Victoria. This organisation assists families, employers and industrial organisations on matters concerning industrial deaths. Other initiatives include Red Nose Day, a well-known fundraising event for Sudden Infant Death Syndrome (SIDS), the AIDS Memorial Quilt Project, a worldwide project that memorialises people who have died from AIDS, the Pink Ribbon Breast Cancer campaign (www.breastcancercampaign.org) and the 'Movember' campaign to raise awareness on men's health issues (www.movember.com). These are all examples of successful political campaigns which are helping to raise public awareness and change attitudes and meanings.

A practice reflection

In my work as a counsellor/advocate at a community-based organisation for refugees and asylum seekers, I worked with a woman from a minority group in a Middle Eastern country who had come to Australia as a refugee, having f ed persecution and murder of family members by the oppressive ruling regime. A former professional in her country of origin, 'Farah' (not her real name) suffered various health problems, including a physical disability. As a refugee to Australia, she was socially marginalised. Unable to continue to pay private rent, she was offered public housing by the Off ce of Housing, only to be placed at the bottom of a f fteen-year waiting list after rejecting the f rst offer for its unsuitability due to her disability.

Dominant discourses about Farah's status as a refugee contributed to her feeling 'second best' and quite powerless. An important part of my work with her was to help her to see how perceptions of refugees were impacting on her experiences and opportunities. I wove between supporting her to develop her own agency by taking action for herself, and using my own power emanating from my white, middle-class professional privilege, as discussed by Baines (2007b). Through all of this, it was important to bear witness to Farah's grief over the multiple losses she had experienced throughout her life. Using critical ref exivity, I was mindful of the dominant Western discourse that emphasises counselling for people experiencing ongoing grief and questioned the applicability of this approach. Working carefully with Farah's own values and meanings, we discussed her sadness about events that had occurred, but importantly placed priority on her material conditions, which were a primary anxiety. I am acutely aware that in popular counselling discourses, material aspects can sometimes be minimised or avoided as not being the 'proper' domain of counsellors, a dualism that in particular can create ambiguity and inconvenience for service users. I bore witness to Farah's grief, which as Tew (2002) suggests can be profoundly empowering, but simultaneously worked with an advocacy housing organisation to successfully reinstate Farah's name at the top of the Off ce of Housing's waiting list, which subsequently allowed her to obtain suitable accommodation.

I ref ected on whether there was potential for Farah herself to become actively involved in any activities with others in order to work towards improving housing policies and practices or challenging mainstream discourses that marginalise refugees. Because Farah was satisf ed with achieving one of her main goals of appropriate public housing and had strong social connections with her own cultural community, she was not driven to do this. Working from a critical social work perspective, I am aware that, while it may be an option for service users to join with others in like situations to agitate for change, this may not be possible, feasible or desirable for them, and I must respect this and seek other opportunities to foster changes. One of the ways I choose to do this is by raising awareness through education about the social, cultural, political and material dimensions of grief experiences. This particular practice example aff rms the need for critical social workers to be f exible, to listen to those who are grieving and to not adhere strictly to one particular way of working.

Conclusion

The f eld of loss and grief is a complex and contested area in which to work. This chapter has illustrated the political and socially constructed nature of grief and grieving processes, and has highlighted some of the inherent contradictions. Critical social workers can assist grieving individuals by working in sensitive, respectful and culturally appropriate ways and by remaining critically self-ref exive. They can nurture individuals' resistance to disabling dominant discourses, and help them to support themselves by assisting them to make meaning of their experiences and negotiate the contradictions that they encounter. Assisting those who grieve to link up, where appropriate, with others in groups can help create and strengthen communities of support. Work with individuals and groups can ensure that people who are grieving have access to information, to needed material and emotional resources, and to justice. Critical social workers, along with or on behalf of grieving individuals and groups, can also challenge unjust attitudes and processes that precipitate grief or discriminate against those who grieve, and contribute to the strengthening of the social fabric that is known to be so important for supporting us all when grief strikes.

17

addressing violence and abuse in a gendered world

Heather Fraser and Christine Craik

Violence and abuse are social problems that adversely affect societies, groups, families and individuals. From a critical social work perspective, many forms of violence and abuse are examined, and attention is given not only to the effects they can have on individual lives but also on collective health and wellbeing. Recognising institutional violence as well as interpersonal forms of abuse (such as child abuse, intimate violence, 'queer' and elder abuse), 'we' show that violence and abuse are gendered and sexualised crimes steeped in history, religion and political ideology. Using the term 'we' to refer to the perspectives of the authors (two middle-aged, white, Australian feminists), we also show that susceptibility to violence and abuse is not randomly distributed, but instead connected to social contexts, status and identities, as well as access to resources.

Connecting the personal with the political, we examine how some forms of violence and abuse—and some groups of victims/survivors—are liable to be ignored, trivialised and/or discredited. Yet we write this chapter in the spirit of *reconstructing*—not just *deconstructing*—social work and social welfare (also see Leonard 1997). Specif cally, this chapter identif es how critical social workers might understand violence and abuse.

The chapter is organised into three parts. First, we identify what we believe critical social work is—and is not—as we discuss how critical social workers are likely to approach violence and abuse. Next, we talk about progressive social change as change that (more actively) recognises the human rights of *all* people, irrespective of gender, age, ethnicity, sexuality, ability and/or geographical location. We concentrate on common forms of violence and abuse, reiterating why a critical social work approach to violence and abuse is needed. In the third section, we foreground gender-based violence as a 'case study' because it constitutes such a large proportion of all violence and abuse committed.

Viewing violence and abuse critically

Critical social work is a name given to a broad constellation of approaches interested in the concepts of *power* and *language, discourses* and *progressive social change*. Critical social workers are a broad coalition of people who share some common interests, values and hopes about how power might be exercised in the future, and language used to narrate different ways of being in the world (McMaster & Swain 1989; Dominelli 1996, 2002c; Pease 1996, 1997, 2004; Ife 1997, 2001; Milner 2001; Brown 2003; Thompson 2003; Weeks 2003; Baines 2007a).

As indicated in Chapter 3, 'critical social work' is a term inclusive of many others who use other referents (or names) for their work, such as: 'anti-oppressive', 'anti-discriminatory', 'human rights-oriented', 'feminist', 'anti-racist', 'structural', 'radical', 'liberationist', 'narrative and strength based' and/or 'anti/post-colonial' (Leonard 1997; Mullaly 2002, 2007; Briskman 2003b; Fisher 2004; Briskman et al. 2008). This means that across these perspectives there is diversity of opinion. Yet, for all the differences, we (the authors) believe that f ve broad views about violence and abuse tend to be shared:

- that violence and abuse are widespread social problems that can generate any number of other social problems (such as substance abuse, further violence, mental health problems and so on) (DVIRC 2006)
- that violence and abuse have a range of causes and effects, with different implications for social groups (such as women, children, the aged, and 'queer') (Pease 1996; McMaster 1997; CASA House 2006; Couch et al. 2007)
- that stories told about violence and abuse inf uence who is held accountable for violent and abusive acts (Wood 2001; Gilchrist & Price 2006; Briskman et al. 2008)
- that attempts should be made to eliminate violence, or at least reduce it (Plummer 2003; Weeks 2003; Ayres & Gerarda Brown 2005) and
- that peace and non-violence are worthy values to uphold (Ife 2001; Fisher 2004; Klosterman & Stratton 2006; Ramon et al. 2006).

As critical social workers, we are inf uenced by ideas from critical theory and scrutinise social institutions, groups and practices for unfairness (Thompson 2003; Brown & Strega 2005; Couch et al. 2007). We therefore understand violence and abuse from socio-cultural, interpersonal and intrapersonal points of view (also see DeLois & Cohen 2000; Mullaly 2002). While attending to questions about group dynamics and individual personalities, we do not ignore the implications of gender, class, 'race', sexuality, age and/or ability (CASA House 2006; Gilchrist & Price 2006). That is why we use def nitions of violence and abuse that allow collective and socially sanctioned forms of domination, control and manipulation to come to light (Mullaly 2007).

Taking our lead from survivors, we are concerned about all forms of violence and abuse, including those based on emotional, psychological, intellectual, spiritual, f nancial, material or physical domination, or a combination of the above (Memmott et al. 2001; Department of Justice Canada 2007; Gilchrist & Price 2006). While we realise that violence has historically been used to refer to acts of physical aggression, and that abuse has often referred to chronic interpersonal patterns of exploitation and degradation, we appreciate the potential slippage between the two terms and prefer to show interest in how def nitions are deployed, and what they attempt to capture, or omit (Fraser 2008).

Across a diverse range of f elds and modalities, critical social workers pay attention to common patterns of violence and abuse, including those that are counter-intuitive or unintended (Fraser & Briskman 2005; Briskman et al. 2008). Working with many 'shades of grey', we appreciate that violence and abuse are often complex, contradictory phenomena, especially when they occur in family and intimate relationships (Fisher 2004; CASA House 2006; Fraser 2008). We appreciate this when we work with people affected by abuse (victims/survivors and perpetrators), realising that some perpetrators 'accept responsibility' and are able to sustain non-violent change (Jenkins 1990; Fisher 2004), while others are not. Similarly, we appreciate that while some victims/survivors will feel shame and blame, and even chronic depression (Allers et al. 1992), others will not, that the legacy of abuse symptoms (such as sleeplessness, poor concentration, self-loathing and self-censorship) can vary, as can the utility of classif cations such as 'post-traumatic stress disorder', 'battered woman's syndrome' and 'learned helplessness'. That is why we are cautious of the idea that victims/survivors are 'needy' or become 'hostage' to their captors and/or suffer from 'false consciousness' if they are not able to 'free themselves' of the abuse. We are cautious because we know how these theories can be used to patronise victims and/or sully their reputations (Gilchrist & Price 2006).

Guided by concepts such as equality, safety, community, humanity and freedom, critical social workers try to imagine alternative ways of being in the world (Plummer 2003; Baines 2007a). Alternative ways are important because they help to envisage worlds where violence and abuse are not regular features of so many people's lives (Bagshaw et al. 2000; Rose 2000; Hart 2002; SECASA 2004a; UN CEDAW 2007). Yet alternative visions (or stories or scripts) are not always well received. By conservatives and liberals alike, they are sometimes criticised for being 'utopian', 'naïvely optimistic' or 'magical' in thinking. Our use of 'nebulous', 'feel good', 'modernist concepts' (such as needs, rights and equality) and our deployment of 'essentialising categories' (such as 'men', 'women', 'straight', 'queer', adult and child) may also be criticised for overgeneralising or 'totalising' people's lives (Mann 1994). However, these criticisms are valid only if we adhere too rigidly to these categories, and to the exclusion of all other factors.

Critical social workers are advocates of progressive social change who work towards egalitarian and democratic social processes. We realise that for our arguments to be heard and 'taken seriously', we may have to argue them more strongly than those reiterating 'tradition' or 'balance'—that is, those who try to 'trim' the difference between human rights and their abuses (Eagleton 2003). Because we correlate objectivity not with 'even-handedness' but *fairness*, we may be accused of being too partisan or 'subjective' by conservatives and liberals alike (Eagleton 2003). Even so, we try to contain any frustration or anger we might feel and harness it to challenging injustice. Equanimity is required because it would be more than 'ironic' if change that purported to promote peace, safety and non-violence were to be aggressively or *violently* pursued.

Apart from being stonewalled by expressions of fatalism (that 'nothing will change' because 'that's the way it's always been'), we may also have to confront the dilemmas of objectivity that Eagleton (2003: 134) describes:

> Objectivity requires a fair degree of passion—in particular, the passion for doing the kind of justice which might throw open your most deep-seated prejudices to revision . . . It demands imagination, sympathy and self-discipline. You do not need to rise majestically above the fray to decide that in a specif c situation somebody else's interests should be promoted over yours.

Critical social workers try to practise non-violence in our day-to-day work (McMaster 1997; Pease 1997; Fisher 2004), monitoring ourselves (Myerhoff & Ruby 1992) and our work cultures for acts of aggression, bullying, harassment and discrimination. Our underlying aim is to try to work respectfully with others, including those different from ourselves (Ife 2001; Bishop 2002). We ref ect on the language used to frame situations because we know that language helps to construct reality (Myerhoff & Ruby 1992). We pay attention to the forms of abuse most likely to be denied, ignored or justif ed (Hart 2002; Mayo 2005; CASA House 2006). We are open to recognising new forms of abuse and forming alliances to tackle them. That is why we respect the work done to recognise sexual abuse perpetrated by priests and other clergymen against parishioners, mostly children. It is also why we have supported victims/survivors, their families and religious communities more generally, as they call to account those who have participated in the public denials and cover-ups (Rossetti 1996; Fortune & Longwood 2004).

While critical social workers value peace, we do not try to 'keep the peace' if it means turning a blind eye to violence and abuse (Rose 2000; Klosterman & Stratton 2006). Having the presence of mind to recognise violence when we see it, we remain alert to the possibility that some forms may still be hidden or underestimated (Rose 2000; Hart 2002; CASA House 2006). We have learnt this through revelations of the abuse inf icted on many Indigenous children, stolen from parents and maltreated in orphanages and children's homes in Australia up until the 1970s (HREOC 1997; Memmott et al. 2001). We learnt it from the people subjected to the Child Migration Scheme, which existed between Britain, Australia, New Zealand, Canada and Zimbabwe up until the 1970s (Child Migrants' Trust 2001). Through the People's Inquiry into Detention in Australia, we were able to see some of the f ner detail of the violence and abuse inf icted on asylum seekers (Briskman et al. 2008). And through inquiries into the health and wellbeing status of transsexuals, we can more carefully appreciate how oppression can operate (Couch et al. 2007). With so many others, these examples are sobering reminders of what can happen when people remain, or become accustomed to or acculturated by, justif cations for violence and abuse (Segal 1999; Wood 2001; Robinson 2008).

Working towards social change, not just personal change

Critical social workers resist complacency and naïve and overly optimistic thinking. That is why we challenge the idea that equality has arrived or that we have entered a 'post-patriarchal', if not 'post-feminist', period (Ebert 1996; Segal 1999; Wood 2001). Aware of the importance of challenging heterosexism and publicly exposing homophobia (Robinson 2008), we recognise the diversity of interests within the category of GLBTI (gay, lesbian, bisexual, transgendered and intersex), while questioning the validity of narrowly constructed gender categories and roles (Burge 2007; Couch et al. 2007).

Concerned about rising numbers of refugees around the world, we challenge the legitimacy of invasions and warfare, even when they are done in the name of 'border control' and 'anti-terrorism' (Cox & Pawar 2005; Briskman et al. 2008). Thinking laterally, we also recognise how other social practices impact on our environments. We do not ignore the potential violence caused by 'environmental issues' such as rising carbon emissions and global warming, a likelihood of a peak oil crisis across the world, and potential wars over the global water and food supply (Smith 2008).

We participate in debates about basic human rights across the world, such as access to decent water, food, housing, work and income (Ife 2001). We are conscious of debates about 'competing priorities', namely those related to 'protecting the environment' with 'exploiting the environment', in the name of economic progress (Ife 2001; Cox & Pawar 2005). Well aware of the problems of the rapid growth of global capitalism, we realise that the 'rape of the earth' is connected to dominating and exploitative social relations, productive of many forms of violence and abuse (Smith 2008).

Critical social workers are concerned about oppression and socially sanctioned abuse (Mullaly 2002, 2007; Baines 2007a). Yet we know that the work involves much more than dividing the world into 'good' or 'evil', victim or enemy, so that the latter can be condemned (Fisher 2004). We know that people do not always abide by conventions, nor do what they are told (Burge 2007). We know that exceptions are possible and possibly numerous, that some people can triumph over hardship, and that their stories can be inspirational.

We realise that concepts, categories and classif cations (such as class, ethnicity, gender, age, sexuality, ability and geographical location) can be unstable and need to be used with care (Leonard 1997; Mulvey et al. 2000; Burge 2007). Sometimes this has involved facing new forms of abuse, including those perpetrated by women and suffered by men (Mulroney & Chan 2005). Aware that social contexts, status and identities (alone) do not explain the full range of violence and abuse (Mulvey et al. 2000), we appreciate the individually felt aspects of social problems while still drawing on 'unstable' concepts (such as needs and rights). We still use collective terms such as 'needs' and 'rights' because they help us to see, explain and take action against violence and abuse in ways that do not over-pyschologise (Segal 1999). These concepts help us to imagine change beyond personal def ciency, pathology and 'maladjustment' (Goffman 1963; Anastas 2007).

In all its diverse forms, 'social change' is an important but volatile concept with a wide range of ambitious possibilities. Progressive social change may be even more volatile, given that it usually means challenging prevailing social norms and practices, including those that assume that prof t trumps human needs, that competition beats collaboration, and that conformity is preferable to diversity (Burge 2007). For critical social workers, however, prof t, competition and conformity are not revered or promoted because they perpetuate steep social hierarchies and legitimate systemic forms of abuse, such as poverty and oppression (Mendes 2007). Instead, we value human needs, collaboration and diversity as we strive to promote emancipatory practices that will not, for instance, see children, women and 'queers' revictimised through the legal system following abuse, or rural communities further disadvantaged through 'environmental crises' such as droughts because of the stripping of public infrastructure. Progressive social change means supporting rural, remote and urban communities alike, including those trying to rebuild after emergencies and disasters (Yanay & Benjamin 2005). It is helped by efforts made to document progressive social change in action (Yanay & Benjamin 2005; Mendes 2007).

With respect for diversity, we try to be 'inclusive' and democratic (Briskman 2003b; Pease 2004; Briskman et al. 2008). We know this is ambitious, but we pursue it nonetheless—and across many modes and f elds of social work. We notice it in action when we see sexual assault services open their doors to male victims/ survivors (SECASA 2004a; 2004b), including those experiencing same-sex abuse. Respect for democracy and diversity is evident through the multitude of alliances formed to support the rights and needs of newly arrived refugees. We see it when religious and secular groups come together to support Indigenous communities (Briskman et al. 2008). It appears through the support given to people affected by industrial foreclosures and unpaid redundancies (ABC 2002). It is evident when social workers join with women service users to co-author research about violence and abuse while promoting women's friendship and solidarity (Gilchrist & Price 2006). Respect for diversity is also evident in work done with court-mandated violent men (Fisher 2004), and social work carried out with people at war with one another (Lev-Wiesel et al. 2008). Overall, the work is often done with people with scarce material resources and the most socio-cultural and political obstacles to overcome (Baines 1997, 2007a; Sev'er & Yurdakul 2001; Koenig et al. 2003).

Given its scope and aspirations, critical social work can be emotionally taxing and intellectually demanding work, especially in the area of violence and abuse. These demands are intensif ed by the need for critical social workers to speak out against violence and abuse, and in ways that do not—even inadvertently—*blame the victim* (Ryan 1976) or scapegoat victimised communities.

Realising the importance of viewing social problems as *social*, not just personal, problems, critical social workers are motivated to stand up against injustice, sometimes against allies, workmates, bosses, friends or family members (Fisher

2004). We do this even though we know that questioning (hetero)sexist privilege, or deconstructing currently popular ideas about 'attachment', 'trauma', 'victimisation', 'recovery' and 'resilience', may not win us friends or favours. At the same time, we appreciate the need to be strategic with language. We value attempts to f nd new ways to represent growth after hazards and trauma, without suggesting that if such growth is absent, it ref ects some kind of inadequacy or failure on the part of victims (Lev-Wiesel et al. 2008).

Mounting arguments that we know are often out of step with traditional (hierarchical, asymmetrical) social arrangements, we know we run the risk of having our arguments distorted and/or being called obstructionists or troublemakers (Eagleton 2003). We know that we are more likely to be charged with unearthing strong emotions and/or testing longstanding loyalties than those reiterating 'tradition' (Goffman 1963; Maushart 2001; Couch et al. 2007). We forge ahead not out of some heroic motivation, but because working in the f eld of violence and abuse has brought us up close to hurtful social practices that have long traditions (Herman 1992; Jackson 1999; Maushart 2001; Wood 2001; Couch et al. 2007).

Historical discourses about provocation, culpability and blame have had a long and lingering hold over the popular imagination, and have perpetuated 'normative' beliefs (or beliefs that narrowly def ne what is normal and abnormal) which have then been used to rationalise or excuse violence (Oakley 1981; Pease 1997; Fraser 2008; Robinson 2008). These beliefs are evident when particular communities or cultures are cast as 'naturally inclined' to be violent (e.g. 'cultures of poverty'), or as having a naturally high threshold for violence (e.g. 'they are used to it'). They surface through the claims that some groups 'can't help' being violent, and even enjoy the violence (see Segal 1999). They have a nasty habit of blaming victims and absolving perpetrators, as evidenced through the historical assumption that men are naturally aggressive, and women and Indigenous people 'get used to' violence, or even take some kind of masochistic pleasure in being abused. For abuse survivors, attacks on their characters and credibility may have profound effects, sometimes for generations (Allers et al. 1992; HREOC 1997; Child Migrants' Trust 2001).

Traditional, patriarchal and asymmetrical gender discourses are founded on the beliefs that, (1) the sexes are naturally 'opposite' and 'attracted to each other'; (2) fathers are the natural heads of families and households (Oakley 1981); and (3) women are natural wives (to men) and primary caregivers to all members of the family (Waring 1999; McPhail et al. 2007). They include corollaries, such as men having active 'sex drives' and 'instinctual' aggression and women being inherently passive and supplicating (or accommodating) (Segal 1999; McPhail et al. 2007). They are used to promulgate (or push) dominant sexual scripts for romance and family, including those idealising 'masterful, decisive and strong' men pursuing beautiful women who still protect their sexual reputations with the view of ultimately creating nuclear family units of reproduction and consumption (Oakley 1981; Fraser 2008). They are dominant because they are applied not just to people for whom they f t but to all people, including those for whom they do not (bene)f t, and who they may actively harm. For so-called 'sexual deviants', their effects have been palpable (Couch et al. 2007; Robinson 2008).

While working with some of the most personal dimensions of abuse, critical social workers still maintain a watchful eye over patterns of abuse, including common forms of and targets for abuse. The proliferation of research into violence and abuse has certainly helped. It has taught us that people classif ed as 'sexually deviant' are more vulnerable to being abused and implicated in, if not blamed for, the abuse after it has occurred (Bell & Binnie 2000; Willett 2000; Couch et al. 2007). We know that women are more susceptible to abuse than men, and that when they are abused, they are often incriminated (Flood & Pease 2006; McPhail et al. 2007).

Age is also a well-known risk factor for abuse, with the very young and old particularly vulnerable to abuse, especially from 'loved ones' (CASA House 2006). Women, children, the disabled and frail-aged, and people classif ed as queer also have a much higher risk of violence and abuse than able-bodied heterosexual men (Bell & Binnie 2000; Willett 2000; Mullaly 2007). Violence among ethnic minorities is also usually higher than it is for middle- and upper-class Anglo-Europeans. We know that the risk of being abused increases for people with threatened or 'spoiled' identities (Goffman 1963; Breakwell 1986; Willett 2000), including those who are working class, disabled or from 'culturally and linguistically diverse' backgrounds (Oakley 1981; Ebert 1996; Plummer 2003; Mooney Cotter 2004). We also know that the levels of violence and abuse are usually higher for people who are Indigenous, resource poor, not formally educated, and living in rural or remote communities (Memmott et al. 2001).

In 'peacetime', the bodies of women, children, homosexuals, the elderly and/or disabled are susceptible to denigration, objectif cation and violation (Herman 1992; Wood 2001; Couch et al. 2007). In wartime, human bodies may become even more of a battleground, with rape, abduction and humiliation common practices of armed conf ict, and increasing numbers of civilian casualties (Cox & Pawar 2005), most of whom are female (UNIFEM n.d.).

In short, critical social workers appreciate that while we may have 'come a long way' with respect to sexual equality, we still have a 'long way to go' (Flood & Pease 2006; Mendes 2007). We know that, while some women are the benef ciaries of global capitalism, many more live in the economic margins, if not in poverty, with decreasing educational and employment opportunities (Young 1997; Fraser 2008). We also know that to this day many women across the world, and across social classes, f nd their lives disrupted and/or disf gured by violence, particularly spousal violence (IFSW 2005) and sexual assault (CASA House 2006).

Recognising global violence against women

As Ban Ki Moon, the United Nations Secretary-General, said on 8 March 2007:

> Violence against women and girls continues unabated in every continent, country and culture. It takes a devastating toll on women's lives, on their families, and on society as a whole. Most societies prohibit such violence—yet the reality is that too often, it is covered up or tacitly condoned (UNIFEM n.d.).

In Australia, the United Kingdom and the United States, between 20 and 30 per cent of women experience domestic violence (UNIFEM n.d.). In other countries, the estimated f gures are higher. Take, for instance, Bangladesh, Peru and Tanzania, where around 50 per cent of the women are abused (Koenig et al. 2003; WHO 2008b), or rural Ethiopia, where 71 per cent of women are thought to suffer some form of physical abuse from spouses (WHO 2008b).

From international research, we know that women of the 'developing world' or 'Third World' are exposed to a wider range of violence and abuse, including those associated with 'indentured' (or slave) labour, honour killings, dowries and female circumcision (Ghansham 2002; WHO 2008b). Five thousand women every year are estimated to be victims of 'honour killings', with perpetrators justifying their actions on the grounds that the violation of the woman's chastity (through premarital sex) was an affront to their family's honour (Sev'er & Yurdakul 2001; WHO 2008b).

Attacks against women for 'failing' to protect their sexual reputation are widespread across the world, and have a long history (Fraser 2008). In Pakistan, Turkey, Jordan, Syria, Egypt, Lebanon, Iran, Yemen, Morocco and other Mediterranean and Gulf countries, however, 'honour killings' have been most prominent (WHO 2008b). With these crimes, another 7000 women are killed each year, especially in Southern Asia, because of dowry disputes (UNIFEM n.d.), with an unknown number of deaths wrongly classif ed as 'suicides'.

Even when laws and other social policies are enshrined to protect women's rights and prevent gender-based violence, discriminatory and harmful social practices may endure, and may therefore become the focus of critical social work attention. As Hitchcock (2001) writes:

The anti-dowry laws in India were enacted in 1961 but both parties to the dowry—the families of the husband and wife—are criminalised. The laws themselves have done nothing to halt dowry transactions and the violence that is often associated with them. Police and the courts are notorious for turning a blind eye to cases of violence against women and dowry associated deaths. It was not until 1983 that domestic violence became punishable by law.

Critical social workers are interested in international issues of gender and sexual equality because we appreciate that the notion of community extends beyond our individual 'habitus' and national borders (Cox & Pawar 2005; IFSW 2005). We also realise that some of the issues that affect the 'Third World' have now embedded themselves in the societies of more aff uent nations through the rapid expansion of migration and global capitalism (Cox & Pawar 2005; Mendes 2007). 'Female circumcision', early marriage, foeticide and human traff cking are good examples.

With no single health benef t from the procedure but many possible risks (WHO 2005), an estimated 130 million girls and women around the world have undergone 'female circumcision', or female genital mutiliation (FGM) as it is otherwise known. Even when formally outlawed, an estimated two million girls each year are thought to have it done (WHO 2008b). In many regions of Africa, the Middle East and Asia, including some parts of India, Indonesia, Malaysia and Sri Lanka, FGM is still considered an acceptable cultural or religious practice (UNIFEM n.d.).

Prevalent throughout the world, especially in Africa and South Asia, early marriage involves young girls being pressured, if not forced, into early marriage and sexual relations. As well as jeopardising their general health, this (i.e., early marriage) increases their risk of exposure to HIV/AIDS, and limits the girls' chance of completing school (UNIFEM n.d.).

Foeticide, or the abortion of a foetus simply because it is female, is also practised in many parts of the world, so much so that it has been held responsible for creating gender imbalances in Asia, particularly India (UNIFEM n.d.). In India, foeticide has been illegal for the past twelve years but among the urban middle classes it is still practised widely (Hitchcock 2001; Ghansham 2002). Apparently, the Indian government is offering f nancial incentives to families which give birth to girls and raise them until they are 'marriageable' (UNIFEM n.d.).

While precise data are hard to come by, human traff cking is estimated to range from 500 000 to two million people per year (Cox & Pawar 2005; UNESCO 2004; WHO 2008b). The majority of victims are poverty-stricken females (see IFSW 2005), some of whom are kidnapped by human traff ckers, while others are lured to 'developed countries' such as Australia through false promises of overseas jobs and educational opportunities (UNESCO 2004; UNIFEM n.d.).

Conclusion

Locally, nationally and internationally, critical social workers are concerned with how social problems such as violence and abuse interact with social patterns, dynamics and identities. Caring for and about individuals and groups alike, we do not ignore the social contexts of people's lives, including those that make people more or less susceptible to violence and abuse. To do so would be to ignore the vast body of knowledge about violence and abuse, both historical and contemporary, that correlates violence and abuse with gender, class, ethnicity, age, ability and sexual identities.

As with other social problems, critical social workers attend to the social, cultural and political dimensions of violence and abuse. We recognise that sexism, misogyny, ageism, heterosexism and homophobia continue to pattern many people's socio-emotional landscapes. We know that laws, policies and social conventions have a long history of benef ting heterosexual men, especially middle-class, white, able-bodied ones. And we know that even when these laws are dismantled they may be reproduced through dominant discourses, which inf uence the types of relationships we are likely to have, the resources we are likely to be able to access when relationships 'go wrong' and the stories that are told about our love lives along the way.

As we have suggested, critical social workers are well aware that there is no magic to working for peace and the elimination of violence and abuse, but hard and often confronting analyses. Whether it is about violence and abuse, or some other social problem such as poverty and unemployment, we know that being critical means recognising that people often live in environments that are unfair, and need to be challenged. As we do so, we try to envisage and then institute fair(er) alternatives by promoting the values of equality, safety and humanity in intimate relationships and beyond.

PART IV

locating critical social work in shifting worlds

18

critical practice in a changing context

Catherine McDonald

Due to a range of developments in the contemporary context, critical social work runs the unfortunate risk of becoming increasingly hard to do. While this may seem a disheartening introductory statement to make (especially in a book such as this), it can nevertheless credibly be argued that there are many factors at play in the environment which render it diff cult to engage 'critically'. It is this situation I wish to ponder—especially in the f rst part of this chapter. Nevertheless, for an optimistic vocation such as social work it is not good enough to merely argue that doing what we want to do is becoming increasingly diff cult. Rather, it is important that I also point to the spaces and cracks where practising critically has some real potential. Before turning to these tasks, I wish to make what I suggest are important and (I hope) relevant comments about the project of critical social work itself, particularly as it might be taken up by some emerging practitioners.

I am a little suspicious of the discursive effects of the promotion of critical social work—in educational settings in particular—when students are not, at the same time, taught about the realities of contemporary welfare. Divorced as universities are from the contested and often outright diff cult nature of contemporary human services, educators run the danger of promoting 'false clarity' (Bourdieu 1979: 52) and 'bogus optimism' (Garrett 2007a: 369) on the part of students. Social work, critical or otherwise, inevitably deals with a radically reconstituted welfare system, the contours and effects of which are often not fully understood from the vantage point of university students. This situation is not aided by the relative lack of contemporary contextual background in many social work practice texts. As a consequence, students learning about social work may inadvertently be taught about practice in organisational contexts more attuned to an imagined (or should I say remembered) world of the halcyon days of social work's high point in the 1960s and the 1970s. Unfortunately, social workers are currently operating in a human services environment which is at worst overtly hostile and at best indifferent to our endeavours as a collective group as well as to our core interests and objectives. Furthermore, it is a context in which many human service organisations are struggling to function—indeed, to survive—increasingly hedged into particular roles and modes of operations through the ubiquitous use of purchase of service contracts by governments.

Increasingly, the various sub-f elds of the human services are now constituted as quasi-markets which draw their logic and their operational models from bodies of thought alien to those which inform past and present social work and the post–Second World War Keynesian welfare state. These bodies of thought are known as public choice theory and agency theory (Buchanan & Tulloch 1962; Niskanen 1971; Buchanan & Tollsen 1972; Olson 1965; Williamson 1985). From these perspectives, for example, the role of values and ideology is utterly irrelevant. Values such as commitment to social justice, commitment to the notion of professionalism and sets of professional ethics—all of these have little place in public choice and agency theory. For a values-rational profession such as social work, this development is disastrous because it denies a fundamental core of what social work is. Further, public choice prescriptions for the business of welfare seek to constrain both the power and the autonomy of social workers. Similarly, public choice prescriptions for government seek to limit the power and discretion of public servants by, for example, exposing public functions to competitive tendering. The major tactic is the relocation of government welfare functions outside of government (contracting out) and by the creation of quasi-markets. By such processes, public choice-inspired reforms have redesigned the post–Second World War welfare state into an entirely new form.

Social work generally (and I suggest that critical social work is no exception) is aligned to sets of social, economic and political conditions represented by the Keynesian welfare state which no longer exist (McDonald 2006). As such, it is currently experiencing a form of institutional slippage which social work appears to have diff culty even addressing, much less responding to. By institutional slippage, I am suggesting that the institutional order that provided the foundations for social work to f ourish has all but disappeared and a new institutional order has arisen which shows little sign that it will wane in the foreseeable future. This is the crux of the problem confronting critical social work (and also the dominant mode of professional social work). The new institutional order of the contemporary workfare state does not foster the sorts of orientations to welfare, to human service organisations and to service users that were promoted in the old post-Second World War Keynesian welfare state.

Failing to acknowledge the dramatic restructure of welfare can result in a form of magical thinking wherein people have diff culty accepting the realities of the contemporary world, and as a result cannot engage in ways that f nd real purchase. And it is this purchase that critical social workers need to f nd if critical social work is going to survive. Effective critical social work in the current workfare world of welfare has three essential components: a critical analysis; critical ref exivity combined with a critical consciousness; and critical politics. The f rst component asks that we attend to theoretical accounts which attempt to appreciate the operations and impact of an advanced capitalist accumulation system—the driver of the shift to workfare. The second asks that we leaven that with an (inevitably inadequate but nevertheless necessary) appreciation of the complexities of power and our inescapable contribution to the construction of identities which have greater and lesser degrees of distinction. It also asks that we focus on the knowledge assumptions that are brought to bear in everyday practice. The third characteristic insists that we engage in whatever way we can with the resultant injustices in a manner which attempts to redress them.

Due to space limitations, in this chapter I address the f rst and third of these, noting that I address the second more comprehensively elsewhere (see McDonald 2006: Chapter 5), as do other chapters in this volume. I do so by f rst applying what is known as a post-Fordist or regulationist approach to understanding the contemporary conditions—in particular, the shift from a welfare state to a workfare state under conditions of advanced capitalism (Jessop 2002). I do so because post-Fordism provides a quite dramatic and sweeping analysis, and as such it shakes us out of any complacency that might exist about what is going on now, in twenty-f rst century capitalist Australia. Nevertheless, it is an approach which has limits which I note in due course—a process which allows those 'spaces and cracks' alluded to in my introductory paragraph to become clearer. To address the third condition of practising critically, I turn to French theorist Pierre Bourdieu for both a powerful analytic arsenal to deploy in my world of practice and for an example of an intellectual who never forgot that engagement in the politics of the day was his duty. I do so not to suggest that either post-Fordism or Bourdieu's work are the 'answer'. Rather, I use both to demonstrate that to practise critically in the way I have suggested above, I need a deep appreciation of a range of critical social theories. In other words, I am suggesting that critical social work is also an intellectual practice of signif cant complexity.

From welfare to workfare: a post-Fordist account

Post-Fordism takes its analytical orientation from the Marxist notion of the recurrent crises of capitalism. Post-Fordists consider the role played by political and cultural institutions and relations in attempts to regulate the instability of advanced economies. They stress, for example, the role of such institutions as the state in attempts to balance patterns of production and social demand. They recognise that the pattern of accumulation and growth in advanced economies is secured as much by *social regulation* as it is by *economic regulation* (Peck 2001; Peck et al. 2007). In this way, post-Fordists direct our attention to different parts of the overall mode of social regulation, such as the welfare state.

Post-Fordists concern themselves with the structure of *regimes of accumulation* and *modes of regulation*. Regimes of accumulation are periods of growth characterised by whatever it is that ensures a compatibility between what is produced and what is consumed in an economy. Under a Fordist regime of accumulation, for example, production and consumption are both characterised by mass standards (exemplif ed by the ubiquitous model T Ford motor vehicle—ergo Fordism). A mode of regulation functions more or less as a support framework for the growth regime. It pulls together and directs the wide variety of actions taken by a range of actors (for example, social workers) into a kind of regulatory network (for example, the welfare state). Accordingly, a capitalist mode of production and reproduction is manifested in a regime of capitalist accumulation. Distinctive historical periods in the development of capitalism can be discerned. Each successive wave of capitalist development has its own regime of accumulation and associated mode of economic, political and social regulation. In other words, each regime has regime-specif c modes, methods or processes of socialisation, and regime-specif c methods or processes of promoting social cohesion and integration. Both of the latter are necessary strategies to ensure economic growth (or capital accumulation).

Post-Fordism takes its starting point at the period of capital accumulation between the late 1930s and the mid-1970s, known as the golden age of *Atlantic Fordism*. This period was a period of unprecedented and sustained economic growth in Western industrialised nations, predicated on the development and maintenance of mass production and mass consumption. It was also a period noted for its political and social stability. There are a number of central features which account for that. First was the establishment of a social pact between capital and labour after the 1929–33 Depression, ref ecting agreement about basic social institutions (the welfare state and a managed market economy). Second, the *welfare state* developed, designed to deal with the dysfunctions of the market economy, to establish a minimum wage and thus place a f oor underneath consumption, and to promote 'norms' of mass consumption. Third, there was a general acceptance of the need for state regulation and intervention in the economic sphere. In other words, there was a commitment to a set of economic policies designed to sustain demand, to secure full employment and promote economic growth. Fourth, mechanisms were developed to control the increasingly international economic order.

The success of mass production (Fordism) required simultaneous transformation and regulation of consumption to ensure mass markets. While transformations in the methods of production were at the heart of the regime of accumulation, to be sustained it also needed transformations in all social institutions. Therefore, the state and the family were reconf gured to facilitate particular modes of social conduct conducive to mass consumption. Post-Fordists, for example, link a particular family form and a particular order of gender relations with the Fordist regime of accumulation (Jessop 2002a). This family form (the nuclear family) serves as a powerful mode of social regulation enhancing and embedding the capital accumulation regime. The nuclear family, it is argued, played a key role, both as a locus for privatised consumption and as a site for social and emotional integration. In its simplest terms, women were largely excluded from the labour market, remaining within the private sphere of the family. In doing so, one of their primary roles was to act upon and transfer the norms of mass consumption. Another was the reproduction of the labour force. Around this family form, a whole series of other social institutions both supported and extended this order of gender relations. The welfare state, for example, clearly supported this pattern of relations by overtly constructing women as dependent upon men (O'Connor et al. 1999).

As a regime of accumulation and as a particular social order, all went well for a signif cant period of time. Inevitably, the seeds of crisis embedded in the regime eventually grew into full-blown contradictions, resulting in a crisis of accumulation. The indicators were stagf ation (sustained high levels of inf ation); an increased share of capital going to labour through high wages and a large welfare state which shifted the underlying balance of class forces in favour of organised labour in the economic sphere; the rise of the new social movements increasingly critical of capitalism; and, perhaps most importantly, the combination of the f nancial crises, the oil shocks and declining prof ts.

The last of these was catastrophic for Fordism as it became progressively exhausted. The declining rate of prof t was both the vital indicator of decline and the straw that broke the camel's back. Critical voices began to be raised, disparaging of the dominant economic policy prescriptions of the time while continuing to champion the superiority of capitalism. Wages were said to be too high, wage-f xing processes were considered too rigid, and the rights of labour were considered to have gone too far. As a consequence, it was claimed, workers were pricing themselves out of jobs and labour mobility was seriously impeded.

Consequently, from the 1970s onwards, it became increasingly 'evident' to policy-makers that minor reforms to the system would not solve the crisis, and a new model of socioeconomic organisation needed to be established which would support continued prof t growth. This new 'model' of global capitalism (with national variations and diverse fortunes) has now emerged, and in the process has altered the three key elements of Fordism. The f rst is accelerated economic globalisation. Australia is f rmly part of the global economic order, particularly in terms of its reliance on commodity exports. Second, capital has succeeded in appropriating signif cantly higher shares of prof ts by using a number of strategies, all of which have reduced the power of labour (confrontations with the trade union movement; deregulation of the labour market; deregulation of the wage f xing system; workplace restructuring; and employment of less well-organised labour such as women and migrants). The Australian trade union movement, for example, was seriously destabilised by the Howard government and trade union membership has reached historic lows. Further, centralised wage f xing—once the hallmark of the Australian welfare state and the major means of redistribution from capital to labour—has been undone. Third, state intervention has shifted away from promoting the goal of social redistribution. In Australia, for example, the goal of state intervention in the form of welfare provision has shifted from social redistribution to promoting workforce participation.

The resulting restructuring of social and economic life results in a number of discernible outcomes (Sassen 1991): the rise of global cities divorced from their local and national economies (for example, Sydney); an accumulation of government and corporate debts to recondition and reservice these global cities, resulting in a decline in infrastructure in other areas within the same country (for example, the massive building projects that accompanied the 2000 Sydney Olympics); a loss of manufacturing jobs and a steady increase in service sector employment (for example, the steady decline of the car manufacturing industry in Australia); a polarised wage structure; deterioration in economic and social conditions for low wage workers; the demise of the compact between labour and capital; the rise of a post-Fordist consumerist middle class with a large disposable income consuming 'new' goods and services (personal services, lifestyle goods), creating demand for another type of low-wage worker to service them; and greater demand for the products of sweated industries and outwork.

The post-Fordist city is marked by spatial polarisation (Brenner & Theodore 2001), illustrated by the notion of the dual or quartered city, a metaphor which aptly characterises the emerging urban forms in Australian cities. The evolving city centres, for example, with their considerable upmarket investment, are not places for the poor. Marcuse (1989) has developed a representation of the idea of the 'many cities within a city' thesis. He identif es the economic city, the prestigious off ce blocks where the 'big decisions' are made; luxury housing spots, enclaves of isolated buildings and blocks occupied by the rich; the city of advanced services, characterised by downtown clusters of professional off ces enmeshed in a complex communicative network; the gentrif ed city, for those professional and managerial groups that are 'making it'; the suburban city, for single family housing, the middle professional and managerial groups and the skilled artisans which can be found both at the outer reaches of the city or near the centre; the tenement city, constituting cheaper single family areas and including areas of social/public housing occupied by lower paid workers; the city of unskilled work, located in relatively cheap industrial units, warehouses and sweatshops providing goods and consumer services in the city; and the abandoned city where the 'victims', the poor, the unemployed, the homeless and the excluded congregate, a city coloured by a subculture of drugs, alcohol and street crime.

This shift to the new mode of production, with its far-reaching spatial, political and social implications, is also encapsulated by the notion of a shift from a welfare state to a workfare state. Clearly, social welfare is centrally implicated, as are social workers, and it is to this that I now turn. The welfare state has, as has been suggested, been supplanted by the workfare state, as a result of which the def nitions of welfare have changed, the institutions and institutional arrangements responsible for its delivery have changed, and the practices in and through which welfare is delivered have changed (Jessop 1999). Social policy is now focused on transforming the 'identities, interests, capacities, rights and responsibilities' of its citizens so that they may become active agents in the pursuit of a competitive edge in a global economy (Jessop 1999: 353). The coalition of interests that underpinned the welfare state has fragmented, and this fragmentation has led to demands for a more differentiated form of economic and social policy—that is, approaches to policy that treat different groups of people in different ways. Currently in Australia, for example, the unemployed are the objects of a particular model of employment services policy which constitutes them as lesser citizens than those in the workforce, subject to various forms of coercion and threat (McDonald & Marston 2005).

The workfare state is geared to promote permanent innovation and f exibility in an open economy. It has abandoned full employment for full employability (in which a government seeks to engage the unemployed in job-preparation and job-seeking instead of providing actual employment) as it seeks to promote structural and systemic competitiveness. Welfare services, once delivered as part of a parcel of citizenship rights, are now pulled apart and bundled together in new ways as additional means to benef t business, demoting the individual citizen to second place in the dynamic. Finally, there has been (to shifting degrees) devolution of policy and its operations to sub-national levels along with a transfer of delivery of services away from the state to non-state sectors.

It should be quite clear by now that all social workers, critical or non-critical, need to think about what can be learned from post-Fordist political economy in regard to welfare generally and for social work in particular. In the f rst place, it is a framework which encourages appreciation that much of what is occurring in the broader economy and society—in the human services and to the welfare state in particular—is a result of the *role* of the welfare state and the human services within the economy. Post-Fordism would suggest to critical social workers that the various contexts of practice have all the characteristics of an industry undergoing signif cant restructuring.

The characteristics of that environment have altered signif cantly, designing out 'spaces' where critical social work could be practised. The quasi-market and its associated contracts, for example, increasingly specify exactly what type of service intervention contracted agencies will undertake and have all but removed organisational autonomy to work in ways individual organisations see f t. Critical social work, for example, is not a mode of intervention or practice nominated in government purchase of service contracts. Further, work practices associated with modernist practice in welfare states have changed, promoted by the relentless and ubiquitous spread of particular and highly controlling management principles and techniques to human service organisations. Those spaces of practice where traditionally critical social work was undertaken have remorselessly been reconf gured through processes of aggressive instrumentalism. The non-prof t sector, once relatively autonomous and as such a primary site of critical social work, has been tightly drawn into the service delivery system or structure shaped by the state. Now critical social workers f nd themselves operating in a 'shadow state' (Wolch 1989) and social workers, wherever they are, serve as the 'little f ngers of the state' (Nyland 1993: 100).

Wages and conditions are increasingly exposed to market forces. Signif cant inequalities have developed in the welfare workforce as a whole. State services have reduced their commitment to training and development, particularly if they are no longer the chief provider. Issues of training, licensing and credentialling in these groups arise. Service-delivery outcomes for disadvantaged people are characterised by even greater inequality of provision than existed under the welfare state as the market processes differentiate between types of providers and groups of service users. In all, a post-Fordist analysis would suggest that the spaces for critical social work practice have relentlessly been designed out of the contemporary human services delivery system, leaving little pockets lurking under the radar of the newly conf gured post-Fordist neo-liberal state.

As I suggested earlier, a post-Fordist framework clearly provides a powerful and disturbing analytical framework which should make us sit up and take notice. Further, there is evidence readily available that many of the processes noted have actually taken place in the context of the Australian version of the welfare state. That said, before retreating into total despair it is worth noting the limits to post-Fordism, which give us a sense that there is room to wriggle. Post-Fordist accounts have three primary problems (Barnett 2008). First, they can be overly deterministic and pretty much fail to take human agency into account. Agency is, of course, the very lifeblood of practising critically (as it is the lifeblood of social work). That said, my position is that critical practice is a bounded form of agency, and what can be done is inevitably constrained by institutional realities. Good critical practice is doing the possible in a manner cognisant of the context.

Second, post-Fordist accounts provide a rather thin version of what counts as political action—one that is obsessed with hegemonic neo-liberalism and which only conceptualises the state as acting in the interests of capital. In reality, the state is far more complex, messy and differentiated than that—and, as such, remains a site of political action by outsiders. Again, this is very important because it is within the messy bits of political engagement by diverse interest groups that critical practice can emerge strongly. Critical practice involves eyeing up the state and working out where, strategically, inf uence can be inserted into the game of politics and government. Third, and relatedly, it inevitably focuses on the role of elites as the primary agents of change. Their focus, for example, is on neo-liberal think tanks and on what they position as the cascading of their ideas unchallenged through all levels of government. A more pluralist approach to the state would suggest that the post-Fordist position probably oversimplif es the more complex and differentiated realities of how ideas enter the state 'ideas bank' and what happens to them once they are in. Furthermore, post-Fordist accounts homogenise states, presenting them as helpless in the face of the onslaught of global economic forces. In fact, states retain signif cant autonomy and national politics remain important in forging the shape and character of welfare policies (Clarke 2003). Finally, and as Clarke (2003: 207) also notes, the state was never the stable Fordist edif ce promoted by post-Fordism. It was always, and will in all likelihood continue to be, unstable—a site of ongoing contestation. The dynamism of that complex edif ce we call 'the state' opens up, in turn, more opportunities and possibilities for action. For example, critical as we may be of the current Labor government's social inclusion agenda, it nevertheless provides excellent cover for critical social workers to engage in both macro practice and the policy level and micro practice in social inclusion-inspired programs in areas of socio-economic disadvantage.

Finally, I would suggest that acknowledging each of these limits allows us to see the cracks in the edif ce of the contemporary context, and provides us with the wriggle room critical social workers probably need to keep going. This leads to my next set of comments, comments which involve picking up the political intent and analysis of post-Fordism in a more nuanced way—through the work of Pierre Bourdieu.

Orienting to the possible: Pierre Bourdieu

Why Bourdieu? For me, the answer to that lies in several characteristics of his distinctive yet hard-to-neatly-categorise position on the social and political world. First, politically Bourdieu was intently focused on what he termed the 'scourge of neo-liberalism' (Bourdieu 2001: vii), that 'planetary vulgate' or biblical text of the contemporary era, crisscrossing the globe like transcontinental traff c (Bourdieu & Wacquant 2001; Wacquant 1999). He held tightly to a politics which rejected the entire package of economic and social policies that have accompanied neo-liberalism as a project. He fulminated against neo-classical economic policies which position the freedom of the market over the wellbeing of citizens. He was enraged, for example, by an approach to economic management which deliberately uses policy-induced unemployment to control inf ation. He was infuriated by accompanying social policies which then (amazingly) blame the unemployed for their plight and which authorise coercive and punitive responses. For Bourdieu, key parts of the contemporary workfare state have turned into a 'war machine against the poor' (Garrett 2007b: 237). He fervently believed that intellectuals (which, I suggest, critical social workers should aspire to be) should work tirelessly to reinstate a state which focuses its interests on the wellbeing of the people, rather than the interests of capital.

The second reason I turn to Bourdieu lies in his theoretical approach and associated 'conceptual arsenal'—both of which are highly informative for critical social work practice (Garrett 2007a, 2007b). Theoretically, Bourdieu's perspective acknowledges that there are irrepressible structures that are linked to the capitalist accumulation regime, but he also recognises agency, specif cally, actors' ability to effect change in their daily lives (Houston 2002). In Garrett's (2007b: 226) words, Bourdieu's 'intellectual project . . . was to overcome the opposition between the subjectivist emphasis on individual consciousness and the objectivist preoccupation with social structures'. Clearly, then, Bourdieu provides theoretical legitimisation of the will to act and capacity to engage central to both the politics and the purpose of critical social work practice.

Further, he was centrally interested in understanding how it is that social systems reproduce hierarchy and domination. Using culture as the crucible, in his acclaimed work *Distinction* (1979) as well as in the classic *Outline of a Theory of Practice* (2003), he developed the notions of habitus, the f eld and capital: an interconnected set of concepts of signif cance for social workers. As will become clear, their signif cance lies primarily in that taken together, his approach allows us to see how, embodied in the lives of the people we work with and in ourselves, are the means of both domination and resistance.

Habitus refers to characteristic sets of dispositions people have—that is, ways of being, tendencies, proclivities, inclinations. These serve to integrate past experiences in and to the present. It is an internalisation of the past which, when enacted in the present as a projection of self, propels that self into the future. Habitus is formed through a person's life experience; it is second nature to a person, forgotten and unnoticed. Nevertheless, it is habitus which shapes how a person goes about living their lives. People propel their habitus in *fields*, physical and social spaces, characterised as much by the physical properties as by f eld-specif c social relations. These social relations shape for people what is right and wrong, what is acceptable and not, what is valuable and what is worthless.

Different f elds allow the accumulation of different forms of *capital*. As Wacquant (1998: 221, cited in Garrett 2007a) notes 'the system of dispositions people acquire depends on the position(s) they occupy in society, that is, on their particular endowment of capital'. Naturally, possession of capital results in power and authority in a given f eld. The strength of Bourdieu's notion of capital is that he nominated different types, thereby introducing much-needed nuance in the face of complexity in the social world. In addition, this nuance opens out the possibilities of practice. There is the obvious *economic capital* in the form of material and f nancial resources. There is *cultural capital*: educational credentials, engagement and familiarity with high culture such as art, classical music, literature. Further, cultural capital is embodied in the modes of dress and presentation, enunciation and accents ref ecting different class dispositions. Then there is *social capital*, those resources, contacts and networks that people acquire through membership of a particular group. Different types of capital (and different mixes) are more or less fungible. That is, they translate into value at different rates. Economic capital is directly fungible; cultural capital and social capital are less directly fungible; but are nevertheless both deeply implicating in 'f xing' a person in society's social hierarchy with the associated capacity to acquire (or not acquire) wealth and privilege.

As suggested earlier, habitus—operating in f elds characterised by the presence or absence of people with different types and mixes of capital—provides a nuanced framework for thinking about how capitalism creeps in and through the living of lives and how, in turn, that living reproduces social structures. It also provides us with a framework to see the cracks, mobilise agency and promote resistance. It allows us to value what is not valued (for example, different modes and forms of cultural and social capital). It opens up all sorts of avenues for working creatively with people beyond the immediate and traditional concern with addressing f nancial or other forms of hardship. It encourages us to speak to people's strengths as those are authentically experienced. Most importantly, and in relation to myself as someone wanting to practise critically, it makes me attend to my personal mix of economic, cultural and social capital in terms of what my embodied self 'says' to others. In other words, it provides a framework for embodied critical ref exivity.

Conclusion

Bourdieu's work is not simple—then again, neither is post-Fordism. Furthermore, both formulations have their limits. Nevertheless, what each offers is a view of the world, albeit at different 'levels'. Post-Fordism provides a powerful lens through which we can appreciate the workings of advanced capitalism, and as such a means for analysing what confronts us, in this country, at the end of the f rst decade of the twenty-f rst century. Bourdieu's work takes us conceptually to the other end of that spectrum—down to people living their lives in the spaces and places of contemporary Australia. Both of these bodies of theory provide fruitful insights into what we, as critical practitioners, wish to engage with and how we might actually go about that. Good critical social theory is always a challenge. My position is that good critical practice means that we must engage with the complexities of the bodies of theory that we claim inform us, and we must not ever resort to reductionism and oversimplif cation. We must, as Bourdieu asked of himself, turn away from false clarity and engage with the world in which we have a duty to work with all of its convoluted intricacies. Fortunately, we have help.

19

enacting critical social work in publicly funded contexts

Nick Halfpenny

In recent years, the issue of restriction, compliance and control and their impact on social workers has been the subject of considerable comment (Harris 2003; Baldwin 2004; McDonald 2006). Changes to the structure, delivery and composition of welfare services have had a profound effect on practice within the welfare sector. In considering this contemporary context of social work, it is useful to recall that, in 1965, Wilensky and Lebeaux noted that 'any worker that tries to be a good humanitarian and a good agency representative at the same time is in for a torment of conscience' (1965: 321–2). The authors remind us that competing accountabilities are nothing new to the social work profession and social workers themselves—that the interests of service users, community service organisations, governments and their agencies, professional associations, individual social workers and the wider community rarely align. The intersections of justice, accountability, availability and equality occur brief y—if at all.

The rise of 'risk culture' in the human service represents a tectonic shift in social work. The concept of 'risk' has become a def ning principle that informs the organisation and delivery of (welfare) supports and services (Green 2007). It is a particular approach that seeks to 'manage out' the uncertainty that is so much a part of human service practice/s (Baldwin 2004: 48). This chapter seeks to explore two contemporary concepts woven with the thread of 'risk' and the issue of what constitutes the elements of critical social work practice needed to negotiate the contemporary context. Focusing on the organisation and practice of child and family welfare services in Victoria, this chapter charts recent restructuring and reform in publicly funded services to explore the issues of accountability and control for social workers. As noted by Smith (2001: 289), 'in their daily work with children and families social workers are constrained by a panoply of regulation guidance and procedure'. The chapter charts the two interrelated streams of reform (managerialism and contractualism, and systems of assessment and compliance) and the ways in which they have altered the landscape of welfare practice for social workers. Central to the critical approach is a focus on how dominant ways of thinking and seeing impact on people's lives (Pease et al. 2003: 2). Critical social work involves the capacity to identify these trends, and disrupt the narratives by highlighting the assumptions and the privileges of these discourses to further the interests of service users. The case studies illustrate the contemporary regimes of control that social workers are required to negotiate and are followed by a consideration of how social workers can critically engage with, and respond to, these emergent trends. As McDonald so usefully reminds us (2006: 213), 'it is wrong in the contemporary conditions to assume that goodness of heart and purity of intent are suff cient characteristics to ensure desirable outcomes for the people who use social work services and for the profession'.

Publicly funded welfare services

An analysis of publicly funded welfare services begins with an acknowledgement of the role of non-government organisations in the delivery of services. Unlike other jurisdictions that have a history of welfare service provision by public agencies and government departments, in Victoria the non-government sector has a strong tradition of delivering welfare services in partnership with government (Tierney 1963; CSV 1992: 1–12; Saunders 1994: 155; Hoatson et al. 1996: 133; Gleeson 2008). The role of non-government organisations acting as 'subsidiaries' of government to deliver welfare services is ref ected in funding arrangements which see the largest twenty non-government organisations receiving a majority of their funding from government sources (Blacher 1997: 43; Industry Commission 1995: xix). Despite the key role such community welfare organisations have played in the delivery of welfare services, material regarding the size, disposition and economic contribution of the sector is uneven (Lyons 1993: 27). The sector consists of a diverse range of religious and community-based service organisations (Lyons 2001). In relation to child and youth welfare services, successive governments in Victoria have a long history of subsidising the non-government agencies to provide welfare services such as residential care (Tierney 1963: 28–33; Hiskey 1980; Markiewicz 1996) and granting statutory powers to non-government organisations in areas such as the investigation of child abuse and neglect (Jaggs 1986; Swain 2000). While the prevalence of social workers employed with non-government agencies suggests this sector has played a key role in the development of the profession of social work (McDonald 1999; Fook et al. 2000), there has been relatively little research undertaken about the particular role of social workers practising in this setting.

Managerialism, contractualism and the human services

The following section seeks to elaborate on the concepts of 'managerialism' and 'contractualism'. From a critical perspective, I acknowledge that, in and of itself, neither concept refers to anything that is tangible. What they share is a reliance on human actors to make them 'real'—the politicians, bureaucrats, managers, social workers, and so on to actively accept and put these ideas into practice. These concepts are tools of description rather than concrete forces of change.

Since the early 1980s, Australia's public sector policy-making and program delivery have been reshaped by the application of ideas of 'managerialism' (Muetzelfeldt 1992; Meagher 2000; Baldwin 2004; Tilbury 2006). The restructuring of Australia's patterns of governance and the organisation of human service delivery have altered the conditions and practice of the areas where social workers are employed (Alford & O'Neill 1994; Harris 2003; Baldwin 2004; Tilbury 2006). To begin with, let's consider the concept of 'managerialism'. Put simply, the term as applied to human services is used to describe an array of reforms and restructuring techniques with the general aim of aligning practices more closely with market, and market-like, modes of organisation (Muetzelfeldt 1992; Meagher 2000; Harris 2003). Central to the restructuring that has occurred in human services since the 1980s has been the reform of organisational structures and policy processes both within and outside publicly funded welfare services. Applied to public welfare, the concept of 'managerialism' is typically used as a banner term for a bewildering range of organisational reforms, public policy priority changes and the restructuring of the relationships between agents of public service delivery and their 'clients'.

Meagher (2000: 74) argues that 'the language and practice of the Australian public policy have become increasingly organised around the assumption that economic development in the form of more competitive and dynamic markets will achieve all national economic and social aims.' These reforms were aimed at improving the eff ciency of private, government and non-government organisations (Alford & O'Neill 1994; Considine 1988; Lyons 1998).

The key characteristics of managerialist reforms can be summarised as follows:

- work determined by clear objectives denoted by managers
- role specialisation
- hierarchical line management and some devolution of decision-making to managers down the line of control (Baldwin 2004: 48)
- higher levels of technical control (Harris 2003: 64).

For Tilbury (2006), the managerialist way of doing things has become a 'new orthodoxy' in welfare practice. Such characteristics sit in sharp contrast to the values associated with critical social work. For example, Llewellyn (1998: 38), in a discussion of costing and caring in the f eld of social work, says:

> the values of accountability and responsibility can still sit in stark contrast to the inherent indecision and ambiguity of social work practice. Where 'real' social work (the professional counselling task) has to defend itself against the encroachment of managerialism it can f nd itself exposed as lacking in substance and as being devoid of objectives.

Such a movement suggests an undervaluing of those factors or issues that defy quantif cation. For O'Connor et al. (2000: 1):

> social work and the human services are currently undergoing fundamental and rapid change. The mission, focus, structure, funding, organisation and governance of social welfare and community services are being reshaped by these changes. The existence of a welfare state that provides even the minimum level of support for all citizens is under question.

Such critiques paint a rather dark and foreboding picture of the environment currently occupied by social work professionals.

The 'second wave' of human service restructuring: 'contractualism'

The 1990s saw the emergence of a 'second wave' of reforms in the welfare services with the increased use of contracts to regulate the direct service functions of non-government organisations—characterised as 'contractualism' (Alford & O'Neill 1994; Lyons 1998).

The foundations of contractualism, with the assumption of the individual as primarily guided by the 'rational' choice of self-interest, are found in public choice (or agency) theory (Alford & O'Neill 1994; Hancock 1998; Yeatman 1998b). Such ideas are well represented by the advocates of public sector restructuring. In their inf uential book *Reinventing Government*, David Osborne and Ted Gaebler (1992) famously def ned their preferred model of public administration as the government 'steering not rowing'. The simplicity of the metaphor belied its powerful impact on public policy. Formally separating service provision from policy and funding through the mechanism of contracts became *de rigueur* in public administration (Alford & O'Neill 1994; Ramia & Carney 2001).

While the debate has quietened in the succeeding years, the practice of funding and service agreements to govern the conduct of community service organisations delivering publicly funded welfare services has continued. This restructuring and reform have had a concrete and far-reaching effect for the social worker practising in publicly funded welfare agencies. For social workers, this restructuring has not been battles fought off distant shores—the work of frontline social workers has been part of this transformation. The operationalisation of the concepts of managerialism and contractualism is plain to see across practice settings as particular theories of practice become fused with managerialist and contractualist imperatives; to simply describe the reforms as a discourse that has been entirely externally imposed would be a mistake. As a number of authors have argued, social work is not a united profession based on an unambiguous discourse or body of professional knowledge (Gibelman 1999: 298; Baldwin 2000). Just as the modernist project of social work professionalism has been brought into question, there is also a demonstrable alignment between certain modernist sciences within the human service f eld and the unifying discourse of managerialism. As Harlow (2003) suggests, there are particular discourses of social work that 'f t' more comfortably with the prevailing managerialist themes in social work. In the next section, I outline the impact of the practices associated with increased technical control on the practice of social workers.

The emergence of practice tools and the intersections with managerialism and contractualism

To the critical eye, there is certainly a nice f t between certain human service disciplines and the project and practice of managerialism (Baldwin 2000: 112–16; Searing 2003; Carey 2007). As Epstein (1999: 11) notes, 'social work has been instrumental in turning therapy into social policy'. Similarly, Kingf sher (1998:

132) points out that a feature of human service work is the tendency to 'construct clients from otherwise signif cantly more complicated human beings'. There are examples of a number of developments from within the human service f eld that have been prompted (at least in part) by the discourse of managerialism. I shall use the example of the Looking After Children (LAC) framework to explore this issue in more detail.

The Looking After Children (LAC) Framework[1]

The LAC Framework was developed in the United Kingdom as a response to the very poor outcomes for young people in out-of-home care. The framework is used as a case-management tool for young people placed in the care and protection of the state. It is a framework that is informed by a discourse of children and young people, and particular ideas of the role and functions of 'the good parent'. The framework articulates seven 'life domains' that inform a series of related tools and processes.[2] The life domains are health, education, identity, family and social relationships, social presentation, emotional and behavioural development, and self-care skills. From a critical perspective, it is an approach that can be situated as one of the 'technologies of intervention' (Foucault 1984, cited in Epstein 1999), with the emphasis on 'observation, measurement, assessment and administration'. Such a technique applied to a population seeks to 'discipline, regulate, administer and arrange' (Epstein 1999: 14).

Beyond the United Kingdom, the framework and tools have been applied in a number of countries, including Canada and Australia. Much like the Westminster system of government, the LAC Framework has been adapted and applied in different ways in the jurisdictions that have taken it up. In the Australian state of Victoria, the application of the LAC Framework is mandatory for all children and young people entering out-of-home care—a service that is provided by non-government agencies in Victoria. As set out below, the LAC Framework is applied in Victoria using a series of documents to be completed by human service workers in consultation with children, young people in the out-of-home care system and their families within specif ed timeframes. The application of the LAC tools by community welfare organisations is mandatory for all young people entering out-of-home care through the child protection system.

As a system of case management, the LAC Framework revolves around the completion of four separate practice tools (or 'records'): the Essential Information Record (EIR), the Care and Placement Plan (C&PP), the Review of the Care and Placement Plan (C&PP) and the Assessment and Action Record (A&AR). The information recorded in each tool is structured around the seven 'life domains'. The LAC Framework specif es timeframes within which each record is to be completed. The EIR is completed at the time of referral and updated regularly (at least every six months); the C&PP is to be completed within fourteen days of a child or young person entering an out-of-home care placement; the process of f lling out the A&AR begins immediately following the f rst C&PP and is completed over the following six weeks; the RC&PP follows the completion of the A&AR and informs the development of a new C&PP. The LAC records are lengthy documents[3]—for example, the C&PP is approximately 24 pages long, while the A&AR can run to more than 62 pages for a young person aged f fteen or over. The thread of accountability runs heavily through these documents—all needs that are identif ed have a corresponding section outlining how they will be responded to, who is the person responsible and a completion date.

While there is an administrative logic to the approach, timelines and the linkages between the records, the above description highlights the fact that the LAC documents represent a detailed and highly structured practice tool for social worker. The framework contains a high level of prescription both in term of the content of the tools and the timelines within which they are to be completed. Given the widespread application of the framework, the critical response to the LAC Framework has been relatively muted. The debate has been characterised as one between 'relatively uncritical advocacy of LAC or its wholesale critique' (Yeatman & Penglase 2004: 233). Garrett (1999a, 1999b, 2002, 2003) has provided a spirited critique of the key assumptions underlying the system. He highlights the problematic position of the LAC system and its use both as a tool for research and as a practice tool for social workers (1999a: 296). For Garrett, the LAC framework is attempting to be a servant of two masters, each with priorities that, to a certain extent, sit in opposition to one another. Such a tension leads to the argument that the application of the tools involves pressuring social workers to devote a disproportionate amount of their work towards recording information contained in LAC tools rather spending time with their clients (Munro 2001).

Garrett (2002) also notes the silence of the tools on the issue of class and power, factors that appear to be more salient characteristics requiring redress for the population of children and young people entering out-of-home care systems. In a similar vein, Yeatman and Penglase (2004) raise questions about the eff cacy of individualised planning approaches such as the LAC Framework in providing client-centred services beyond narrow service contexts. Perhaps more tellingly, Garrett (1999a) argues that LAC documents are rooted in assumptions that are potentially oppressive and contain powerful subtexts about acceptable and unacceptable behaviour. For example, Garrett highlights the tools' 'unquestioning bias towards adult authority f gures (teachers and managers) . . . that is rooted in normative assumptions and social conformist imperatives' (1999a: 301).

Such normative assumptions can be found in the 'Social Presentation' section of the Assessment and Action Record for young people aged f fteen and over:

> Do you know how to adjust your behaviour and conversation to different situations (eg at work, TAFE, or school, with friends, teachers or managers, at home or with people you don't know very well)? (Assessment and Action Record 15+: 45)

Also, to the question of a young person's behaviour:

> *Objective 1: The young person's appearance is acceptable to young people and adults.* Respondents are asked to provide a response along a continuum from 'acceptable to young people and adults' to 'not acceptable to either'. (Assessment and Action Record 15: 46).

The LAC tools themselves are somewhat resilient to change. In keeping with the oeuvre of the time, the LAC tools associated with the framework are licensed. The tools' licensing obligations can prove to be a disincentive to the easy adaptation of the tools. In Australia, the University of New South Wales and Barnardos Australia hold the LAC International Licence. The use of the tools and any changes that an agency would like to make to the tools will attract a fee.

From the point of view of the critical social worker, the LAC Framework and associated tools can be seen as representative of a wider trend that is positioning social work as an increasingly technical task. Serving the interests of service users/clients involves questioning the assumptions that run through these regimes of practice.

Compliance and assessment in the human services

Beyond the sector and organisational restructuring, and the encroachment of prescribed techniques of practice, recent years have seen the application, evolution and expansion of performance standards applied to community service organisations. The basic premise of such standards is to ensure service providers conform to or meet a set of basic standards. The key features are generally associated with services of a high quality. In some quarters, such standards were seen as a useful antidote or improvement of techniques associated with managerialism and contractualism (that is, the focus on outputs and performance monitoring). Such standards have evolved to the point where they represent a rigorous form of surveillance on community service organisations by funding bodies. A range of regimes of standards are presently applied to community agencies by state and federal government agencies (aged care, health, disability, housing, family and community services, homelessness and community care, to name a few). One of the key diff culties for social workers is the evidentiary requirements associated with demonstrating compliance with such regimes of standards.

The registration standards for community service organisations in Victoria

In 2007, the Registration Standards for Community Service Organisations (CSO) were introduced in Victoria. The standards apply to all agencies funded to provide out-of-home care and family services in Victoria. There are eight standards representing different dimensions of organisational practice that can broadly be def ned as governance; organisational processes; human resources; service environment; case practice; building capability; service responsiveness; and service integration. Each standard has a series of sub-standards—for example, Standard 5.4a states: 'The CSO [community service organisation] adopts a partnership approach when working with children, youth and their families which is responsive to the children's age, gender, culture, communication needs and developmental stage and works to understand their needs and views in the context of the family, community and culture.'

Agencies are required to conduct an annual self-assessment against each of these standards, providing four different 'types' of evidence to demonstrate compliance for each sub-standard. The four evidence types are:

1. *Approach*—for example, documented policy, procedures or guidelines.
2. *Understanding*—evidence of staff understanding of policy, procedure or guidelines.
3. *Action/Implementation*—evidence of policy 'in action', such as in client f les.
4. *Feedback*—evidence of systems to gather 'stakeholder' feedback on the policy, procedure or guidelines.

Such a system of standards and assessment is not amenable to a more qualitative consideration of practice and outcomes—by design or default, it encourages a process of evidence-gathering in relation to human service practice that is forensic rather than fulsome—an approach Parton (2003: 2) describes as 'attempts to rationalise and scientise increasing areas of social work activity'.

In addition to the annual self-assessments, each agency will undergo an independent audit every three years. Based on the legislation, agencies found to not comply with the standards can be subject to interventions such as the appointment of administrators or deregistration and the loss of government funding. Such standards represent the further evolution of the concepts of managerialism and contractualism with the emphasis on external control on internal processes. Not surprisingly, compliance with the LAC Framework (documentation and timelines) is a key source of evidence for the practice-related standards in the Registration Standards.

For the social worker, it is not suff cient to do something—there must be evidence of the doing! This type of compliance regime has direct and profound implications for social workers. It brings to another level the issues of compliance, control and risk management. The problem associated with such forms of performance monitoring is explained by Zifcak (2001: 95) thus: 'the disciplinary shift from social to economic science that has been involved has dictated a movement away from evaluation towards measurement'—for example, gauging the existence of plans, the number of contacts with clients and so on, rather than focusing on more qualitative aspects of the client experience. Porter (1995) provides a useful reminder that 'the quantitative technologies used to investigate social and economic life work best if the world they aim to describe can be remade in their image' (1995: 43). For Jones (1993, cited in Power 1998: 93), current approaches to public administration represent the ascendancy of administrative rationalities over substantive justice goals. As Power (1999: 123) asserts:

> The audit society is a society that endangers itself because it invests too heavily in shallow rituals of verif cation at the expense of other forms of organizational intelligence. In providing a lens for regulatory thought and action audit threatens to become a form of learned ignorance.

The effectiveness of services is governed by systems of audit, performance monitoring and other 'technologies of trust' (Porter 1995; Power 1999), rather than the less concrete, more immeasurable, forms of service outcomes. Power (1999: 136–7) concludes that:

> it is clear that trust can never be eradicated in social arrangements. The audit society is not simply a distrusting society; rather, it ref ects a tendency not to trust trust.

> This means a systematic tendency towards uncritical trust in the eff cacy of audit processes, a trust which results in the absence of evaluation of audit process itself.

Power suggests that trust in systems of audit has displaced conf dence in the judgement and discretion of professionals—the predominance of quantif cation over intuition (Power 1999: 134–8).

Public policy and critical practice

The capacity to critically engage with such manifestations of public policy is a def ning feature of social workers working towards meaningful transformation for the benef t of service users. As the above sections have sought to illustrate, social workers are often faced with service environments characterised by compartmentalisation and the individualisation of client work—characteristics that can undermine the ability to challenge more entrenched social and political inequities. While the above sections have sought to outline some of the key challenges for critical social work practice, there are reasons for considerable optimism. To infer that social workers in the current climate are merely enactors of public policy is to ignore the complexity of frontline work—to deny the oppositions between the 'lived in', messy and contingent nature of welfare practice and the banality and repetition that accompany much of the work. The analysis tends to remove the worker from the sphere of welfare work and decision-making almost entirely. The dire predictions of the death of practice discretion in the face of prescriptive and actuarial (evidence-heavy) models for social work tend to ignore one thing: the social worker.

Attempts will continue to codify and systematise practice, but the inherent uncertainties of social work will allow scope for discretion and worker agency (Evans & Harris 2004). Lipsky's (1980) seminal work on the autonomy of frontline bureaucrats is of continued relevance to social work. As Baldwin (2000: 173) reminds us:

> [I]t made little difference whether there was a well-organised rationalist managerial technology in place or not . . . Discretion will happen because human beings will create their own reality through relationships . . . discretion is essential as well as inevitable.

In the concluding section, I outline pathways through the milieu that are charted by a number of authors (Gardner et al. 2006; McDonald 2006). I also consider two interrelated strategies that can both heighten the critical engagement with the contemporary reform approaches.

Peer collaboration and alliances with service users

With the increasing prominence of non-government agencies (community service organisations) in the delivery of publicly funded welfare services as outlined above, there are dangers associated with the fragmentation of practice settings. Peer networks and collaborations can be a useful antidote to break down the prevailing constraints of dispersed practice settings. This approach can democratise practice by opening it up to colleagues and service users to share experiences to develop and support shared approaches to a more critical practice—developing a collaborative approach to resist attempts to locate service users and/or social workers solely within programmatic or diagnostic categories.

Critical reflection and action

The capacity to engage in critical ref ection is the single most important attribute for social workers practising today. Gardner et al. (2006: 229–31) outline a useful summary of the key characteristics of critical ref ection. Particularly salient to the issues outlined in this chapter are the characteristics the authors identify that centre on opening up the politics of human service organisation and practice to critique—embracing approaches that build the capacity to question underlying assumptions and dominant discourses, and their manifestations in practice.

The current conditions of welfare work require of social workers an ever-increasing literacy regarding the public policy implications for social work practice and ways in which to negotiate these changes. To an extent, the value of critical ref ection is very much dependent on the resultant action. Social workers are well positioned to highlight alternative interpretations in order to challenge the assumptions that run through many public policy initiatives. In a climate that often deploys a narrow concept of 'evidence-based' approaches to inform human service policy and practice, social workers have a duty to both contest the meanings of 'evidence' and contribute more nuanced and robust understandings of how social policy can work in the interests of services users.

Conclusion

Blank canvases do not exist, and have never existed, in social work. The longing for a practice context free of constraint and obligation is a chimerical pursuit. To retreat from or simply dismiss the contemporary challenges outlined in this chapter is counterproductive. The capacity to engage with service users to work towards transformation has always been the 'core business' of social work. In the contemporary context this is neither simple nor unproblematic. Social workers should be able to demonstrate the eff cacy of the work they do with service users, but not in a manner that is counter to the interests of justice, equity and transparency.

20
framing critical social work practices with rural and remote communities

Uschi Bay

One of the key challenges for social workers in rural and remote Australian communities is to understand the interaction between geographical location, place-based policy, livelihood strategies and various forms of inequality. There are many myths and cultural meanings attributed to the 'rural' and 'remote' in Australia. Both terms can be understood as a social construction where meanings and identities have been constructed over time (Lockie & Burke 2001: 8). One common social construction 'equates "the rural" with "traditional", "organic" communities of homogeneity and social cohesion' (Miller 1996: 95; Mowbray 2005). Current Australian government policies aim to facilitate def cits in urban, rural and remote communities' 'social capital'. Governments see their role as facilitating local communities to build their 'capacity' through 'community-based initiatives' and 'partnerships' (Shortall & Shucksmith 2001: 122). This governmental approach appears to be intensif ed for Aboriginal remote communities, whose livelihood strategies and funding support from federal government are framed in terms of a 'return-on-investment model' requiring Aboriginal communities to identify long-term economic outcomes before being provided with government funds (Rea & Messner 2008: 88). Recent neo-liberal policy and a discursive emphasis on 'social capital' tend to romanticise rural and remote communities, with the unfortunate effect of depoliticising social problems and potentially reinforcing current inequalities and locational disadvantage (Shortall 2004; Mowbray 2005).

It is within this socio-political and discursive framework that social workers engage with rural and remote communities in their various job roles. Many social workers are engaged in direct practice, or provide specialised services to communities on an outreach basis (Cheers et al. 2007) in rural and remote settings. Some social workers are engaged as community developers and are facilitating rural revival or researching remote Aboriginal community livelihood strategies (Alston 2002; Ingamels 2008). Critical social workers bring to these job roles a structural and discursive understanding of power relations at the individual, cultural and structural levels (Mullaly 2002; Thompson 2006). Critical social workers pay attention to the specif c effects of various socio-political and discursive frameworks on various groups, including the gender, age, race and ablement dimensions. Regardless of the specif c social work job requirements, a critical overview and analysis of the impact of current policies on oppressed and marginalised populations in rural and remote communities are necessary for critical social work practice. Critical social workers aim to work towards social justice, and use an understanding of the mechanisms of oppression to explore specif c power relations within, between and external to rural and remote communities, in order to redress these oppressive relations at the individual, cultural and structural levels (Mullaly 2002; Thompson 2006).

I will brief y outline some aspects of the recent socio-political context of Australian rural and remote communities and some of the ecological, economic and social challenges confronting these settlements. The recent and very popular 'social capital' discourse inf uencing government policy and practices in rural and remote communities is critically reviewed, to illustrate the kind of structural and discursive analysis critical social workers can undertake to prepare for engaging with specif c communities. I apply a socio-political and discursive analysis to some of the current pressures on remote Aboriginal settlements in 'desert Australia' to comply with Western economic ways of life, regardless of their social, political, cultural and historical context. These socio-political and discursive analyses inform critical social work practices with rural and remote communities and assist social workers to engage effectively with communities, individuals and various sub-groups (Ingamels 2007).

Effects of globalisation and neo-liberal economic policies on rural and remote communities

Rurality, for most people, means a 'geographic location beyond the city, characterised at the very least by sparser population density, paucity of service infrastructure and a relationship with primary industry' (Briskman 1999: 4). The concept of rurality is often associated with how people who live rurally make their livelihoods; the usual conception is of primary industries like farming, f shing, forestry, hunting and mining. However, less than a quarter of rural residents are now employed in primary industry (Lockie & Bourke 2001: 6). This indicates one of the major shifts in livelihood strategies in rural and remote areas in Australia. For instance, in the period from 1970 to 1990, the total number of farms in Australia decreased signif cantly by over 64 000 farms (Higgins & Lockie 2001: 178). The pressure to compete in international markets and increase productivity was particularly intense for middle-range farms, rather than small farms where off-farm work by various family members, particularly women, could supplement annual income. These changes to livelihood practices have gender implications, as Alston (2002) indicates. Critical social workers aim to understand what these changes mean in relation to social justice outcomes, through an analysis of power relations, and engage with various community groups to identify and redress mechanisms of oppression or exploitation occurring within specif c rural and remote communities.

Overall, there has been a 'sharp exodus of population from inland towns to regional sponge cities and to the coast' (Alston 2002: 2). This has raised some conjecture over whether small inland rural towns will inevitably decline and whether small remote Aboriginal communities will be viable in the long term. This question of whether small rural and remote settlements will inevitably decline needs to be analysed from a critical social work perspective in relation to how global, national, regional and local policies have impacted adversely on small communities in relation to the opportunities and rights residents of these settlements have and can exercise. This issue becomes particularly poignant in relation to small Aboriginal homeland settlements in remote desert Australia. It could be argued that, to some extent, the decisions about rural and remote communities' viability and Australian governments' support for different ways of life in these non-urban settings represent a major ideological, political, historical, cultural, social and ecological battleground. These questions bring into focus the signif cance of these issues for Australian citizens' rights to self-determination over their livelihood strategies and diverse ways of life.

Rural and remote communities in Australia have been facing a number of global, national and regional changes. These major changes in economic policies and f uctuations in the global market have impacted on the prices of goods grown, made or mined in rural Australia. There have been worldwide changes in agricultural production, deregulation of the dairy industry and trials of genetic engineering, as well as moves to organic farming practices (Stewart & Lockie 2001). Major shifts in how property ownership rights are understood at the national and regional levels, and the development of new land use rights agreements, have brought additional challenges to various groups living in rural and remote areas. Native title, water rights and policy, and vegetation management legislation are all affecting relationships and livelihoods in rural and remote communities. Critical social workers, in working with specif c communities, need to analyse the impact of these major changes on the power relations within particular settlements and between related settlements, and generate an analysis with relevant groups about the implications for various sub-groups within the community.

In addition, due to Australian governments' privatisation and competition policies, many rural communities have 'experienced the loss or rationalisation of key services, such as hospitals, schools, police stations and welfare services' (Tonts 2005: 195; Harris 2007). This list can be extended also to include privatisation of postal services, differential rollout of telecommunications services (impacting on access to online educational services), bank closures and rationalisation (generally reductions, cancellations or non-introduction of new services) and public transport services. These recent changes in national economic policy appear to have made the situation in rural and remote areas more diff cult.

Alston (2002) indicates that rural areas are over-represented among the most disadvantaged. 'Poverty in rural Australia both on-farm and off-farm is generally higher, more widespread and more chronic than in urban areas' (Bourke 2005: 98). Usually, rural areas have much higher rates of unemployment. At times, rural areas seem to offer more affordable housing; however, living costs like food, transport, access to health and education are much higher. When working with rural and remote groups across various settlements, critical social workers need to engage in conversations about these broader socio-political factors impacting on the lives of people, to facilitate generating an analysis of the current predicaments and opportunities for various groups in these communities.

It is within this socio-political, economic and ecological context that neo-liberal government policy has positioned local rural and remote communities as able to address their problems through 'self-help' action. This renewed emphasis on localism, according to Bryson and Mowbray, 'effectively paves the way for low cost communitarian solutions' (2005: 93) rather than reducing inequalities through macro-level reforms. Bryson and Mowbray's analysis suggests that these 'low cost communitarian solutions . . . exonerate the state, businesses and the market from responsibility' (2005: 93). Critical social workers can engage with people affected by these changes to explore how this specif c policy discourse tends to shape people's understanding of the problems and their aspirations. This kind of analysis undertaken within a contextual socio-political framework assists social workers to highlight at a personal, cultural and structural level how communities have lowered both their aspirations and their expectations of governments, markets and business.

Analysing 'social capital' discourse

It is currently very common for researchers, policy makers, social service providers and community developers to use the notion of 'social capital' when working with rural and remote communities (Cocklin & Dibden 2005; Davies et al. 2008). The prominence of the 'social capital' discourse means that critical social workers need to engage critically with how the notion of 'social capital' discursively functions and its effects on various marginalised and oppressed groups. The notion of 'social capital' tends to refer to local community groups' level of trust, reciprocity, mutuality, shared norms of behaviour and a sense of belonging and commitment to a place—an intangible 'something', the 'glue' that makes communities function (Kay 2006). This kind of use of the notion of 'social capital' needs to be understood in relation to the recent broader neo-liberal policy attempts to realign the relations between governments, markets and communities. This realignment tends to shift the responsibility for social problems to individuals and communities, even though these problems are not usually within their local control.

The discourse of 'social capital' shifted governance from sectoral policies like agriculture to supporting more spatial (rural) policies (Shortall 2004). Rural and remote place-based policies tend to focus on rural areas' capacity to support themselves through 'capacity-building', 'community-based initiatives' and 'partnerships' (Shortall 2004: 109). Australian state governments have been making claims about 'strengthening communities, rebuilding social capital and addressing human needs in innovative ways' (Mowbray 2005: 255). One recent community-building scheme promoted its role as being to help 'small communities take charge of their destinies' (Mowbray 2005: 255). The concept of 'social capital' implies a notion of community that is about 'trust and reciprocity' about harmonious social relations of mutual support and benef t (Fraser 2005). It is this idea of 'community' that can 'all too easily obscure the social reality of communities and pre-empt the necessity to locate community in its wider socio-economic context' (Shaw 2007: 28). When the ideal of community comes to be treated as social fact by policy-makers, it is likely to be detrimental to rural and remote communities. One of the key concepts critical social workers bring to an analysis of the 'social capital' discourse is this awareness of how the concept of 'community' can be used ideologically in ways that repress analysis of power relations, both within the settlement and outside it.

A neo-liberal policy framework tends to present structural problems as local problems, and aims to encourage local communities to take action to redress these issues. Recently, this has meant Australian governments have been focusing their efforts on facilitating local communities to build their 'social capital' rather than addressing spatial inequality and poverty through multidimensional policy processes. When governments argue that it is a community's lack of 'social capital' that is impeding the community's economic and social viability, then this claim in effect blames the community for policy and ecological changes that are not within the community's control or agency. The way the current discourse of 'social capital' functions to blame communities makes it even harder for various groups in a community to make claims on governments for resources. Critical social workers can assist various community groups to identify how the discourse of 'social capital' and 'community' functions to disempower groups within the communities.

Critical social workers are clear that the term 'community' 'is def ned and applied in a myriad of ways' (Fraser 2005: 286), and that it 'remains deeply problematic' (Berner & Phillips 2005: 23). In the 'social capital' discourse, the term 'community' tends to subsume all differences and the plurality of interests; 'community' is treated as a 'single unitary 'subject', which oversimplif es reality (Shaw 2007: 28). By ignoring the conf icting interests between various groups in a community, those most powerless to inf uence the community agenda are further disempowered. It is important for the critical social worker to think about who is constituted as 'the community' and how the community's interests are understood. It can be detrimental to already disempowered groups in a community if social workers only listen to dominant interests (Gray 2005). How power relations are operating within rural and remote communities, and how less inf uential residents are affected by current policy discourses, is important for critical social workers to identify, recognise and articulate through various conversations, reports and in negotiations about policy implementation. An anti-oppressive approach to critical social work practice prioritises understanding the effects of a policy discourse within a socio-political framework like neo-liberalism on marginalised groups, and works to generate a specif c local analysis with and across various groups, including those groups usually left out of decision-making processes in particular settlements with the aim of resisting the ongoing negative effects of such discourses.

Surviving the 'dying town syndrome'

The discursive frame legitimating federal, state and local government concern with 'building community and connections' is based on positing 'social capital' as the missing link between what makes a successful community and what creates a def cit community. In Australia, some small rural towns are represented as taking action to 'survive the dying town syndrome' through building their social capital. Small towns, through various Community Capacity Building Initiatives or through various pilot schemes under the 'Building a Future for the Country' project developed by the Community Employment Council of Central Victoria, funded under the Regional Assistance Program by the Commonwealth Department of Employment, Workplace Relations and Small Business, have taken up the invitation by state and federal governments to take action (see Case study 20.1).

Case study 20.1: small town revival

A small rural town in the state of Victoria suffered a decline in population with the closure of mines, local government amalgamations and residents moving away for education, employment and business opportunities. Local agribusiness had been affected by the devastating effect of bushfires and the drought since the 1990s. The small town was offered a chance to be involved in a pilot scheme under the 'Building a Future for the Country' initiative funded under the Regional Assistance Program by the Commonwealth Department of Employment, Workplace Relations and Small Business.

The community residents formed a group that surveyed residents of the town and began a process of setting up sub-committees to rebuild and fit out community facilities. It planned to establish a youth activities centre, to develop a tourism industry plan, and to encourage business and product development and a food cooperative. The model used by the small-town group aimed to allow for the widest possible participation by community residents.

Mowbray (2005) considers these community projects to be typical consensual community development activities that do not challenge the broader governmental context for dealing with problems of inequality and poverty. These consensual activities are understood through the notion of 'social capital' to mitigate small rural towns' locational disadvantage by making the most of their existing resources and by importing some additional f nancial and human resources. These activities are not to be discounted for their value to individuals and to building a sense of community and a sense of belonging. Self-help can be an excellent tool, and collective self-help can be an effective way of pooling resources for mutual benef t (Berner & Philips 2005: 27).

There are, however, important limitations to 'self-help' to be considered by critical social workers. The internal dynamics of communities are complex in themselves, and meanings imposed by policy-makers based on external expectations of rural and remote communities' social cohesion can disenfranchise some individuals and groups to their detriment. Critical social work principles require that these detrimental effects are identif ed, recognised and articulated to address marginalisation and oppression.

Communities are systems of conf ict as well as cooperation; social policy and economic macro policies that focus only on cooperation may further harm groups who have the least power in setting community agenda or gaining access to resources by expecting the articulation of singular unitary community interest. Recognition of the diversity and complexity of people and needs in communities is recognised by critical social workers, who also aim to provide spaces for these marginalised voices to be heard, as part of a critical approach to community work.

Desert settlements

'The history of Aboriginal settlement patterns since colonisation has been impacted by successive, albeit overlapping, stages in Aboriginal affairs' (Young & Guenther 2008: 178). These policies ranged from protectionism and assimilation to self-determination in the last century. Many of the larger settlements in desert Australia were the result of government or church groups setting up reserves or missions without regard to proximity to markets, employment or other resources. There are about 30 towns of 1000 to 30 000 people each, mainly of non-Indigenous people, and 1200 settlements of twenty to 500 people that are mainly Indigenous in 'desert Australia'. Of the 33 186 Indigenous people in the desert, more than 4000 live in communities of fewer than 50 people, and they are highly mobile across the region (Young & Guenther 2008).

The 'emergence of distinct settlement structure on Aboriginal lands involving the formation of numerous, dispersed, small and discrete Indigenous communities', described by Taylor et al. (2006: 41–2), suggests a 'homelands movement'. 'The large number of small communities with fewer than 50 people are a clear manifestation of the homelands movement—enabled through land rights and native title legislation and the infrastructure support that could be leveraged throughout the 1980s' (Young & Guenther 2008: 178).

The homelands movement has ensured ongoing connection to country and facilitated 'a safer, healthier and culturally more satisfying lifestyle, free of the social stresses, alcohol abuse, petrol sniff ng and domestic violence of some of the larger communities and towns' (McDermott et al. 1998, cited in Young & Guenther 2008: 178). The homelands movement has also raised challenges for governments and communities around the provision of 'basic services deemed necessary for healthy and safe living—housing, water, sanitation and power supply' (Young & Guenther 2008: 178). The provision of education opportunities is also challenged by Aboriginal mobility patterns in desert Australia, which appear to meet both Aboriginal social identity needs and a need to engage with mainstream agencies that 'enforce the rules for receipt of income support' (Young & Guenther 2008: 179). The non-Aboriginal professional workforce is also highly mobile and transitory, as workers appear to make temporary moves to 'desert Australia' for career gains; this pattern of inward and outward migration also affects service provision in remote settlements.

Over the last few years, the intentional development of remote Aboriginal communities livelihoods strategies was framed by the Howard government's 'return-on-investment model where the conditions of investment and the prerequisite returns are clearly def ned before the provision of funds' (Government of Australia 2006a, cited in Rea & Messner 2008: 88). This places enormous pressure on remote Aboriginal communities to prove evidence of the long-term economic outcomes of livelihood strategies, a pressure that puts additional burdens on groups that are already underresourced by governments, business and markets. The expectation is that remote communities will design and develop livelihood strategies in ways that f t an economic model which takes little account of the political, social, cultural, geographic and historical contexts of these settlements. Critical social workers' emphasis on understanding the processes and structures that perpetuate domination and oppression highlights the importance of the socio-political analysis that contextualises these demands on remote Aboriginal communities.

Many of the events that happen in desert Australia are outside local control. For instance, mineral prices are set globally and are currently set high, and desert Australia has no inf uence over this (Stafford Smith 2008: 8). Tourism is affected by transport costs, sentiments and trends, all out of local control. Some aspects of local desert businesses like Aboriginal art may present opportunities for more local control over prices. 'The dramatic "state of emergency" declared by Australian prime minister John Howard in June 2007 is but one extreme example' of centralised decision-making (Stafford Smith 2008: 8). This means that remote communities do not have local control over many of these livelihood strategies and, according to Stafford Smith (2008: 131), have to 'orient themselves to manage for the variability' and the unpredictability of these changes.

One recent example of Aboriginal people having to orient themselves to major changes in their livelihood strategies was the abolition of the Community Development Employment Projects scheme by the Howard government and the reinstatement of the project by the Rudd government after it took off ce in November 2007 (see Case study 20.2).

Case study 20.2

The Community Development Employment Projects (CDEP) scheme historically grew out of a recognition that Aboriginal applicants from remote areas did not qualify for unemployment benefits, because they did not have a 'work history' (Sanders 2004: 1). Aboriginal people in remote areas do have a work history; however, 'the abolition of paternalistic training allowances and their partial replacement with award positions resulted' in a rapid increase in Aboriginal unemployment in remote Australia (Altman 2007: 1).

CDEP was introduced in the mid-1970s to deal with the dilemma of not being able to refuse unemployment benefits to people even if they could not realistically apply the 'work test' due to living in geographically remote areas where mainstream work 'may never become available' (Sanders 2004: 2). The program paid community councils rather than individuals so that work projects could be funded. This gave the Aboriginal community-based organisations a greater degree of funding security and flexibility than many other programs in activities undertaken according to local aspirations (Sanders 2004; Altman 2007). It also worked well for individual Aboriginal participants because it meant that they did not have to engage in the demanding administrative and exacting bureaucratic compliance requirements. The scheme worked well for governments because it was cost-effective and was based on 'active work participation, in many small communities remote from labour markets and commercial opportunities'. In some remote places, CDEP participation is the only source of employment and income (Altman 2007: 1). In 2004, despite 36 000 Aboriginal people and over 200 Indigenous organisations participating in CDEP, it was under threat.

In July 2007, the CDEP was abolished for Northern Territory communities under the Howard Liberal–National federal government intervention (see Chapter 8 for more details). The effects of abolishing the local CDEP organisations in the Northern Territory meant that enormous strain was put on the viability of 560 remote Aboriginal communities with populations of less than 100, almost all located on Aboriginal land. Altman considers that abolition of the CDEP in effect considerably disempowered remote Aboriginal communities.

In July 2008, the new federal Labor government reintroduced the CDEP. However, Indigenous Affairs Minister Jenny Macklin said that: 'The last thing we want is for people, especially young people, having their only aspiration to have a job on CDEP. We want their aspirations to be to get a properly paid job' (AAP 2008).

Asking Aboriginal people in remote communities to compete for 'real jobs' is part of a mainstreaming policy strategy that imposes Western economic and social norms on them. This emphasis on 'real jobs' for Aboriginal people living in remote areas indicates a return to an assimilationist policy, a form of cultural imperialism that reinforces current power relations and measures the subordinate groups against dominant norms (Mullaly 2002). Differences in complying with the norms become construed as def cits. Mullaly (2002: 46) indicates that, through cultural imperialism, 'the other' is made deviant, dangerous and inferior through negative stereotypes.

The recent press has painted remote Aboriginal communities as places where 'things are *really* bad'—and compared with Australia-wide standards, remote communities are badly underfunded. The Australian Medical Association is calling for a Royal Commission to examine why governments are underfunding Aboriginal communities (Briskman 2007a: 233). It is within this context of material deprivation that calls are made for remote Aboriginal communities to be entrepreneurial in exchange for government funds. Failure to comply is all too easily blamed on the incapacity of communities to develop 'social capital'. Critical social workers need to be alert to the effects of such policy discourses to not collude with policies that increase the hardship of people who are being exploited, dominated and oppressed. Cultural imperialism further functions to devalue an oppressed group's life. For critical social workers, recognising and valuing diverse forms of life and livelihood strategies are crucial parts of Australian citizens' right to self-determination.

Critical practice strategies for working in rural and remote communities

Critical social workers informed by an anti-oppressive approach need to engage in an ongoing quest to understand the socio-political and historical dimensions of interlocking patterns of power and inf uence. A discursive analysis adds to this understanding by highlighting how communities are being positioned and position themselves in relation to these wider socio-political contexts. The recent neo-liberal framework shifted responsibility to individuals and to rural and remote communities in ways that deny historical, ecological, economic, cultural and socio-political contexts and their impacts on various community groups in Australia, who are marginalised and oppressed. Critical social workers aim to engage with local communities to collectively generate understandings of the mechanism of oppression at the personal, cultural and structural level

(Thompson 2006: 27). This process has to be undertaken sensitively with specif c regard to the effects that gender, race, age, ethnicity and ablement have on various sub-groups within a community. An analysis of how power relations operate and impact on people's life chances and livelihood strategies is an important part of critical social work practice.

Critical social workers aim to use processes that are egalitarian, dialogical and participatory in generating with sub-groups in communities a socio-political, historical and cultural analysis of how they and the community as a whole are positioned in policy discourses. The effects of specif c discursive frameworks need to be collectively identif ed, articulated and recognised to develop an alternative framework for the construction of problems and solutions. Critical social workers can assist communities in undertaking these processes. The workers' skills in policy analysis, community development processes and the linking of personal, cultural and structural analysis of oppression mean that a wider gaze can be developed with community groups.

Ingamels (2007: 1) suggests that if our analysis takes a 'narrow gaze we might point to successful outcomes of the immediate kind' in these kinds of rural and remote community-building schemes. A wider gaze might help us to understand how these community-building and rural revival activities 'more broadly undermine local people' (Ingamels 2007: 1) by neglecting power relations within communities, and also within the broader governmental policy arena. Community-building schemes are promoted as helping 'small communities take charge of their destinies'; however, 'a critical analysis reveals nothing of the kind' according to Mowbray (2005: 255). What is not considered problematic is that 'local community action is often local class action instigated by the articulate and wealthy residents' (Blackstock 2005: 43).

There is a tension between consensual community development work in rural and remote communities and social action approaches (Weeks et al. 2003). To work with a community requires treating all sub-groups respectfully, regardless of their social and political position. It is crucially important that critical social workers using a community development approach adopt a democratic style of communication that facilitates equality of decision-making, respects differences and does not push one correct view on to the situation (Kenny 2006: 248). Critical social workers communicate across various sub-groups in a community, some of whom will have much more power in decision-making, access to resources and inf uence over the community's agenda and the agenda of external policy-makers. It is within these socially stratif ed power relations that critical social workers aim to empower marginalised groups and to f nd ways to work collectively 'against domination and manipulation' (Kenny 2006: 250). How power is used to 'nourish grassroots bottom-up activity, in the context of disadvantaged and powerless communities' is an ongoing challenge (Turner 2007: 13).

Conclusion

Critical social workers need to take into account the many socio-political, historical and ecological diff culties faced by rural and remote Australian communities in forging livelihood strategies and culturally diverse ways of life. It is important to continuously quest to understand the specif c mechanisms of oppression operating within a rural and remote community, and across related settlements. One of the key processes is to collectively generate with various groups an understanding of how the community and sub-groups within a community are being positioned through policy discourses, like 'social capital'. It is also important to analyse together how people are positioning themselves within these discourses to understand how relations of power are being produced and reproduced within rural and remote settings.

An anti-oppressive and empowerment approach to working in rural and remote communities requires that critical social workers engage with the socio-political dimensions of interlocking patterns of power and inf uence at the personal, cultural and structural levels. It is important to work at the pace of the community in generating these analyses and with great sensitivity to power differences, as well as differences in relation to race, gender, ethnicity, age and ablement. One important indicator of empowerment is whether all the sub-groups in the 'community' have a say over their own resources, 'set their own agendas based on their knowledge, their lived experience and their language' (Kenny 2006: 167), and do so in meaningful ways.

21

for a solidarity-based practice in the globalising context

Jacques Boulet

What does it take and feel like to 'act-think-local-global' as a social worker in the present global environment? I initially evoke the historical context, and then brief y examine aspects of globalisation and international social development, linking them with critical social work. I discuss notions of 'development' and human rights and their relevance for social workers and for the lives of those the profession touches in globalising—but still very local and diverse—contexts. Final thoughts are devoted to the role of social work education in a globalising and internationalising context, suggesting an alternative value-base for the profession, based on modes of reciprocal and solidary relationship.

The chapter offers only fragments of a context for thinking about 'global-local praxis', responses to my constant baff ement when facing so much human capacity for destruction but also an expression of hope in our willingness to see things through. It is based on my participation in the international solidarity movements for the past 45 years, working and living across f ve continents, f rst as a volunteer 'development worker' in the Congo in the mid- to late 1960s; and from the early 1970s as an academic and activist participant in international and local networks. Generally, I have been chronically astounded by the contradictions I have entered into when trying to 'do' something about global inequalities and injustices—and have felt worse when *not* trying to do so. The spirit of the chapter, therefore, leans more towards the sharing of 'wisdom' than the development of a 'body of knowledge'; it is written in a spirit of humility and deep gratitude to all those who let me share in their wisdom, knowledge and friendship ever since I started social work education in 1962, in my home country of Belgium.

A global perspective

While I barely refer to social work 'practice', the following has everything to do with social work 'practice', its theory and the changing context in which it occurs. Furthermore, attempting to appropriately elaborate 'global' processes and events in their interrelated objective and (inter)subjective dimensions requires much more space and many more layers of analysis. The 'critical' tradition of social work evocation of the 'personal' being 'political' maxim and of the 'structure–agency' dialectic—as this book illustrates—requires a great deal of intellectual effort when applied to the local and the 'known'; how much more overwhelming it is, then, to apply such principles to the expectation to 'think/act both globally and locally'. Consider issues like 'post'- and 'neo'-colonialism; the tragic history and present of the International Monetary Fund (IMF), World Trade Organization (WTO) and Structural Adjustment Policies; 'development aid'; famine, drought, water and resource politics; and traff cking of women and children. Add all the things the various science 'disciplines' have to say about the matter and you will start to appreciate what it might entail to link 'globalisation' and 'international social development' with critical social work practice and theory. Often only passing attention is given to such matters in professional social work and in social work education (Boulet 2001), as it is in our everyday lives.

Yet the September 11, 2001 attacks on the World Trade Center and the Pentagon, and the associated loss of life and other global (especially ecological) events since then—which have occupied so much media space and our emotional energies and conversations—bring 'home' the global in rather unsubtle and urgent ways. Suddenly, events usually occurring in places 'out there'—referred to as 'underdeveloped', 'Third World', 'un-civilised', at their closest located in 'our backyard' but generally well away from our doorstep—such events have now come 'home' to roost as some lesser-heard but harder-edged commentators opine. Attempts by our 'civilised' political, economic and opinion leadership to name these events 'terrorism' and get on with the business of eradicating it and exterminating their (assumed) perpetrators have come to sound unconvincing, especially when allowing ref ection about such events and empathy for their victims—or when applying knowledge, skills, attitudes and ethics associated with critical social work.

Indeed, how do we come to grips with the fact that, across the globe, all our pasts, presents and futures are inseparably bound up together? This occurs in a range of situations:

- whether sheltering from NATO missiles in drought-stricken Afghan or Iraqi mountainsides, wondering where our next meal will come from or whether we'll still 'be' when it comes
- or whether refusing entry to and residence in Australia to those fleeing the missiles, detaining them as 'illegal asylum seekers' on poverty-stricken Pacific islands, badly needing the cash we pay them to do that job
- or whether remembering that those arriving here two centuries ago—rejects and refugees-of-sorts from nations denying them present and future—took the land from its original owners, simply calling it 'nobody's land': *terra nullius*
- or whether—as Australian volunteers or contractors—erecting shelter against the blazing sun and bitter winter cold for Afghans, motivated by Christian or human rights and social justice ideals or just to make a living
- or whether contributing to support the volunteers, our tax-deductible donation derived from salaries made from or shares invested in the manufacture or sale of the missiles raining on Afghans and Iraqis
- or whether we, stressed social workers in Melbourne, Australia, recuperate on a Sunday afternoon with some retail therapy at global-Swedish IKEA, sipping a cappuccino before joining the throngs to pick a lounge suite to replace the barely three-years-old and out-of-fashion one, soon to move to the Vinnies' op shop frequented by—eventually 'legal'—Afghan and Iraqi refugees
- and finally, whether local community, educational and other services become unavailable because our ('developed'-Western) government decides that economic rationalism requires their privatisation and marketisation, or because the IMF/WTO forces our ('developing'-Southern) government to use our meagre economic resources to repay loans (plus interest) back into the pockets of those amongst us who, already having too much, gamble it away on the stock market.

Such are the challenges of inserting a global perspective into a reflective framework for critical social work practice and theory.

Social and community work in an international context

The field of international 'development' has seen remarkable transformations since the 1960s. Then, the term 'development cooperation' still captured reasonably well the attitude and motivation of those wanting to address the increasing evidence of past and ongoing ravages imposed on the 'developing' or barely postcolonial world. For a while, 'development' and 'cooperation' seemed to provide converging points for governments, NGOs and activists, with a strong emphasis on community development, education and rapid industrialisation, under the benevolent aegis of the f edgling sub-systems of the United Nations (including, rather timidly then, the World Bank and the IMF).

That convergence quickly shattered from the early 1970s; 'neo-colonialism' and 'imperialism' became standard concepts in the verbal repertoire of those of us in the developed West who were critical of the 'underside' of development 'aid'—of the 'Bad Samaritans' (Chang 2008) and their rather self-interested ways. Cast in the context of the (thawing) Cold War, the emergence of new social movements and a vigorous critique of globalising capitalism, our support for national liberation struggles in the dependent countries took shape, also generating initial traces of a critique of the development enterprise itself.

By the late 1970s, nagging doubts about the universal applicability of our analyses of the dependency syndrome began to rise. Features of the socialist project became suspect as the global roles of the Soviet Union and China grew more ambiguous—not to mention the growing evidence of the human price of their 'development' models. Our modernist certitude about the rightfulness and inevitability of the violence used by some liberation movements was shaken and we were appalled at the 'bourgeois' excesses of their leaders and governance systems after their victorious struggles. In line with emerging postmodern thought, our awareness grew of how much we had projected our own desires, frustrations and impotent rages into our support for the liberation struggles in dependent countries and we started to understand how much we—Western Marxists, humanists, feminists, environmentalists, critical/radical social workers—had homogenised and appropriated peoples' struggles against their specif c local oppressions. 'We' seemingly had expected 'them'—as if 'by proxy'—to f ght 'our' struggles against global oppression and alienation, a struggle we had found ourselves unable to persevere with—let alone win—in our own societies (Hobsbawm 2002).

Meanwhile, from the early 1970s and somehow by stealth, the onslaught of the neo-liberal, economic-rationalist reconstruction of the global 'order' spread, under the ideological-political hegemony of capitalism and the military-political powers sustaining it and sustained by it. While those of us 'on the left' were having great deductive arguments about the best ways to address both the global inequalities and the locally specif c, 'derived' problems, the logic and real-life practices of the political economy of capitalism were inexorably directing the worldwide course of events. Aided and abetted by the global bodies (World Bank, IMF/WTO), facilitated by the demise of the once dominant power of the 'second' world, the Soviet Union and its associates, (re-)imposition of Western hegemony on the rest of the world took its course virtually unopposed (Tabb 2002). Thatcher's 'There is No Alternative'—in short, TINA (Chang 2008)—sounded like the triumphant f nal nail in the coff n of 'the old order', where states and social movements still carried weight. Or so it seemed.

Indeed, the last twenty years certainly have sobered United States President Bush-the-elder's triumphal 1989 declaration after the 'fall' of the Soviet Union that a 'new world order' was to break loose, bringing 'wealth and solidarity' on the basis of 'market-oriented policies, democratic polities and individual rights', leading to the 'well-being of billions of people' (Lechner & Boli 2000: 7). As I write, many assumptions underlying the positive globalisation mantra have meanwhile 'melted down' with the global economy. We probably should have known earlier what provisos were attached to the New World Order when, at the occasion of the 1992 Rio Earth Summit, President Bush Senior enunciated that 'the lifestyle of the United States would not be up for discussion at Rio' (Sachs 1995).

Depending on where one is positioned along the continuum of political ideology and 'real' wealth and poverty, judgements about the outcomes of policies implemented by the second Bush at the end of his second term will vary, and they occupy a great proportion of the daily news we are fed via print and other media: dozens of wars, conf icts, genocide and oppression; shocking and growing inequalities; persistent ill-health epidemics; hunger and malnutrition contrasting with anorexia and obesity; the lack of shelter and of subsistence/income-generating work; ecological and economic disasters. It is a depressing list, inexorably leading to a question necessarily central to social work with any critical claim: how long does it take for Western moral indignation to tip the balance towards establishing the mere conditions for livelihood for all and to move away from short-term, self-interested economic and ideological calculation?

On the other hand, there have been successes scored by a groundswell of alliances of activist groups everywhere, including the 1999 blocking of the implementation of the OECD's Multilateral Agreement on Investments, worldwide attempts at preventing the further entrenchment of the WTO's policies geared at maintaining existing inequalities and leading to further deterioration of the environment (Tabb 2002; Chang 2008). The globalising resistance movements and events (Tabb 2002) will, hopefully, become historical markers on the road to a more accountable and just world. Given the growing reality of our hybrid communities everywhere and reaching deep into the centres of global power, it is more likely that whatever goes on anywhere will be transported across the globe right into the heart of Western capitals, thus making it less likely that the divide-and-rule strategy of those in power will remain unchallenged.

Thus, when the 2001 'terrorist attacks' on the symbols of Western hegemonic power carried the challenge violently and destructively right across the doorsteps previously thought to keep 'us' immune from 'them', the precariousness of our global 'arrangements' was suddenly brought 'home'. Add growing awareness of our human-made ecological fragility ('global warming') and the 'economic meltdown' occurring as I write these words and we are—possibly—w itnessing the strengthening of the conditions in which the groundswell of resistance mentioned before may lead to a more fundamental shift in global relationships and realities.

Yet, given the power of the 'guardians of public information', domestic repression and political populism inside Western nations may also increase, and recent and present events may cast the spell of suspicion and complicity on those of us who ask for more complex thinking about them. It will also likely bring more devastation to those groups, peoples and nations already suffering most from the present inequalities and exploitative relationships on a world scale and in their more local contexts.

Still, the multifaceted and multifaced resistance against the destructive aspects of globalisation, already receiving aff rmation from some 'serious' commentators during the early years of the new millennium, has now a veritable chorus of critics on its side. Amartya Sen—economics Nobel Prize winner—speaking in Melbourne in 2001, said:

> The world in which we live is both remarkably comfortable and thoroughly miserable. Faced with this dual recognition . . . [t]here is . . . a partial but effective congruence between the stubborn optimist and the incorrigible pessimist. The optimist f nds resistance unnecessary, whereas the pessimist f nds it useless. The opposing views unite in resignation . . . The protest movements against the global economy are often ungainly, ill-tempered, simplistic, frenzied and frantic, and yet they do serve the function of questioning and disputing the complacency about the world in which we live (*The Age*, 16 May 2001: 17).

About seven years after this pronouncement and several ecological and economic crises 'wiser', we now witness a minor f ood of works by 'converted' global economists and leaders of global institutions (Soros 1998, 2008; Stiglitz 2006; Bello 2008; Green 2008). Acceptance seems to grow that the neo-liberal, economic rationalist credo concocted during the early 1970s probably was not that fail-safe—indeed, it is now acknowledged that 'the Unholy Trinity of the IMF, the World Bank and the WTO' have imposed a 'level-playing f eld [which] leads to *unfair* competition *when the players are unequal*' [emphasis in original] (Chang 2007: 218).

Agreeing with Sen's suggestion in the above quote that interrogating the context of globalisation is a necessary task, critical social work and community development should ref ect on the very terminology and intervention modalities we use to critically understand and address the complex paradoxes hidden behind everyday phenomena associated with such context.

Reflections on the notion of development

The term 'development' is used in a variety of social work contexts ('child or lifespan development', 'organisational' or 'community development') and is often applied as a comparative marker of and for the assessment of the level of economic prowess and the level of wellbeing and welfare across nations and groups of people. The Western perspective on development suggests, rather arrogantly, that it represents the most successful of all past and present models of and for human existence, and that it is unproblematic overall, in spite of some minor—and largely unavoidable—side-effects. In addition, its semantic f eld does not easily allow variations of meaning, let alone alternative or competing ones, to be accepted as viable purposes for human living, individual and collective. Esteva's initial blast (in Sachs 1993: 8–9)—that 'Development occupies the centre of an incredibly powerful semantic constellation. There is nothing in modern mentality comparable to it as a force guiding thought and behaviour . . . [It] gave global hegemony to a purely Western genealogy of history, robbing peoples of different cultures of the opportunity to def ne the forms of their social life'—has meanwhile been joined by a plethora of other voices (Korten 1990, 1995, 2006; Verhelst 1990; Ndione 1992, 1994; Latouche 1993; Crush 1995; Escobar 1995; Sachs 1995; Tabb 2002). It has also been joined by work associated with the concept of Human Scale Development and 'real-life economics' (Max-Neef et al. 1991), as well as by the post-colonial (Said 1993), feminist (Mies & Shiva 1993) and ecological (Dow & Downing 2006; Stern 2006) voices.

My own examination of the 'hegemonic existential syndrome' of Western development/progress thinking, informed by postcolonial discourses, led to a framework which may assist in ref ecting on how the suggestive-ideological power of the development/progress belief system closes off our own minds, as it is dialectically supported by and in turn supports the existing 'objective' societal- and global-structural arrangements from which we Westerners benef t most. It also helps explain a great deal about the psycho-social predicaments with which Western social work deals in its daily practices. Having more fully developed it in the f rst edition of this book (2003), I summarise it here in the hope that it may support critical ref ection and dialogue within those committed to the critical tradition in social work.

Within the Western development/progress syndrome, I identify six 'praxis'-clusters (praxis being understood as a dialectically related set of ideological, normative and philosophical moments and associated and often distorted life-practices) which give meaning to and around which we organise our daily lives, our institutional arrangements and the overall structures and processes of our societies. Formulated as 'biases', the clusters can be summarised as follows:

1. The *economistic* bias and the focus on paid work as the main, central meaning-giving human activity, based on the assumption of the centrality of (capitalist) economic-utilitarian processes and relationships to both society and individual and the reductive conception of the human being as merely a 'homo economicus'.
2. The *political* bias of 'formal' representation and the focus on democracy as 'abstract' delegation, rather than 'participation', including the belief in the necessity of centralism and delegation as the proper and only way to cope with issues on a global scale, largely justifying existing forms of domination.
3. The Judeo-Christian *ideological* bias towards and focus on 'humans' as the species central to (the rest of) the universe, anthropocentrism being endemic to our Western conception of the self, both individually and collectively and often combined with Darwinist, creationist and other supremacist assumptions.
4. The *socio-cultural* bias towards the primary focus on the individual as the only relevant and autonomous ontological-existential category and as the only seat of morality, reducing the 'social' to a mere contractual arrangement or to an abstract political construct.
5. The masculine-patriarchal *gender* bias, leading to the degendering of the economy, the body politic and the systematic devaluing of women's work and actions, and of all non-commodif ed, non-paid or nurturing work.
6. The systematic *discursive/practical reversal of the material and spiritual dimensions* of our social-individual reproduction or recreation; the West as a merchant in commodities, artefacts and spiritual systems, dogmas and beliefs and the loss of 'connectivity' with other humans, the non-human and of spirituality.

I will return to some of these 'biases' and propose some alternatives, notably those we may want to (re-)learn from those peoples and cultures we have come to understand as 'less developed' than ourselves.

Human rights and social work

Over the past twenty years, Jim Ife (1995, 1997, 2008a) has attempted to establish Australian social work as a 'human rights profession', and another contribution can be found in this volume. I will therefore restrict my comments here to human rights' relevance for internationalisation. Ife posits (1995: 72) that 'rights not only provide a universal moral framework for the legitimation of a social justice perspective', but also support 'a model of empowerment-based practice'. Still, 'many of the ideals of the Universal Declaration are only imperfectly realised in the Australian context' (1995: 181), and Ife lists a series of domestic issues—Aboriginal peoples' rights, ecology, the social versus the individual (and their associated rights), public versus private, needs- versus rights-based policies, laws and interventions—which highlight the contradictory and potentially irresolvable tensions which emerge when dealing with 'rights-based' approaches to policy and practice. Ife nevertheless takes a f rm stand on the side of the 'universality' of rights, providing a moral and a legal basis for the pursuit of social justice (1995: 70), warning against 'a too ready acceptance of a relativist position', as this would be too easily misused to excuse oppressive practices.

Subsequently, Ife (2008a) has provided analyses of the nature of human rights, referring to the tensions existing between what is commonly referred to as the 'three human rights generations': the 'negative rights' establishing individual liberties; the 'positive rights' concerned with social justice, participation and freedom of want; and the 'collective rights' on regional, national and international levels (Berting et al. 1990; United Nations & Centre for Human Rights 1992: 6). Unfortunately, not much help is given with the 'universalists' versus 'relativists' dichotomy, which often leads to 'I-know-where-you-come-from' pigeonholing—based more on assumption than understanding—and which prevents establishing a more useful and creative tension between the universal and the specif c dimensions of rights. This tension is particularly important when considering issues we have been exploring, and which relate to the imposition of the Western mode of thinking and behaving on other people(s).

During the massive United States-initiated and supported human rights campaigns of the late 1970s, the years of the presidency of Jimmy Carter, the focus on human rights was often denounced as a political instrument of both the 'rich' Western nation states and of the various capital interests which made and still make up global capitalism:

> So when the capitalist world, and especially its richest countries, are faced with the real problems of their survival, the diplomacy of human rights is quickly forgotten,

> for it is in fact a luxury for the rich countries. And the United States only accept to pay themselves this luxury as there are no more fundamental emergencies which solicit their attention (Jouve 1979: 91).

If, as is often claimed, human rights are indivisible, why is it that the right to a life without poverty, the right to development and to work, are recognised or pursued with much less vigour, if at all, by those same countries? The successive UN 'Summits' (particularly the Social Development [Copenhagen 1995] and Environment [Rio 1992] Summits and their ten-year follow-up meetings) have incisively demonstrated the double standards applied by many human rights protagonists. This is especially so when viewed against the background of the crisis—even if denied by some (e.g. Weiss 1998)—of the nation-state, the traditional *bête-noire* against which human rights of the 'individual' were to be established and maintained. Paradoxically, it is also demonstrated when realising that UN agencies themselves (IMF/WTO and World Bank) are doing a lot of the damage.

Kilby (1994: 20) equally indicates that the human rights abuses being detected and discussed seem solely to refer to civil and political rights and the various conventions which enshrine them. By contrast, rights of the 'second generation'—those relating to social, economic and cultural matters, including the right to development—are 'largely ignored and often openly f outed by donor and recipient countries'. Kilby refers to the fact that some of the 'small script' which comes together with Structural Adjustment Programs 'directly contravenes the Conventions' relating to these rights: the 'right to a free elementary education is fast disappearing; freedom from hunger and the equitable distribution of the world's food resources is not happening; and the access for all to medical services is declining'. And, if anything, the situation has become worse since the time of Kilby's writing (Murphy 2003; Chan 2008).

Addressing the tension between universality and specif city, Wendy Brown (1995: 97) confronts a set of paradoxes about rights, 'the central one of which is the question of the liberatory or egalitarian force of rights [which] is always historically and culturally circumscribed'. Brown maintains that 'rights have no inherent political semiotic, no innate capacity either to advance or impede radical democratic ideals'. On the other hand, they 'operate in and as an a-historical, a-cultural, a-contextual idiom . . . and they necessarily participate in a discourse of enduring universality rather than provisionality or partiality'. Brown (1995: 134) warns against making rights too 'specif c' and against 'attaching them' to the 'current constitutive injuries' of certain groups of people. She fears that such strong specif city (for example, focusing rights on 'the hungry', 'the poor' or 'the disabled') 'may draw on our least expansive, least public, and hence least democratic sentiments'. She advocates inserting rights within the context of 'an egalitarian political community' so that—'in the abstraction from the particulars of our lives'—they can be made valuable in the 'democratic transformation of these particulars'.

It is useful contribution, but inconclusive as to how practical applications and systematic translations from the universal to the culturally, geographically, socially and gender-specif c are to be made. Critically evaluating Brown's hopes attached to the universalising of human rights, we should listen to Emmanuel Wallerstein, urging us to understand the present and future of human rights as part and parcel of the 'Insurmountable Contradictions of Liberalism':

> Liberalism today is cornered by its own logic. It continues to assert the legitimacy of human rights and, a bit less loudly, the rights of peoples. It still doesn't mean it . . . The self-contradiction of the liberal ideology is total. If all humans have equal rights, and all peoples have equal rights, then we cannot maintain the kind of inegalitarian system that the capitalist world-economy has been and always will be . . . And if this system has no legitimacy, it will not survive (1995: 1175–7).

This is a useful reminder in the aftermath of the 'terrorist attacks' and in the context of the 'eradication of terrorism' euphoria seemingly engulf ng the 'free' (and rich) part of the world.

Looking more specif cally at social work and welfare policy, the debate around the universality of needs, claims and rights remains somewhat subdued in the local discourses (apart from Jim Ife's work), and it may be useful to revisit some previous contributions. Drover and Kerans (1993: 11) are critical of an unqualif ed adherence to and promotion of universal rights as they are based on 'respect due to an abstract, generalised, disembedded and disembodied other'. They see such universalism as 'substitutionalist' rather than 'interactive' and—with Benhabib (1989)—suggest that it rests on a 'paradigmatic' assumption of the human as, generally, white, male, propertied adults and that 'people who def ne themselves or are socially def ned in other ways are understood as lacking'. Drover and Kerans (1993: 11) conclude that a 'ref ection on welfare cannot rest content with the received distinction between the right and the good, nor that between public and private'.

Various attempts have been made during the last decades to reconceptualise the relationship between 'basic/universal' and 'relative' understandings of need, especially those deriving from the feminist debates about the ambiguity of the concept. Nancy Fraser (1989), borrowing from Geertz's (1973) characterisation of ethnography as the 'thick description' of reality, proposed to distinguish between 'thin' and 'thick' needs as two ends of a spectrum, thus avoiding the oppositional dichotomisation inherent in the universal–relative conceptual pair:

> [The] 'thin' notion of need is abstract, objective and universal . . . developed to show that need has 'moral weight', that it implies an obligation on the part of others to meet it, hence it provides the moral foundation for the non-market allocation of resources' [while the] 'thick' understanding of need is rooted in an attempt to understand the cultural context in which people name their needs . . .

They further state, adopting Benhabib's post-colonial stance (1989: 415–16), that the purpose of a thick, interpretive approach is critical rather than prescriptive, and points to the 'ideological limits of universalistic discourse—the unthought, the unseen and the unheard in such theories'. And this 'can only happen within a framework which is dialogical, where those without power are heard out as carefully as any other' (Fraser 1989). Drover and Kerans (1993: 11) conclude that such a framework needs to focus on 'the politics of need interpretation', as claims arising from the particularities of everyday experiences and incommensurate with others will be contested.

What I am suggesting here is the possibility that 'universal-thin' descriptions of rights, while having their usefulness as 'benchmarks' for minimum conditions and claims across the spectrum of cultures and social specif cities, are to be complemented by 'specif c-thick' negotiated understandings of what they 'mean' for the locally concrete situation within which they are to be implemented, with the aim of improving people's lives and of responding to their 'fundamental-yet-specif c' needs. There is, therefore, a need for 'important postmodernist investigations [which] will not be rejecting modernist assumptions [for example, those expressed in universalist or essentialist terms] as such but rather problematising them in some "positive" rather than "negative" way' (McLennan 1994: 120). And as Paolo Carozza (2003: 38) suggests: 'The principle of subsidiarity . . . gives us a conceptual tool to mediate the polarity of pluralism and the common good in a globalized world and helps us make sense of international human rights law.'

Finally, enlarging on Brown's suggestion to insert the rights-needs discourse into the discourse about democracy and equality, Caroline New (1996: 94), discussing eco-feminism, proposes that such theoretical work:

> would encourage the creative critique of current political forms and methods. It would require the extension of the practical critique of dualism to the overlapping dimensions of class, ethnicity, and so on. It would offer . . . alongside irreducibly

real sectional interests, the ethical vision of grounded human solidarity, of human interests in reversing the current destructive trend.

Clearly, the need for such a vision will increase, given our ecological predicaments and f nite global/local resources (Barlow 2007; Harcourt 2008).

Some possibilities for critical and solidarity-based social work

Given the traditional presence of the 'needs debate' in critical social work discourse, the suggested integration of such investigations would offer the 'rights debate' a useful beginning framework, to which the work of Manfred Max-Neef (1991) would equally powerfully contribute, based on a strong ontological, epistemological and methodological foundation towards 'dreaming' better futures for humanity and the cosmos of which it is part.

'Subsidiarity'—the 'principle that each social and political group should help smaller or more local ones accomplish their respective ends without, however, arrogating those tasks to itself' (Carozza 2003: 38)—is to be given a higher prof le (Lowell 2006: 5), and considerations of a new 'public ethics'—asking for a reconsideration of the linkages between governments and governance, civic participation and activism, global civil society and global accountability—are urgently needed. Ebrahim and Weisband (2007: 317) demand that 'the ethical implications of global interdependencies are realized in practical terms by means of *accountability networking* as an organizational form'. They suggest (2007: 321), quoting David Held (2004), the development of a 'cosmopolitan multilateralism' based on '*the principles of global subsidiarity*', leading to global accountability, which combines participatory praxis with f uid concentric circles of governance ensuring 'inclusiveness, subsidiarity, and, by implication, greater accountability'. To that end, 'sovereignty can and should be dispersed horizontally and vertically, to multiple levels and loci of authority, each exercising distinct and determinate power over kinds of human practice and resources' (2007: 331). With Kuper (2004), they assert that: '*Principles of Distributive Subsidiarity and Democracy* [would] connect the lines between citizen activism, networks, accountability, and postmodern public ethics.'

I also suggest (Boulet 2007) that it would be timely for us to revisit the 'notions of solidarity and partnership [as they] are inherently inappropriate to describe most processes covered within the ambit of mainstream development aid . . . [and have become] detached . . . from anything development "experts" [and social workers] live their lives like and from anything remotely relevant for the real lives of the real people to be "aided"'.

I assert elsewhere (Boulet et al. 2008) that we generally need to redevelop our ways of thinking about relationships of reciprocity and solidarity and could learn enormously from Indigenous intelligence (Resurgence 2008) and the submerged work on gift-relationships (Godbout & Caillé 1998; Mauss 2002; Papilloud 2004; Healey et al. 2006) to replace their often implicit structural-functionalist assumptions. As social work should rightfully be called a 'relational' profession, a critical and solidarity-based social work approach should not be satisf ed with a notion of relationship resting on the paradigm positing self-centred individuals engaged in utilitarian market exchanges at its heart.

Conclusion

I conclude these ref ections with a call on critical social work educators to take the task of 'globalising' their respective curricula seriously and comprehensively. This call is based on the following four broad philosophical-practical grounds, and I offer them as a possible guide to ref ect on existing curricula and their associated teaching and learning formats and practices, and the content associated with them (Boulet 2001):

- The global–local futures of all of us—North–South and East–West—are all bound up together; from our factual interconnectedness through communications to the inexorability of the socio-ecological consequences of our individual and collective acts.
- We, in the dominant North or West, have a responsibility to recognise and redress past injustices to the peoples of the non-West/North and their ongoing consequences.
- Social work and welfare thinking has traditionally and generally assumed, and continues to assume, that the necessity of addressing the unequal distribution of resources can be diminished by the possibility of an ever-expanding availability of resources. The f niteness of resources and, therefore, of 'growth', however, inexorably forces us to shift our focus to global–local political and economic mechanisms and relationships of redistribution.
- Finally, looking at the decay of ethical/moral grounding increasingly revealed throughout our Western/Northern ways of living, acting and thinking, and our apparent inability to properly understand our common predicament, learning from the wisdom and practices of those who are 'differently civilised' is becoming a necessity for our common survival. For social workers, that would def nitely include the need to learn from colleagues from other places and cultures.

notes

Chapter 1: Introducing critical theories for social work in a neo-liberal context

1 See Fraser (1991) for an attempt to integrate feminist perspectives with critical theory.

Chapter 2: Tracing the origins of social work practice

1 *Editors' note:* A number of our contributors have used the word 'black' and we are aware that there is an ongoing debate about usage of this term. For this reason we have ensured that as much as possible use is sparing, context-specif c and denotes the ongoing colonialism that reproduces racialised hierarchies.

Chapter 3: Theorising new developments in critical social work

1 Wood and Middleman (1989) and later Goldberg Wood and Tully (2006), drawing on postmodern ideas, revised Middleman and Goldberg's earlier work. Essentially the interpretation of structural social work embedded in these writings is premised on a view that social problems are based in a social environment that lacks adequate or appropriate resources and leaves the structures of society intact.

2 Healy (2005a: 198) notes the need for development of postcolonial perspectives in social work theory and practice to bring greater insights to how colonialist ideas have inf uenced modernist and anti-racist approaches.

3 Poststructuralism is a term often equated with postmodernism, but more particularly is related to deconstruction of language and meaning, viewing truths as constructed in language and discourses (Macey 2000: 309).

Chapter 4: From evidence-based practice to critical knowledge in post-positivist social work

1 The concept of 'critical knowledge-informed practice' is my own formulation, one that is yet to be fully developed. I am proposing that critical social workers elaborate this as an alternative knowledge base for social work practice.

Chapter 8: Reversing colonial practices with Indigenous peoples

1 Practical reconciliation stems in part from a formal reconciliation process that ran for ten years from 1991 in order to improve relationships between Aboriginal and Torres Strait Islander peoples and the wider community. Although hailed as a success by some for increased

understandings, the process was critiqued for its failure to deliver tangible outcomes that redressed the socioeconomic divide.

Chapter 9: Reconstructing social work practices with families

1 With thanks to Nikki Butler, Lee Darroch and Sue Beecher for comments on the Aboriginal and practice content.
2 Dependent children are those aged under f fteen years or full-time dependent students under 24 years of age.
3 Thanks to Tracy Castelino for permission to use her case scenario of Bruce, Gina and Talia.
4 All names are pseudonyms and the case scenarios are f ctional.
5 Complementary to the Lakidjeka service is the Dhum Djirr Aboriginal Family Decision Making Program, also managed through the Victorian Aboriginal Child Care Agency. This program promotes the view that responsibility for bringing up children is shared by parents together with extended family, community and Elders (VACCA 2008).

Chapter 10: Examining the meaning of childhood in critical social work practice

1 Apart from cited quotes that are referred to in this chapter, I have also used inverted commas around some concepts. The usage of the inverted commas is sometimes a convention of social constructionism whereby the author wants to draw attention to the critical perspective being taken for some concepts. In the chapter, I have sought to critically question and disrupt the concepts of the 'child', 'adult' and 'parent'.
2 See, for example, the European Network of Ombudspersons for Children. (2007, <www.ombudsnet.org/enoc/members/member.asp?id=3085>); Children's Ombudsman Off ces in the United States (2008, <www.ncsl.org/programs/cyf/ombuds.htm>); the National Children's Bureau, UK (2007, <www.ncb.org.uk/Page.asp?originx2572po_27291116328194w8n1361462404>).

Chapter 11: Using critical reflection to improve feminist practice

1 As this case study represents a critical ref ection on my practice, it necessarily focuses on my interpretations and experience. It does not attempt to represent the experiences of the service user or other professionals involved.
2 A pseudonym has been used to preserve conf dentiality and protect the identity of the service user.
3 Many of the ideas in this chapter have been informed by unpublished research that I am currently undertaking for my PhD thesis, 'Critical postmodernism and social change: Using critical ref ection to reconstruct possibilities for change orientated social work practice in the context of the legal system's response to victim/survivors of sexual assault', at La Trobe University, Melbourne.

Chapter 12: Challenges and directions for profeminist practice with men

1 The emphasis in this chapter is on what men can contribute to ending sexism. Following Pringle (1997), I do not believe it is appropriate for men to suggest what women should do to challenge patriarchal gender relations. Furthermore, a number of feminist commentators have already proposed feminist strategies for working with men. See, for example, Cavanagh and Cree (1996), Dominelli (1999) and Orme et al. (2000).

Chapter 14: Disabling discourses and enabling practices in disability politics

1 For references that reveal the complexity of insitutionalisation, see Walmsley (2005) and Johnson (1997).

Chapter 16: Weaving together the personal and the political in loss and grief

1 In a recent Australian sociological study examining the place of the cemetery within concepts of grief, Bachelor (2002) reveals that, annually, around 33 million visits are made to Australia's 2300 cemeteries.

2 Holocaust survivors from Europe, people f eeing regimes in which ethnic cleansing has been practised (for example, Cambodia and Burma) and more recently, those f eeing civil wars and highly repressive regimes such as those in Afghanistan and Sudan, are examples of these movements.

3 For a useful account of the patterns of care in traditional, modern, late modern and postmodern societies, refer to Walter (1999: 185–7).

Chapter 19: Enacting critical social work in publicly funded contexts

1 For a more detailed history of the development of the Looking After Children Framework in the United Kingdom, Australia and elsewhere see, for example, Parker et al. (1991); Kufeldt et al. (2000); Wise (2002, 2003).

2 For further information regarding the Looking After Children Framework process, visit <www. lacproject.org>.

3 With the exception of the Assessment and Action Record, these documents are now completed electronically in Victoria. The page numbers of the previous hard copies are listed to convey a sense of the breadth of the information contained in the tools and the work involved for social workers.

references

AAP 2008, 'Macklin says CDEP reforms on the way', *SBS World News Australia*, Thursday, 10 July.

AASW 2002, *AASW Code of Ethics 1999*, 2nd edn, Australian Association of Social Workers, Barton, <www.aasw.asn.au/adobe/about/AASW_Code_of_Ethics-2004.pdf> [7 October 2008].

——2008, Australian Association of Social Workers, *Draft Australian Social Work Education and Accreditation Standards*, 2 September.

ABS 1996, 'Australian Bureau of statistics: housing stock: housing conditions of indigenous people 4102.0', *Australian Social Trends*, 24 June.

——2005, *Australian Bureau of Statistics 1286.0—Family, Household and Income Unit Variables*, 1 June.

——2006, *Australian Bureau of Statistics 2006 Census Data*, Australian Bureau of Statistics, Canberra, 10 September 2008.

——2007, *Australian Bureau of Statistics 6287.0—Labour Force Characteristics of Aboriginal and Torres Strait Islander Australians, Estimates from the Labour Force Survey*, 22 May 2008.

——2008a, Australian Bureau of Statistics 4442.0—Family Characteristics and Transitions Australia 2006–07, 6 June.

——2008b, *2008 Year Book Australia*, Australian Bureau of Statistics, Canberra.

ACF 2008, *Australian Childhood Foundation*, <www.childhood.org.au/research/reports.asp>.

Achenbaum, W.A. 1997, 'Critical gerontology', in *Critical Approaches to Ageing and Later Life*, eds A. Jamieson, S. Harper and C. Victor, Open University Press, Buckingham, pp. 16–20.

Age of Majority n.d., <http://en.wikipedia.org/wiki/Age-of-majority> [11 June 2008].

AIC (Australian Institute of Criminology) 2001, *Young Australians and Domestic Violence*, Trends and issues, no. 195, AIC, Canberra.

AIHW 2002, *Older Australia at a Glance*, 3rd edn, Australian Institute of Health and Welfare & Department of Health and Ageing, Canberra.

——2003, *Australia's Welfare*, Australian Institute of Health and Welfare, Canberra.

——2007a, Australian Institute of Health and Welfare: Child Protection Australia 2005/06, *Child Welfare Series no. 40*. cat. no. CWS 28, <www.aihw.gov.au/publications/index.cfm/title/10527> [19 September 2008].

——2007b, *Older Australia at a Glance*, 4th edn, Australian Institute of Health and Welfare, Canberra.

Alberti, S. 2000, 'Changing the system through casework: a critical incident analysis', in *Breakthroughs in Practice: Theorising critical moments in social work*, eds L. Napier and J. Fook, Whiting & Birch, London, pp. 38–48.

Albury, R. 1998, 'The status of human embryos', *Journal of Australian Studies*, no. 59, pp. 129–38.

Alford, J. and O'Neill, D. 1994, *The Contract State: Public management and the Kennett government*, Centre for Applied Social Research, Deakin University, Geelong.

Alinsky, S.D. 1971, *Rules for Radicals: A pragmatic primer for realistic radicals*, Random House, New York.

Allan, J. 2003, 'Practising critical social work', in *Critical Social Work: An introduction to theories and practices*, eds J. Allan, B. Pease and L. Briskman, Allen & Unwin, Sydney, pp. 52–71.

——2005, 'The role of meaning construction in living with grief', in *Social Work in Health and Mental Health: Issues, developments, and actions*, eds T. Heinonen and A. Metteri, Canadian Scholars' Press, Toronto.

Allan, J., Pease, B. & Briskman, L., eds 2003, *Critical Social Work: An introduction to theories and practices*, Allen & Unwin, Sydney.

Allen, J. and Gordon, S. 1990, 'Creating a framework for change', in *Men in Therapy*, eds R. Meth and R. Pasick, Guilford Press, New York.

Allen, S. 1996, 'Sexual assault law reform', *Balancing the Scales*, National Conference on Sexual Assault, Perth, 20–21 June.

Allers, C.T., Benjack, K.J. and Allers, N.T. 1992, 'Unresolved childhood sexual abuse: are older adults affected?', *Journal of Counseling and Development*, vol. 71, pp. 14–17.

Alston, M. 2000, 'Rural poverty', *Australian Social Work*, vol. 53, no. 1, pp. 29–34.

——2002, 'Inland rural towns: are they sustainable?' *Academy of the Social Sciences*, Rural Communities at the Outlook conference, Canberra.

Alston, M. and McKinnon, J., eds 2001, *Social Work: Fields of practice*, Oxford University Press, Melbourne.

——eds 2005a, *Social Work: Fields of practice*, 2nd edn, Oxford University Press, Melbourne.

——2005b, 'Context of contemporary social work practice', in *Social Work: Fields of practice*, 2nd edn, eds M. Alston and J. McKinnon, Oxford University Press, Melbourne, pp. 1–15.

Altman, J.C. 2007a, *Neo-paternalism and the Destruction of CDEP*, Topical Issue no. 14, Centre for Aboriginal Economic Policy Research, Canberra.

——2007b, 'The Howard government's Northern Territory intervention: Are neo-paternalism and Indigenous development compatible?', Topical Issue no. 16, Centre for Aboriginal Economic Policy Research, Canberra.

Altmann, C. 2006, *After Port Arthur: Personal stories of courage and resilience ten years on from the tragedy that shocked the nation*, Allen & Unwin, Sydney.

Alvesson, M. and Willmott, H. 1996, *Making Sense of Management: A critical introduction*, Sage, London.

Alway, J. 1995, *Critical Theory and Political Possibilities*, Greenwood Press, Westport, CN.

Alzheimer's Association 2005, *What is Dementia?*, Alzheimer's Association Australia, <www.alzheimers.org.au/upload/HS1.1.pdf> [5 October 2008].

Amnesty International 2002, 'Children and the death penalty: executions worldwide since 1990', <http://amnesty.org/en/library/info/ACT50/007/2002> [12 June 2008].

Anastas, J.W. 2007, 'Theorizing (in)equity for women in social work', *Affilia, Women and Social Work*, vol. 22, no. 3, pp. 235–9.

Anderson, F. 2005, 'Into the night: Max Crawford, the labyrinth of the social studies enquiry and ASIO's spoiling operations', *Australian Historical Studies*, no. 125, pp. 60–80.

Anderson, P. and Wild, R. 2007, *Ampe Akelyernemane Meke Mekarle, Little Children are Sacred*, Report of the Northern Territory Board of Inquiry into the Protection of Aboriginal Children from Sexual Abuse, Northern Territory Government, Darwin.

Andronico, P. 1999, 'Introduction', in *Men in Groups: Insights, interventions and psychoeducational work*, ed. P Andronico, American Psychological Association, Washington, DC.

Antal, A.B. and Friedman, V. 2003, 'Negotiating reality as an approach to intercultural competence', <http://skylla.wzb.eupdf/2003/iii03-101.pdf> [24 April 2008].

APEA:WA 2006, *Elder Abuse Protocol: Guidelines for action*, Alliance for the Prevention of Elder Abuse, Perth.

Argyris, C. and Schon, D. 1976, *Theory in Practice: Increasing professional effectiveness*, Jossey-Bass, San Francisco.

Ariès, P. 1962, *Centuries of Childhood*, Penguin, Ringwood.

Arulampalam, S., Perera, L., de Mel, S., White, C. and Denborough, D. 2005, 'Stories from Sri Lanka—responding to the tsunami', *International Journal of Narrative Therapy and Community Work*, no. 2, pp. 3–10.

Atkinson, G. and Pease, B. 2001, 'The changing role of Indigenous men in community and family life: a conversation between Graham Atkinson and Bob Pease', in *Working with Men in the Human Services*, eds B. Pease and P. Camilleri, Allen & Unwin, Sydney.

Atkinson, J. 2002, *Trauma Trail, Recreating Song Lines: The transgenerational effects of trauma in Indigenous Australia*, Spinifex Press, Melbourne.

——2008, 'Educare and human rights: an Indigenous Australian response to the effects of colonisation and trauma', in *Activating Human Rights in Education: Exploration and innovation*, eds C. Newell and B. Offord, Australian College of Educators, Canberra, pp. 119–32.

Atkinson, J. and Ober, C. 1995, 'We Al-Li "Fire and Water": a process of healing', in *Popular Justice and Community Regeneration: Pathways of Indigenous reform*, ed. K. Hazelhurst, Praeger Press, Westport, CN.

Attig, T. 1996, *How We Grieve: Relearning the world*, Oxford University Press, New York.

Australian Association of Social Workers (AASW) 1999, *Code of Ethics*, 2nd edn, AASW, Canberra.

Australian Association of Social Workers, Victorian Branch 1973–74, *Newsletter*.

Australian Broadcasting Corporation (ABC) 2002, 'Corporate Collapse', *Compass*, Sunday, 10 March, <www.abc.net.au/compass/s501466.htm> [30 June 2008].

Australian Social Work 2008, vol. 61, no. 2, June.

AVERT 2008, 'Worldwide ages of consent', <www.avert.org/aofconsent.htm> [16 June 2008].

Avis, M. 2006, 'Evidence for practice, epistemology and critical ref ection', *Nursing Philosophy*, vol. 7, pp. 216–24.

Ayres, I. and Gerarda Brown, J. 2005, *Straightforward: How to mobilize heterosexual support for gay rights*, Princeton University Press, Princeton, NJ.

Bachelor, P. 2002, *Life after Death: Understanding bereavement and working through grief—24 real life stories*, Hill of Content, Melbourne.

Bagshaw, D., Chung, D., Couch, M., Lilburn, S. and Wadham, B. 2000, *Reshaping Responses to Domestic Violence: Research into the needs of women, men and young people who have experienced domestic violence*, vol. 1, Off ce of Status of Women, Department of Prime Minister and Cabinet, Canberra.

Bailey, D. 2002, 'Mental health', in *Critical Practice in Social Work*, eds R. Adams, L. Dominelli and M. Payne, Palgrave, Basingstoke, pp. 169–80.

Bailey, R. and Brake, M. 1975, eds, *Radical Social Work*, Edward Arnold, London.

Bainbridge, L. 1999, 'Competing paradigms in mental health practice and education', in *Transforming Social Work Practice: Postmodern critical perspectives*, eds B. Pease and J. Fook, Allen & Unwin, Sydney, pp. 179–94.

Baines D. 1997 'Feminist social work in the inner city: the challenges of race, class, and gender', *Affilia*, vol. 12, no. 3, pp. 297–317.

——ed. 2007a, *Doing Anti-Oppressive Practice: Building transformative politicized social work*, Fernwood Publishing, Halifax, BC, Canada.

——2007b, 'Bridging the practice-activism divide in mainstream social work: advocacy, organising and social movements', in *Doing Anti-Oppressive Practice: Building transformative politicized social work*, ed. D. Baines, Fernwood, Halifax, BC, Canada.

——2007c, 'Extending a radical tradition: building transformative, politicised social work', in *Doing Anti-Oppressive Practice: Building transformative politicized social work*, ed. D. Baines, Fernwood, Halifax, BC, Canada.

——2007d, 'Anti-oppressive social work practice', in *Doing Anti-Oppressive Practice: Building transformative politicized social work*, ed. D. Baines, Fernwood, Halifax, BC, Canada, pp. 1–20.

Baker, M. 2001, *Families, Labour and Love: Family diversity in a changing world*, Allen & Unwin, Sydney.

Baldwin, M. 2000, *Care Management and Community Care: Social work discretion and the construction of policy*, Ashgate, Aldershot.

——2004, 'Critical ref ection: opportunities and threats to professional learning and service development in social work organisations', in N. Gould and M. Baldwin, *Social Work, Critical Reflection and the Learning Organisation*, Ashgate, Aldershot.

Balen, R., Blyth, E., Calabretto, H., Fraser, C., Horrocks, C. and Manby, M. 2006, 'Involving children in health and social research', *Childhood*, vol. 13, pp. 29–48.

Balswick, J. 1982, 'Male inexpressiveness: psychological and social aspects', in *Men in Transition*, eds K. Solomon and N. Levy, Plenum Press, New York.

Barlow, M. 2007, *Blue Covenant: The global water crisis and the coming battle for the right to water*, Black Inc., Melbourne.

Barnett, C. 2008, 'Publics and markets: what's wrong with neoliberalism?' in *The Handbook of Social Geography*, eds S. Smith, S. Marston, R. Pain and J.P. Jones, Sage, London.

Barnoff, L. and Coleman, B. 2007, 'Strategies for integrating anti-oppressive principles: perspectives from feminist agencies', in *Doing Anti-Oppressive Practice: Building transformative politicized social work*, ed. D. Baines, Fernwood, Halifax, BC, Canada.

Bell, D. and Binnie, J. 2000, *The Sexual Citizen: Queer politics and beyond*, Polity Press, Cambridge.

Bell, D. and Klein, R. 1996, *Radically Speaking: Feminism reclaimed*, Spinifex Press, Melbourne.

Bell, V. 1993, *Interrogating Incest: Feminism, Foucault and the law*, Routledge, London.

Bello, W. 2008, *A Primer on the Wall Street Meltdown, Inquirer*, 1 October, <http://opinion.inquirer.net/viewpoints/columns/view/20081001-163889/A-primer-on-the-Wall-Street-meltdown> [18 January 2009].

Benjamin, A. 2007, 'Afterword—doing anti-oppressive social work: the importance of resistance, history and strategy', in *Doing Anti-Oppressive Practice: Building transformative politicized social work*, ed. D. Baines, Fernwood, Halifax, BC, Canada.

Benkov, L. 1994, *Reinventing the Family: The emerging story of lesbian and gay parents*, Crown, New York.

Benn, C. 1981, *Attacking Poverty Through Participation—A Community Approach*, PIT Publishing, Melbourne.

Bennett, B. and Zubrzycki, J. 2003, 'Hearing the stories of Australian Aboriginal and Torres Strait Islander social workers: challenging and educating the system', *Australian Social Work*, vol. 56, no. 1, pp. 61–70.

Beresford, P. 2000, 'Service users' knowledges and social work theory: conf ict or collaboration?', *British Journal of Social Work*, vol. 30, pp. 489–503.

Berner, E. and Phillips, B. 2005, 'Left to their own devices? community self-help between alternative development and neo-liberalism', *Community Development Journal*, vol. 40, no. 1, pp. 17–29.

Berting, J. et al. eds 1990, *Human Rights in a Pluralist World*, Meckler, London and Netherlands Commission for UNESCO, The Hague.

Best, J. 2004, 'Theoretical issues in the study of social problems and deviance', in *Handbook of Social Problems: A comparative international perspective*, ed. G. Ritzer, Sage Thousand Oaks, CA, pp. 14–29.,

Best, S. and Kellner, D. 1991, *Postmodern Theory: Critical interrogations*, Macmillan, London.

Bhaskar, R. 1978, *A Realist Theory of Science*, Harvester, Brighton.

Bishop, A. 2002, *Becoming an Ally: Breaking the cycle of oppression*, 2nd edn, Allen & Unwin, Sydney.

Bishop, B. 1999, *The National Strategy for an Ageing Australia—Healthy Ageing Discussion Paper*, Commonwealth of Australia, Canberra.

Bittman, M., England, P., Sayer, N. and Matheson, G. 2003, 'When does gender trump money? Bargaining and time in household work', *American Journal of Sociology*, vol. 109, no. 1, pp. 186–214.

Blacher, Y. 1997, 'Outsourcing: opportunity or threat—nine misconceptions about competitive tendering', address to the *CWAV Seminar—The Cutting Edge*, Melbourne, pp. 35–45.

Black, B. 2004, 'Contextualising human rights: residents' rights in nursing homes and hostels', PhD thesis, Department of Social Work and Social Policy, Curtin University of Technology, Perth.

——2008, *The Human Rights of Older People and Agency Responses to Elder Abuse*, research report, Centre for Human Rights Education, Curtin University of Technology, Perth.

Blackstock, K. 2005, 'A critical look at community based tourism', *Community Development Journal*, vol. 40, no. 1, pp. 39–49.

Bland, N., Miller, J. and Quinton, P. 2000a, *Upping the PACE? An evaluation of the recommendations of the Stephen Lawrence inquiry on stops and searches*, Police Research Series, Paper 128, Home Off ce, London.

——2000b, *Managing the Use and Impact of Searches: A review of Force interventions*, Police Research Series, Paper 132, Home Off ce, London.

Blaskett, B. 1998, 'Arguing for a social work role in the promotion of ethical social research', *Australian Social Work*, vol. 51, no. 4, pp. 19–25.

Blytheway, B. 1994, *Ageism: Rethinking ageing*, Open University Press, Philadelphia.

Boal, A. 1979, *Theatre of the Oppressed*, Pluto, London.

Bocock, R. 1992, 'The cultural formations of modern society', in *Formations of Modernity*, eds S. Hall and B. Gieben, Polity Press in association with the Open University, Cambridge.

Boldy, D., Webb, M., Horner, B., Davey, M. and Kingsley, B. 2002, *Elder Abuse in Western Australia: Report of a survey conducted for the Department for Community Development—Seniors' Interests*, Curtin University of Technology Division of Health Sciences, Freemasons' Centre for Research into Aged Care Services, Perth.

Bordo, S. 1993, *Unbearable Weight: Feminism, Western culture, and the body*, University of California Press, Berkeley.

Boulet, J. 1996, 'Learning and teaching international social development', in *Advances in Social Work and Welfare Education*, eds J. Ife, S. Leitmann and P. Murphy, School of Social Work, University of Western Australia, Perth, pp. 100–9.

——2001, *International Content in Victorian Social Work Courses: Report of a research project*, AASW & Borderlands Coop, Melbourne.

——2003, 'Globalising practice in the international context', in *Critical Social Work: An introduction to theories and practices*, eds J. Allan, B. Pease and L. Briskman, Allen & Unwin, Sydney, pp. 228–45.

——2007, 'International solidarity and the logic of development aid: Impossible bedfellows?', unpublished paper presented at the 15th ICSD Symposium 16–20 July 2007, Polytechnic University, Hong Kong.

Boulet, J., Healey, L. and Helton, R. 2008, 'Gift relationships and their political-economy of volunteering, community involvement and creating a civil society', *New Community Quarterly*, vol. 6, no. 1, pp. 28–41.

Bourdieu, P. 1979, *Distinction*, Routledge, London.

——2001, *Acts of Resistance: Against the new myths of our time*, Polity Press, Cambridge.

——2003, *Outline of a Theory of Practice*, Cambridge University Press, Cambridge.

Bourdieu, P. and Wacquant, L. 2001, 'New liberal speak: notes on the new planetary vulgate', *Radical Philosophy*, vol. 105, pp. 2–5.
Bourke, L. 2001, 'Rural communities', in *Rurality Bites: The social and environmental transformation of rural Australia*, eds S. Lockie and L. Bourke, Pluto Press, Sydney, pp. 118–28.
Bowers, C.A. and Apffel-Marglin, F. 2005, *How the Ideas of Paulo Freire Contribute to the Cultural Roots of the Ecological Crisis*, Lawrence Erlbaum, Mahwah, NJ.
Bowlby, J. 1951, *Maternal Care and Mental Health*, Monograph Serial No. 2, World Health Organization, Geneva.
Boyden, J. 1997, 'Childhood and the policy makers: a comparative perspective on the globalization of childhood', in *Constructing and Reconstructing Childhood: Contemporary issues in the sociological study of childhood*, eds A. James and A. Prout, 2nd edn, Falmer Press, London, pp. 184–216.
Boyle, M. 2007, 'The problem with diagnosis', *The Psychologist*, vol. 20, no. 5, pp. 290–2.
Bracken, P. and Thomas, P. 2006, 'Democracy, citizenship and the radical possibilities of postpsychiatry', in *Critical Psychiatry: The limits of madness*, ed. D.B. Double, Palgrave Macmillan, Basingstoke.
Breakwell G. 1986, *Coping with Threatened Identities*, Methuen, London.
Breen, R. and Cook, L. 2005, 'The persistence of the gendered division of labour', *European Sociological Review*, vol. 21, no. 1, pp. 43–57.
Brennan, S. and Noggle, R. 1997, 'The moral status of children: children's rights, parents' rights, and family justice', *Social Theory and Practice*, vol. 23, no. 1, pp. 1–26.
Brenner, N. and Theodore, N., eds 2001, *Spaces of Neoliberalism*, Blackwell, Oxford.
Breton, M. 2004, 'An empowerment perspective', in *Handbook of Social Work with Groups*, eds C. Garvin, L. Gutierrez and M. Galinsky, The Guilford Press, New York.
Briskman, L. 2003a, 'Indigenous Australians: towards postcolonial social work', *Critical Social Work: An introduction to theories and practices*, eds J. Allan, B. Pease and L. Briskman, Allen & Unwin, Sydney, pp. 92–106.
——2003b, *The Black Grapevine: Aboriginal activism and stolen generations*, The Federation Press, Sydney.
——2007a, *Social Work with Indigenous Communities*, The Federation Press, Sydney.
——2007b, 'Menschenrechte und Soziale Arbeit—eine globale perspective' (Human rights and social work—a global perspective), *Internationale Perspektiven Sozialer Arbeit*, eds L. Wagner and R. Lutz, Verlag für Interkulturelle Kommunikation, Frankfurt am Main.
——2008, 'Decolonizing social work in Australia', in *Indigenous Social Work Around the World: Towards culturally relevant education and practice*, eds M. Gray, J. Coates and M. Yellow Bird, Ashgate, Aldershot, pp. 83–93.
Briskman, L. and Fiske, L. 2008, 'Teaching human rights at university: critical pedagogy in action', in *Activating Human Rights in Education: Exploration, innovation and transformation*, eds C. Newell and B. Offord, Australian College of Educators, Canberra.
Briskman, L., Latham, S. and Goddard, C. 2008, *Human Rights Overboard: Seeking asylum in Australia*, Scribe, Melbourne.
Briskman, L. and Lynn, M. with La Nauze, H. 1999, *Challenging Rural Practice: Human services in Australia*, Deakin University Press, Geelong.
Briskman, L. and Noble, C. 1999, 'Social work ethics: embracing diversity?', in *Transforming Social Work Practice*, eds B. Pease and J. Fook, Allen & Unwin, Sydney.
Brooks, G. 1998, *A New Psychotherapy for Traditional Men*, Jossey-Bass, San Francisco.
Brown, C. 2001, 'Grief—an Indigenous view', in *Loss and Grief, Our Stories: A collection of stories on loss and grief*, ed. G. McLean, Rose Education, Sydney.
——2003, 'Narrative therapy: reifying or challenging dominant discourse', in *Emerging Perspectives on Anti-Oppressive Practice*, ed. W. Shera, Canadian Scholars' Press, Toronto.
Brown, L. 2006, 'Still subversive after all these years: the relevance of feminist therapy in the age of evidence-based practice', *Psychology of Women Quarterly*, vol. 30, pp. 15–24.

Brown, L. and Strega, S., eds 2005, *Research as Resistance: Critical, Indigenous and anti-oppressive approaches*, Canadian Scholars Press, Toronto.

Brown, T. 2003, 'Critical race theory speaks to the sociology of mental health: mental health problems produced by racial stratif cation', *Journal of Health and Social Behavior*, September, vol. 44, no. 3, pp. 292–301.

——2008, 'Race, racism, and mental health: elaboration of critical race theory's contribution to the sociology of mental health', *Contemporary Justice Review*, vol. 11, no. 1, pp. 53–62.

Brown, W. 1995, *States of Injury: Power and freedom in late modernity*, Princeton University Press, Princeton.

Bryson, L. 1997, 'Ref ections on social work and politics in Victoria in the 50s and 60s', *Victorian Social Work*, vol. 6, no. 2, pp. 8–9.

Bryson, L. and Mowbray, M. 2005, 'More spray on solution: community, social capital and evidence based practice', *Australian Journal of Social Issues*, vol. 40, no. 1, pp. 91–106.

Bryson, V. 2002, *Feminist Debates: Issues of theory and political practice*, 2nd edn, Palgrave, Basingstoke.

Buchanan, J.M. and Tollison, R.D. 1972, *Theory of Public Choice: Political application of economics*, University of Michigan Press, Ann Arbor, MI.

Buchanan, J.M. and Tulloch, G. 1962, *The Calculus of Consent*, University of Michigan Press, Ann Arbor, MI.

Bulbeck, D. 1994, 'Where to now? The contemporary loss of faith in feminism's transformative power', *Social Alternatives*, vol. 12, no. 4, pp. 10–12.

Burge, B.J. 2007, 'Bending gender, ending gender: theoretical foundations for social work practice with the transgender community', *Social Work*, vol. 52, no. 3, pp. 243–50.

Burnside, J. 2007, *Watching Brief: Reflections on human rights, law and justice*, Scribe, Melbourne.

Burrell, G. and Morgan, G. 1979, *Sociological Paradigms and Organisational Analysis*, Heinemann, London.

Burstow, B. 2003, 'Toward a radical understanding of trauma and trauma work', *Violence Against Women*, vol. 9, no. 11, pp. 1293–317.

Butler, B. 1993, 'Aboriginal children: back to origins', *Family Matters*, no. 35, pp. 7–11.

Caffery, T. and Erdman, P. 2003, 'Attachment and family systems theory: implications for family therapists', *Journal of Systemic Therapies*, vol. 2, no. 22, pp. 3–15.

Callery, P. 1998, 'Sex and children in the past and present', in *Children and Sexuality: Perspectives in health care*, ed. T. Harrison, Baillière Tindall, London, pp. 1–18.

Cameron, N. and McDermott, F. 2007, *Social Work and the Body*, Palgrave Macmillan, Basingstoke.

Camilleri, P. 1999, 'Social work and its search for meaning: theories, narratives and practices', in *Transforming Social Work Practice*, eds B. Pease and J. Fook, Allen & Unwin, Sydney.

Camilleri, P. and Jones, P. 2001, 'Doing "women's work": men, masculinity and caring', in *Working with Men in the Human Services*, eds B. Pease and P. Camilleri, Allen & Unwin, Sydney.

Campbell, B. 1988, *Unofficial Secrets: Child sexual abuse, the Cleveland case*, Virago, London.

Campbell, D., Moore, G. and Small, D. 2000, 'Death and Australian cultural diversity', in *Death and Dying in Australia*, ed. A. Kellehear, Oxford University Press, Melbourne.

Carey, M. 2007, 'White-collar proletariat? Braverman, the deskilling of social work and the paradoxical life of the agency care manager', *Journal of Social Work*, vol. 7, no. 1, pp. 93–114.

Carney, T. 1991, *Law at the Margins*, Oxford University Press, Melbourne.

Carniol, B. 1990, *Case Critical: Challenging social work in Canada*, 2nd edn, Between the Lines, Toronto.

——2005, 'Analysis of social location and change: practice implications', in *Social Work: A critical turn*, eds S. Hick, J. Fook and R. Pozzuto, Thompson Educational, Toronto.

Carozza, P. 2003, 'Subsidiarity as a structural principle of international human rights law', *American Journal of International Law*, vol. 97, pp. 38–79.

Carr, D., Loeser, J. and Morris, D., eds 2005, *Narrative, Pain and Suffering*, IASP Press, Seattle.

Carter, B. and McGoldrick, M. 1999, *The Expanded Family Life Cycle: Individual, family and social perspectives*, 3rd edn, Allyn & Bacon, Needham Heights, MA.

Carter, R. 1997, 'Is white a race? Expressions of white racial identity', in *Offwhite: Readings on race, power and society*, eds M. Fine, L. Weis, L. Powell and L. Mun Wong, Routledge, New York.

Cavanagh, K. and Cree, V., eds 1996, *Working with Men: feminism and social work*, Routledge, London.

Cemlyn, S. 2008, 'Human rights and gypsies and travellers: an exploration of the application of a human rights perspective to social work with a minority community in Britain', *British Journal of Social Work*, vol. 38, no. 1, pp. 153–73.

Centre Against Sexual Assault (CASA House) 2006, *Submission to Victorian Government Inquiry into Elder Abuse Prevention, Community Education and Strengthening Service Responses for Victoria*, Royal Women's Hospital, Melbourne, <www.dvc.vic.gov.au/Web19/osv/rwpgslib.nsf/GraphicFiles/CASA/$fle/CASA.pdf> [4 August 2008].

Chambers, B. and Pettman, J. 1986, *Anti-Racism: A handbook for educators*, Human Right Commission Series, No. 1, AGPS, Canberra.

Chan, C., Chan, T. and Ng, S. 2006, 'The strengths-focused and meaning-oriented approach to resilience and transformation (SMART): a body–mind–spirit approach to trauma management', *Social Work in Health Care*, vol. 43, no. 23, pp. 9–36.

Chandler, R. 2005, 'Psychodynamic therapeutic approaches with people who are grieving', *Grief Matters*, vol. 8, no. 2, pp. 30–4.

Chang, H.J. 2007, *The Bad Samaritans: Rich nations, poor policies and the threat to the developing world*, Random House, London.

Chappell, A.L. 1998, 'Still out in the cold: people with learning diff culties and the social model of disability', in *The Disability Reader: Social science perspectives*, ed. T. Shakespeare, Cassell, London, pp. 211–20.

Charles, N. 2000, *Feminism, the State and Social Policy*, Macmillan, Basingstoke.

Charlesworth, M. 1989, *Life, Death, Genes and Ethics: 1989 Boyer Lectures*, Australian Broadcasting Corporation, Sydney.

Cheek, J., Shoebridge, J., Willis, E. and Zadoroznyj, M. 1996, *Society and Health: Social theory for health workers*, Longman, Melbourne.

Cheers, B., Darracott, R. and Lonne, B. 2007, *Social Care Practice in Rural Communities*, The Federation Press, Sydney.

Chenoweth, L. and McAuliffe, D. 2005, *The Road to Social Work & Human Service Practice: An introductory text*, Thomson, Melbourne.

Child Migrants' Trust 2001, 'Submission to the Senate Community Affairs, References Committee, Inquiry into Child Migration', <www.aph.gov.au/Senate/committee/clac_ctte/completed_inquiries/1999–02/child_migrat/submissions/sub132.pdf> [4 April 2008].

Childnet International 2008, 'Parents' Support—Empowering parents with ICT', <www.childnet-int.org/safety/parents.aspx> [16 June 2008].

Children's Ombudsman Off ces in the United States 2008, <www.ncsl.org/programs/cyf/ombuds.htm> [26 February 2008].

Christie, A. 2001a, 'Gendered discourses on welfare, men and social work', in *Men and Social Work: Theories and practice*, ed. A. Christie, Palgrave, London.

——ed. 2001b, *Men and Social Work: Theories and practices*, Palgrave, London.

——2006, 'Negotiating the uncomfortable intersections between gender and professional identities in social work', *Critical Social Policy*, vol. 26, no. 2, pp. 390–411.

Clark, J. 2006, 'Listening for meaning: a research-based model for attending to spirituality, culture and worldview in social work practice', *Critical Social Work*, vol. 7, no. 1, <www.criticalsocialwork.com/units/socialwork/critical.nsf/inToc/29CBE19CA5952C3985257179006FF85B> [5 November 2007].

Clarke, J. 2003, 'Turning inside out? Globalisation, neoliberalism and welfare states', *Anthropologica*, vol. 43, pp. 201–14.

Clarke, M. 1976, 'The limits of radical social work', *British Journal of Social Work*, vol. 6, no. 4, pp. 501–6.

Clegg, S. 1999, 'Professional education, ref ective practice and feminism', *International Journal of Inclusive Education*, vol. 3, no. 2, pp. 167–79.

——2005, 'Evidence-based practice in educational research: a critical realist critique of systematic review', *British Journal of Sociology of Education*, vol. 26, no. 3, pp. 415–28.

Clifford, D. and Burkey, B. 2008, *Anti-Oppressive Ethics and Values in Social Work: Past caring?*, Palgrave, London.

Cocklin, C. and Alston, M. 2003, *Community Sustainability in Rural Australia: A question of capital*, Academy of the Social Sciences in Australia, Canberra.

Cocklin, C. and Dibden, J. 2005, *Sustainability and Change in Rural Australia*, University of New South Wales Press, Sydney.

Coker, A.L., Davis, K.E., Arias, I., Desai, S., Sanderson, M., Brandt, H.M. and Smith, P.H. 2002, 'Physical and mental health effects of intimate partner violence for men and women', *American Journal of Preventive Medicine*, vol. 23, issue 4, pp. 260–9.

Community Services Victoria 1992, *Welfare As an Industry: A study of community services in Victoria*, Victorian Government, Melbourne.

Connell, R. 1982, 'Men and socialism', *Labour Essays 1982*, eds G. Evans and J. Reeves, Drummond, Melbourne.

——1995, *Masculinities*, Allen & Unwin, Sydney.

——2002, *Gender*, Polity Press, Cambridge.

Connelly, J. 2001, 'Critical realism and health promotion: effective practice needs an effective theory', *Health Education Research*, vol. 16, no. 2, pp. 115–20.

Considine, M. 1988, 'The corporate management framework as administrative science: a critique', *Australian Journal of Public Administration*, vol. 47, no. 1, pp. 4–17.

Constantine, M. and Sue, D.W. 2006, *Addressing Racism: Facilitating cultural competence in mental health and educational settings*, Wiley Chichester, Hoboken, NJ.

Cooling, T. 2005, 'The search for truth: postmodernism and religious education', *Journal of Belief and Values*, vol. 26, no. 1, pp. 87–93.

Corbett, L. and Larcombe, W. 1993, 'Lunar landscapes: the dark side of sexual assault and the law', in *Women and the Law*, eds P. Easteal and S. McKillop, Proceedings of a conference held 22–24 September 1991, Australian Institute of Criminology, Canberra, pp. 131–42.

Corrigan, P. and Leonard, P. 1978, *Social Work Practice Under Capitalism: A Marxist approach*, Macmillan, London.

Corrigan, R. 2006, 'Making meaning of Megan's law', *Law and Social Inquiry*, vol. 31, no. 2, pp. 267–312.

Cosgrove, L. 2005, 'When labels mask oppression: implications for teaching psychiatric taxonomy to mental health counsellors', *Journal of Mental Health Counselling*, vol. 27, no. 4, pp. 283–95.

Costello, S. 2004, 'Valuing the complexity of direct social work practice in an era of managerialism', *Women in Welfare Education*, vol. 7, pp. 33–50.

Couch, M., Pitts, M., Mulcare, H., Croy, S., Mitchell, A. and Patel, S. 2007, *Tranznation: A report into the health and wellbeing of transgendered people in Australia and New Zealand*, Australian Research Centre in Sex, Health & Society, La Trobe University, Melbourne.

Cowburn, M. and Pengelly, H. 1999, 'Values and processes in groupwork with men', in *Working with Men for Change*, ed. J. Wild, UCL Press, London.

Cox, D. 1989, *Migration and Welfare: An Australian perspective*, Prentice Hall, Sydney.

Cox, D. and Pawar, M. 2005, *International Social Work: Issues, strategies and programs*, Sage, London.

Craig, L. 2007, 'Is there really a second shift, and if so, who does it? A time diary investigation', *Feminist Review*, vol. 86, pp. 149–70.

Crawford, F., Dudgeon, P. and Briskman, L. 2007, *Developing Therapeutic Communities for Abused Aboriginal Children and Their Families: An Indigenous practitioners' cooperative inquiry*, Curtin University of Technology & Ministerial Advisory Council on Child Protection, Perth.

Cree, V. 2001, 'Men and masculinities in social work education', in *Men and Social Work: Theories and practices*, ed. A. Christie, Palgrave, London.

Cree, V. and Davis, A. 2007, *Social Work: Voices from the inside*, Routledge, London.

Cripps, D. 2001, 'Rights focussed advocacy and elder abuse', *Australasian Journal on Ageing*, vol. 20, no. 1, pp. 17–22.

Crush, J., ed. 1996, *Power of Development*, Routledge, London.

Currer, C. 2007, *Loss and Social Work*, Learning Matters, Exeter.

D'Cruz, H. 2004, *Constructing Meanings and Identities in Child Protection Practice*, Tertiary Press, Croydon.

D'Cruz, H., Gillingham, P. and Melendez, S. 2007, 'Ref exivity: a concept and its meanings for practitioners working with children and families', *Critical Social Work*, vol. 8, no. 1, <www.criticalsocialwork.com/units/socialwork/critical.nsf/inToc/0DB87FD2EA9A59F58525737000638D62> [12 August 2008].

D'Cruz, H. and Jones, M. 2004, *Social Work Research: Ethical and political contexts*, Sage, London.

D'Cruz, H. and Stagnitti, K. 2008, 'Re-constructing child welfare through participatory and child-centred professional practice: a conceptual approach', *Child and Family Social Work*, vol. 13, pp. 156–65.

Dalrymple, J. and Burke, B. 1995, *Anti-Oppressive Practice: Social care and the law*, Open University Press, Buckingham.

Daly, K. and Stubbs, J. 2006, 'Feminist engagement with restorative justice', *Theoretical Criminology*, vol. 10, no. 9, pp. 9–28.

Damousi, J. 2001, *Living with the Aftermath: Trauma, nostalgia and grief in post-war Australia*, Cambridge University Press, Cambridge.

Darlington Social Research Unit 1998, *Caring for Children away from Home: Messages from research*, Wiley, London.

Davies, B. 2003, 'Death to critique and dissent?: The policies and practices of new managerialism and of "evidence-based practice"', *Gender and Education*, vol. 15, no. 1, pp. 91–103.

Davies, B., Gottsche, M. and Bansel, P. 2006, 'The rise and fall of the neo-liberal university', *European Journal of Education*, vol. 41, no. 2, pp. 305–19.

Davies, J., White, J., Wright, A., Maru, Y. and LaFlamme, M. 2008, 'Applying the sustainable livelihoods approach in Australian desert Aboriginal development', *Rangeland Journal*, vol. 30, pp. 55–65.

Davies, L. and Leonard, P., eds 2004, *Social Work in a Corporate Era: Practices of power and resistance*, Ashgate, Aldershot.

Davis, J. and Ridge, T. 1997, *Same scenery, different lifestyle: Rural children on a low income*, The Children's Society, London.

Davis, J.E. 2005, *Accounts of Innocence: Sexual abuse, trauma, and the self*, University of Chicago Press, Chicago.

Davis, M. and Watson, N. 2006, '"It's the same old song": Draconian counter-terrorism laws and the *déjà vu* of Indigenous Australians', *Borderlands ejournal*, vol. 5, no. 1 [5 March 2008].

de Montigny, G. 2005, 'A ref exive materialist alternative', in *Social Work: A critical turn*, eds S. Hick, J. Fook and R. Pozzuto, Thompson Educational, Toronto.

Deegan, P. 1996, 'Recovery as a journey of the heart', *Psychiatric Rehabilitation Journal*, vol. 19, no. 3, Winter, pp. 92–7.

DeLois, K. and Cohen, M. 2000, 'A queer idea: using group work principles to strengthen learning in a sexual minorities seminar', *Social Work with Groups*, vol. 23, no. 3, pp. 53–67.

Dempsey, K. 1997, *Inequalities in Marriage: Australia and beyond*, Oxford University Press, Melbourne.

——2000, 'Men and women's power relationships and the persisting inequitable division of labour', *Journal of Family Studies*, vol. 6, no. 1, pp. 7–24.

Denborough, D. 1996, *Beyond the Prison: Gathering dreams of freedom*, Dulwich Centre Press, Adelaide.

Denborough, D., Koolmatrie, C., Mununggirritj, D., Marika, D., Dhurrkay, W. and Yunupingu, M. 2006, 'Linking stories and initiatives: a narrative approach to working with the skills and knowledge of communities', *International Journal of Narrative Therapies and Community Work*, no. 2, pp. 19–51.

Department of Immigration and Multicultural and Indigenous Affairs (DIMIA) 2002, *Indigenous Australians: A national commitment*, Commonwealth of Australia, Canberra.

Department of Justice Canada 2007, *Family Violence: A fact sheet from the Department of Justice Canada*, <www.justice.gc.ca/en/ps/fm/familyvfs.html> [20 June 2008]

Desai, S. and Bevan, D. 2002, 'Race and culture', in *Loss and Grief: A guide for human services practitioners*, ed. Neil Thompson, Palgrave, Basingstoke.

Devore, W. and Schlesinger, E.G. 1996, *Ethnic-sensitive social work practice*, Allyn & Bacon, Needham Heights.

DHS 2008, *Every Child, Every Chance: Child development and trauma guide*, Victorian Department of Human Services, <www.dhs.vic.gov.au/everychildeverychance> [28 January 2009].

Diamond, J. 2007, *My Father before Me: How fathers and sons influence each other throughout their lives*, W.W. Norton, New York.

Dienhart, A. 1998, *Reshaping Fatherhood: The social construction of shared parenting*, Sage, Thousand Oaks.

Dietz, C. 2000, 'Reshaping clinical practice for the new millennium', *Journal of Social Work Education*, vol. 36, issue 3, pp. 503–20.

Dillon, M.C. and Westbury, N.D. 2007, *Beyond Humbug: Transforming government engagement with Indigenous Australia*, Seaview Press, Adelaide.

Dixon, J. 1993, 'Feminist community work's ambivalence with politics', *Australian Social Work*, vol. 46, no. 1, pp. 37–44.

Doel, M. 2006, *Using Groupwork*, Routledge, London.

Doka, K., ed. 2002, 'Introduction', in *Disenfranchised Grief: New directions, challenges, and strategies for practice*, ed. K. Doka, Research Press, Champaign, IL.

Doka, K. and Martin, T. 2002, 'How we grieve: culture, class, and gender', in *Disenfranchised Grief: New directions, challenges, and strategies for practice*, ed. K. Doka, Research Press, Champaign, IL.

Domestic Violence and Incest Resource Centre (DVIRC) 2006, *When Love Hurts: Working to prevent domestic violence in Victoria*, DVIRC, Melbourne, <www.dvirc.org.au/index.htm> [19 January 2009].

Dominelli, L. 1996, 'Deprofessionalising social work, anti-oppressive practice, competencies & postmodernism,' *British Journal of Social Work*, vol. 26, no. 2, pp. 153–75.

——1998, 'Anti-oppressive practice in context', in *Social Work: Themes, issues and critical debates*, eds R. Adams, L. Dominelli and M. Payne, Macmillan, Houndmills.

——1999, 'Working with men from a feminist perspective', in *Working with Men for Change*, ed. J. Wild, UCL Press, London.

——2002a, *Feminist Social Work Theory and Practice*, Palgrave Macmillan, Basingstoke.

——2002b, 'Anti-oppressive practice in context', in *Social Work: Themes, issues and critical debates*, eds R. Adams, L. Dominelli and M. Payne, Palgrave, Basingstoke, pp. 3–19.

——2002c, *Anti-oppressive Social Work Theory and Practice*, Palgrave Macmillan, Basingstoke.

——2004, *Social Work: Theory and practice for a changing profession*, Polity Press, Cambridge.

——2008, *Anti-racist Social Work*, Palgrave Macmillan, Basingstoke.

Donahoo, D. 2007, *Idolising Children*, University of New South Wales Press, Sydney.

Donnelly, J. 2003, *Universal Human Rights in Theory and Practice*, 2nd edn, Cornell University Press, New York.
Donzelot, J. 1980, *The Policing of Families*, Hutchinson, London.
——1988, 'The promotion of the social', *Economy and Society*, vol. 17, no. 3, pp. 395–427.
Double, D.B. 2006, 'Critical psychiatry and conf ict: renewing mental health practice', in *Critical Psychiatry: The limits of madness*, ed. D.B. Double, Palgrave Macmillan, Basingstoke.
Douglas, P. 1993, 'Men = violence: a profeminist perspective on dismantling the masculine equation', paper presented at the Second National Conference on Violence, Canberra, Australian Institute of Criminology.
Dow, K. and Downing, T. 2006, *The Atlas of Climate Change: Mapping the world's greatest challenge*, Earthscan, London.
Drakeford, M. 2002, 'Social work and politics', in *The Blackwell Companion to Social Work*, ed. M. Davies, Blackwell, Oxford, pp. 288–97.
Drover, G. and Kerans, P., eds 1993, *New Approaches to Welfare Theory*, Edward Elgar, Aldershot.
Duffy, M., Gillig, S.E., Tureen, R.M. and Ybarra, M.A. 2002, 'A critical look at the DSM-IV', *Journal of Individual Psychology*, vol. 58, no. 4, pp. 363–73.
Dunn, K.M. 2003, *Racism in Australia: Findings of a survey of racist attitudes*, National Europe Centre Paper, no. 77, University of New South Wales, Sydney.
Dunne, T. and Wheeler, N., eds 1999, *Human Rights in Global Politics*, Cambridge University Press, Cambridge.
Dupper, D.R. 2003, *School Social Work: Skills and interventions for effective practice*, J. Wiley & Sons, Hoboken, NJ.
Durning, A.T. 1995, 'Are we happy yet?', in *Ecopsychology: Restoring the earth, healing the mind*, eds T. Roszak, M. Gomes and A. Kanner, Sierra Club Books, San Francisco.
Eagleton, T. 2003, *After Theory*, Basic Books, New York.
Easteal, P. 1996a, 'The cultural context of rape and reform', in *Balancing the Scales: Rape law reform and Australian culture*, ed. P. Easteal, Federation Press, Sydney, pp. 1–12.
——ed. 1996b, 'A masculocentric reality: the limits of law reform and choices for the future', *Balancing the Scales*, National Conference on Sexual Assault, Perth, WA Sexual Assault Referral Centre, 20–21 June 1996.
Ebert, T. 1996, *Ludic Feminism and After: Postmodernism, desire, and labor in late capitalism*, University of Michigan Press, Michigan.
Ebrahim, A. and Weisband, E., eds 2007, *Global Accountabilities: Participation, pluralism and public ethics*, Cambridge University Press, Cambridge.
Edgar, D. 1998, 'Reclaiming care for men: family and work futures', in *National Forum on Men and Family Relationships*, Commonwealth Department of Family and Community Services, Canberra.
——2000, 'Families and the social reconstruction of marriage and parenthood in Australia', in *Issues Facing Australian Families*, eds W. Weeks and M. Quinn, Pearson Education, Sydney.
Eekelaar, J., Dingwall, R. and Murray, T. 1982, 'Victims or threats? Children in care proceedings', *Journal of Social Welfare Law*, vol. 4, no. 1, pp. 68–82.
Ehrenreich, J. 1985, *The Altruistic Imagination*, Cornell University Press, Ithaca.
Eisler, I. 2002, 'Comment—The scientif c practitioner and family therapy: a way forward, a strait-jacket or a distraction?', *Journal of Family Therapy*, vol. 24, pp. 125–33.
Eisler, R. 1987, *The Chalice and the Blade*, Harper & Row, San Francisco.
——1996, *Sacred Pleasure*, Doubleday, New York.
——2004, 'Pragmatopia: revisioning human possibilities', *Tikkun*, vol. 19, no. 6, pp. 44–6.
Eisler, R. and Loye, D. 1990, *The Partnership Way*, Harper, San Francisco.
Ellermann, A. 1998, 'Can discourse analysis enable ref ective social work practice?', *Social Work Education*, vol. 17, no. 1, pp. 35–44.

Ely, P. and Denny, D. 1987, *Social Work in a Multi-racial Society*, Gower, Aldershot.

Epstein, L. 1999, 'The culture of social work', in *Reading Foucault for Social Work*, eds A. Chambon, A. Irving and L. Epstein, Columbia University Press, New York.

Erera, P. I. 2002, *Family Diversity: Continuity and change in the contemporary family*, Sage, Thousand Oaks, CA.

Escobar, A. 1995, *Encountering Development*, Princeton University Press, Princeton.

European Network of Ombudspersons for Children. 2007, <www.ombudsnet.org/enoc/members/member.asp?id=3085> [26 February 2008].

Evans, T. and Harris, J. 2004, 'Street level bureaucracy, social work and the (exaggerated) death of discretion', *British Journal of Social Work*, vol. 34, no. 6, pp. 871–95.

Everingham, C. 2003, *Social Justice and the Politics of Community*, Ashgate, Aldershot.

Fabrega, H. Jr 2008, 'On the postmodernist critique and reformation of psychiatry', *Psychiatry*, vol. 71, no. 2, pp. 183–96.

Fairclough, N. 1992, *Discourse and Social Change*, Polity Press, Cambridge.

Fawcett, B., Featherstone, B., Fook, J. and Rossiter, A., eds 2000, *Practice and Research in Social Work*, Routledge, London.

Fay, B. 1987, *Critical Social Science*, Polity Press in association with Basil Blackwell, Oxford.

Faye, B. and Sellick, M. 2003, *Advocare's Speak Out Survey 'S.O.S' on Elder Abuse*, Advocare, Perth.

Featherstone, B. 2005, 'Feminist social work: past, present and future', in *Social Work: A critical turn*, eds S. Hick, J. Fook and R. Pozzuto, Thompson Education, Toronto.

Featherstone, B. and Fawcett, B. 1995, 'Oh no! not more "isms": feminism, postmodernism, poststructuralism and social work education', *Social Work Education*, vol. 14, no. 3, pp. 25–43.

Featherstone, B., Rivett, M. and Scourf eld, J. 2007, *Working with Men in Health and Social Care*, Sage, London.

Feltman, C. 2005, 'Evidence-based psychotherapy and counselling in the UK: critique and alternatives', *Journal of Contemporary Psychotherapy*, vol. 35, no. 1, pp. 131–43.

Ferguson, H. 2008, 'Critical best practice: critical perspectives', in *Best Practice in Social Work: Critical perspectives*, eds K. Jones, B. Cooper and H. Ferguson, Palgrave Macmillan, Houndmills.

Ferguson, I. 2008, *Reclaiming Social Work: Challenging neo-liberalism and promoting social justice*, Sage, London.

Filak, V. and Abel, S. 2004, 'Boys don't cry: cartooning, grieving strategies and gender-based stereotypes in the aftermath of September 11', *Grief Matters*, vol. 7, no. 1, pp. 12–17.

Finch, J. and Groves, D. 1985, 'Old girl, old boy: gender divisions in social work with the elderly', in *Women, the Family, and Social Work*, eds E. Brook and A. Davis, Tavistock, London, pp. 92–111.

Fincher, R. and Wulff, M. 2001, 'Moving in and out of disadvantage: population mobility and Australian places', in *Creating Unequal Futures? Rethinking poverty, inequality and disadvantage*, eds R. Fincher and P. Saunders, Allen & Unwin, Sydney, pp. 158–93.

Findlay, R. 2007, 'A mandate for honesty: Jeff Young's no bullshit therapy', *Australian and New Zealand Journal of Family Therapy*, vol. 28, no. 2, pp. 165–70.

Fine, M. and Turner, J. 1991, 'Tyranny and freedom: looking at ideas in the practice of family therapy', *Family Process*, vol. 30, no. 3, September.

Firestone, T. 1990, 'Accommodation: toward a paradigm–praxis dialectic', in *The Paradigm Dialog*, ed. E. Guba, Sage, Newbury Park, CA.

Fisher, A. 2004, 'Narrative possibilities for unpacking "homophobia": responding to the complexities of men's life journeys', keynote address presented at the *International Summer School of Narrative Practice*, November, Dulwich Centre, Adelaide.

Fisher, J. 1980, *The Response of Social Work to the Depression*, Schenkman, Boston.

Fletcher, R. 1997, *Australian Men and Boys: A picture of health?*, University of Newcastle, Newcastle.

Flood, M. and Pease, B. 2005, 'Undoing men's privilege and advancing gender equality in public sector institutions', *Policy and Society*, vol. 24, no. 4, pp. 119–38.

Flood, M. and Pease, B. 2006, *The Factors Influencing Community Attitudes in Relations to Violence Against Women: A critical review of the literature*, VicHealth, Melbourne.

Fook, J. 1990, 'Radical social casework: linking theory and practice', in *Social Change and Social Welfare Practice*, eds J. Petruchenia and R. Thorpe, Hale & Iremonger, Sydney, pp. 20–47.

——1993, *Radical Casework: A theory of practice*, Allen & Unwin, Sydney.

——1995, 'Science and social work: are they compatible?', unpublished paper presented at the 24th National Australian Association of Social Workers (AASW), Conference, Launceston, 3 July 1995.

——ed. 1996, *The Reflective Researcher: Social workers' theories of practice research*, Allen & Unwin, Sydney.

——1999, 'Critical ref ectivity in education and practice', in *Transforming Social Work Practice: Postmodern critical perspectives*, eds B. Pease and J. Fook, Allen & Unwin, Sydney, pp. 195–208.

——2000a, 'Critical perspectives on social work practice', in *Contemporary Perspectives on Social Work and the Human Services: Challenges and change*, eds I. O'Connor, P. Smyth and J. Warburton, Pearson Education, Sydney, pp. 128–38.

——2000b, 'Deconstructing and reconstructing professional expertise', in *Practice and Research in Social Work*, eds B. Fawcett, B. Featherstone, J. Fook and A. Rossiter, Routledge, London.

——2002a, *Social Work: Critical theory and practice*, Sage, London.

——2002b, *Critical Social Work*, Sage, London.

——2004, 'What professionals need from research: beyond evidence-based practice', in *Social Work and Evidence-Based Practice*, ed. D. Smith, Jessica Kingsley, London.

——2005, 'Challenges and directions for critical social work', in *Social Work: A critical turn*, eds S. Hick, J. Fook and R. Pozzuto, Thompson Education, Toronto.

Fook, J. and Morley, C. 2005, 'Empowerment: a contextual perspective', in *Social Work: A critical turn*, eds S. Hick, J. Fook and R. Pozzuto, Thompson Education, Toronto.

Fook, J., Ryan, M. and Hawkins, L. 2000, *Professional Expertise: Practice, theory and education for working in uncertainty*, Whiting & Birch, London.

Foote, C. and Frank, A. 2000, 'Foucault and therapy: the disciplining of grief', in *Reading Foucault for Social Work*, eds A. Chambon, A. Irving and L. Epstein, Columbia University Press, New York.

Forcey, L.R. and Nash, M. 1998, 'Rethinking feminist theory and social work therapy', *Women and Therapy*, vol. 21, no. 4, pp. 85–99.

Fortune, M.M. and Longwood, W.M. 2004, *Sexual Abuse in the Catholic Church: Trusting the clergy?* Haworth Press, Binghampton.

Foucault, M. 1965, *Madness and Civilization: A history of insanity in the Age of Reason*, trans. Richard Howard, Random House, Cambridge.

——1971, 'Orders of Discourse', *Social Science Information*, vol. 10, no. 2, pp. 7–30.

——1977, *The Archaeology of Knowledge*, Tavistock, London.

——1978a, *The History of Sexuality: Volume 1, An introduction*, trans. Robert Hurley, Random House, Cambridge.

——1978b, 'Politics and the study of discourse', *Ideology and Consciousness*, no. 3, pp. 7–26.

——1979, *Discipline and Punish*, Penguin, Harmondsworth.

——1980, trans. Colin Gordon, Leo Marshall, John Mepham and Kate Soper, *Power/Knowledge: Selected interviews and other writings 1972–1977*, ed. Colin Gordon, Pantheon, new York.

——1984, 'In interview with Paul Rabinow and Hubert Dreyfus', in *The Foucault Reader*, ed. P. Rabinow, Penguin, Harmondsworth.

——1988, 'The concern for truth', in *Michel Foucault: Politics, philosophy, interviews and other writings*, ed. L.D. Kritzman, Routledge Chapman & Hall, London, pp. 255–67.

Fox Harding, L. 1991, *Perspectives in Child Care Policy*, Longman, London.

Frankenberg, R. 1993, *White Women, Race Matters: The social construction of whiteness*, Routledge, London.

——ed. 1997, *Displacing Whiteness: Essays in social and cultural criticism*, Duke University Press, London.

Franklin, R. 1986, *The Rights of Children*, Blackwell, London.

Fraser, H. 2005, 'Four different approaches to community participation', *Community Development Journal*, vol. 40, no. 3, pp. 286–300.

——2008, *In the Name of Love: Women's narratives of love and abuse*, Women's Press, Toronto.

Fraser, H. and Briskman, L. 2005, 'Through the eye of a needle: the challenge of getting justice in Australia if you're Indigenous or seeking asylum', in *Globalisation, Global Justice and Social Work*, eds I. Ferguson, M. Lavalette and E. Whitmore, Routledge, London, pp. 109–23.

Fraser, H. and Strong, D. 2000, 'Teaching structural social work skills to beginning students', *Advances in Social Work and Welfare Education*, vol. 3, no. 1, pp. 27–36.

Fraser, N. 1989, *Unruly Practices: Power, discourse and gender in contemporary social theory*, University of Minnesota Press, Minneapolis.

——1991, 'The uses and abuses of French discourse theory for feminist politics', in *Critical Theory Now*, ed. P. Wexler, Falmer, London.

——2001, 'Recognition without ethics?', *Theory, Culture & Society*, vol. 18, nos. 2–3, pp. 21–42.

Fredericks, B. 1995, 'Recreating the circle with We Al-Li: a program for sharing and regeneration', *Aboriginal and Islander Health Worker Journal*, vol. 19, no. 2, pp. 22–3.

Freedman, J. and Coombs, G. 1996, *Narrative Therapy: The social construction of preferred realities*, W.W. Norton, New York.

Freeman, M. 1983, *The Rights and Wrongs of Children*, Francis Pinter, London.

——2002, *Human Rights: An interdisciplinary approach*, Polity Press, Cambridge.

——2005, 'The historical roots of human rights before the Second World War', in *The Essentials of Human Rights*, eds R. Smith and C. van den Anker, Hodder Arnold, London, pp. 151–4.

Freeman, S. 2005, *Grief and Loss: Understanding the journey*, Thomson Brooks/Cole, Belmont, CA.

Freire, P. 1972, *Pedagogy of the Oppressed*, Penguin, Harmondsworth.

Freire, P. and Faundez, A. 1990, *Learning to Question: A pedagogy of liberation*, WCC Publications, Geneva.

Frost, L. and Hoggett, P. 2008, 'Human agency and social suffering', *Critical Social Policy*, vol. 28, no. 4, pp. 438–60, <http://csp.sagepub.com/cgi/content/refs/28/4/438> [8 November 2008].

Frost, N. and Stein, M. 1989, *The Politics of Child Welfare: Inequality, power and change*, Harvester Wheatsheaf, London.

Fukuyama, M. and Sevig, T. 1999, *Integrating Spirituality into Multicultural Counselling*, Sage, Thousand Oaks, CA.

Fullagar, S. and Gattuso, S. 2002, 'Rethinking gender, risk, and depression in Australian mental health policy', *Australian e-Journal for the Advancement of Mental Health*, vol. 1, no. 3, <www.auseinet.com/journal> [1 June 2008].

Funk, E. 1993, *Stopping Rape: A challenge for men*, New Society Publishers, Philadelphia.

Galloway, G. and Moylan, R. 2005, 'Mungalli Falls Indigenous women's healing camp', *International Journal of Narrative Therapy and Community Work*, nos 3 & 4, pp. 77–88.

Galper, J. 1975, *The Politics of Social Services*, Prentice-Hall, Englewood Cliffs, NJ.

——1980, *Social Work Practice: A radical perspective*, Prentice-Hall, Englewood, Cliffs, NJ.

Gambrill, E. 2001, 'Behavioral social work: past, present and future', *Research on Social Work Practice*, vol. 11, no. 2, pp. 166–75.

Gardner, F., Fook, J. and White, S. 2006, 'Critical ref ection: possibilities for developing effectiveness in conditions of uncertainty', in *Critical Reflection in Health and Social Care*, eds S. White, J. Fook and F. Gardner, Open University Press, Maidenhead.

Garrett, P.M. 1999a, 'Producing the moral citizen: the "Looking After Children" system and the regulation of children and young people in public care', *Critical Social Policy*, vol. 19, no. 3, pp. 291–311.

——1999b, 'Mapping child-care social work in the f nal years of the twentieth century: a critical response to the "Looking After Children'system", *British Journal of Social Work*, vol. 29, no. 1, pp. 27–47.

——2002, 'Yes Minister: reviewing the "Looking After Children" experience and identifying the messages for social work research', *British Journal of Social Work*, vol. 32, no. 7, pp. 831–46.

——2003, *Remaking Social Work with Children and Families*, Routledge, London.

——2007a, 'The relevance of Bourdieu for social work', *Journal of Social Work*, vol. 7, no. 3, pp. 355–79.

——2007b, 'Making social work more Bourdieusian: why the social professions should critically engage with the work of Pierre Bourdieu', *European Journal of Social Work*, vol. 10, pp. 225–43.

Geertz, C. 1973, *The Interpretation of Cultures*, Basic Books, New York.

——1995, *After the Fact: Two countries, four decades, one anthropologist*, Harvard University Press, Cambridge.

Geirsdottir, I.E. and Stefansdottir, G.V. 2005, 'The cost of moving out', in *Deinstitutionalisation and People with Intellectual Disabilities: In and out of institutions*, eds K. Johnson and R. Traustadottir, Jessica Kingsley, London, pp. 130–6.

George, J. 1999, 'Conceptual muddle, practical dilemma: human rights, social development and social work education', *International Social Work*, vol. 42, no. 1, pp. 15–26.

Ghansham, D.M. 2002, *Female Foeticide and the Dowry System in India*, Women's Studies Research Unit, School of Social Work, University of Melbourne, Prepared for Townsville International Women's Conference, July, <www.austdvclearinghouse.unsw.edu.au/Conference%20papers/TIWC/GhanshamDevakiMonani.pdf> [1 August 2008]

Gibelman, M. 1999, 'The search for identity: def ning social work past, present and future', *Social Work*, no. 44, pp. 298–311.

Gibson, D. 1998, *Aged Care: Old policies and new problems*, Cambridge University Press, Cambridge.

Giddens, A. 1984, *The Constitution of Society*, University of California Press, Berkeley.

Gilbert, S. 2001, 'Social work with Indigenous Australians', in *Social Work: Fields of practice*, eds M. Alston and J. McKinnon, Oxford University Press, Melbourne.

Gilchrist, J. and Price, L. 2006, *New Beginnings: A report of practice and co-research supporting women to reclaim friendship in the context of intimate partner violence*, Kyabra Community Association, December, <www.kyabra.org/uploaded_files/New%20beginnings%2026th%20M arch.pdf> [10 October 2007].

Gilligan, P. 2007, 'Well motivated reformists or nascent radicals: how do applicants to the degree in social work see social problems, their origins and solutions?', *British Journal of Social Work*, no. 37, pp. 735–60.

Gillingham, P. 2006, 'ASW—Risk assessment in child protection: problem rather than solution?', *Australian Social Work*, vol. 59, no. 1, pp. 86–98.

Gilmore, K. 1995, 'Violence against women: crimes, not misdemeanours', in *In the Shadow of the Law: The legal context of social work practice*, ed. P. Swain, Federation Press, Syndey, pp. 46–58.

Giroux, H. 1990, *Curriculum Discourse as Postmodernist Practice*, Deakin University Press, Geelong.

Gittins, D. 1998, *The Child in Question*, Macmillan, Basingstoke.

Glasby, J. and Beresford, P. 2006, 'Who knows best? Evidence-based practice and the service user contribution', *Critical Social Policy*, vol. 26, no. 1, pp. 268–84.

Gleeson, D. 2008, 'Some new perspectives on early Australian social work', *Australian Social Work*, vol. 61, no. 3, pp. 207–25.

Glendinning, C. 1995, 'Technology, trauma, and the wild', in *Ecopsychology: Restoring the earth, healing the mind*, eds T. Roszak, M. Gomes and A. Kanner, Sierra Club Books, San Francisco.

Godbout, J. with Caillé, A. 1998, *The World of the Gift*, McGill-Queens University Press, Montréal and Kingston.

Goddard, C. and Briskman, L. 2004, 'By any measure, it's off cial child abuse', *Herald Sun*, 19 February, p. 17.
Goffman, E. 1963, *Stigma: Notes on the management of spoiled identity*, Penguin, Harmondsworth.
Goggin, G. and Newell, C. 2005, *Disability in Australia: Exposing a social apartheid*, University of New South Wales Press, Sydney.
Goldberg Wood, G. and Tully, C. 2006, *The Structural Approach to Direct Practice in Social Work: A social constructionist perspective*, 3rd edn, Columbia University Press, New York.
Golden, T. 1999, 'Masculine Grief', Seminar presentation, Melbourne, 5 July.
——1997, *Swallowed by a Snake: The gift of the masculine side of healing*, Golden Healing, Los Angeles.
Goldsworthy, J. 2002, 'Resurrecting a model of integrating individual work with community development and social action', *Community Development Journal*, vol. 37, no. 4, pp. 327–37.
Goldsworthy, K. 2005, 'Grief and loss theory in social work practice: all changes involve loss, just as all losses require change', *Australian Social Work*, vol. 58, no. 2, pp. 167–78.
Gonzales, J., Ringeisen, H. and Chambers, D. 2002, 'The tangled and thorny path of science to practice: tensions in interpreting and applying "evidence"', *Clinical Psychology Science and Practice*, vol. 9, no. 2, pp. 204–9.
Goodhart, M. 2005, 'Universalism', in *The Essentials of Human Rights*, eds R. Smith and C. van den Anker, Hodder Arnold, London, pp. 353–6.
Goodman, G. and Williams, C. 2007, 'Interventions for increasing the academic engagement of students with autism spectrum disorders in inclusive classrooms', *Teaching Exceptional Children*, vol. 39, no. 6, pp. 53–62.
Gough, L. 2007, 'Walk a day in my shoes: managing unmet need on a daily basis', in *Planning Support for People with Intellectual Disabilities: Issues for case managers and other professionals*, eds C. Bigby, C. Fyffe and E. Ozanne, Jessica Kingsley, London, pp. 84–9.
Graham, H. 1992, 'Feminism and social work education', *Issues in Social Work Education*, vol. 11, no. 2, pp. 48–64.
Graham, M. 2007, 'Gay masculinities', in *International Encyclopedia of Men and Masculinities*, eds M. Flood, J. Gardiner, B. Pease and K. Pringle, Routledge, Milton Park.
Gray, I. 2005, 'Challenges for individual and collective action', in *Sustainability and Change in Rural Australia*, eds C. Cocklin and J. Dibden, University of New South Wales Press, Sydney, pp. 230–46.
Gray, J. 2007, '(Re)considering voice', *Qualitative Social Work*, vol. 6, no. 4, pp. 411–30.
Gray, M. and McDonald, C. 2006, 'Pursuing good practice: the limits of evidence-based practice', *Journal of Social Work*, vol. 6, no. 1, pp. 7–20.
Green, D. 2007, 'Risk and social work practice', *Australian Social Work*, vol. 60, no. 4, pp. 395–409.
——2008, *From Poverty to Power: How active citizens and effective governments can change the world*, Oxfam International, Oxford.
Greenhalgh, T. 1999, 'Narrative-based medicine in an evidence-based world', *British Medical Journal*, vol. 318, pp. 323–5.
Greer, G. 1999, *The Whole Woman*, Doubleday, London.
Griff n, G. 2000, 'Def ning Australian death: religion and the state', in *Death and Dying in Australia*, ed. A. Kellehear, Oxford University Press, Melbourne.
Griff ths, P. 2005, 'Evidence-based practice: a deconstruction critique', *International Journal of Nursing Studies*, vol. 42, no. 3, pp. 355–68.
Grimshaw, P., Lake, M., McGrath, A. and Quartly, M. 1994, *Creating a Nation*, McPhee Gribble, Melbourne.
Gunzburg, J. and Stewart, W. 1994, *The Grief Counselling Handbook: A student's guide to unresolved grief*, Chapman & Hall, London.
Gupta, M. 2003, 'A critical appraisal of evidence-based medicine: some ethical considerations', *Journal of Evaluation in Clinical Practice*, vol. 9, no. 2, pp. 111–22.

Gutiérrez, L., Parsons, R. and Cox, E. 1998, *Empowerment in Social Work Practice: A sourcebook*, Brooks/Cole, Pacif c Grove, CA.
Hacking, I. 1991, 'The making and molding of child abuse', *Critical Inquiry*, vol. 17, pp. 253–88.
Hagman, G. 2001, 'Beyond decathexis: toward a new psychoanalytic understanding and treatment of mourning', in *Meaning Reconstruction & the Experience of Loss*, ed. R. Neimeyer, American Psychological Association, Washington.
Hall, S. 1980, 'Race, articulation and societies structured in dominance', *Sociological Theories: Race and colonialism*, UNESCO, France, pp. 305–45.
Hammersley, M. 1995, *The Politics of Social Research*, Sage, London.
Hancock, L. 1999, 'Health, public sector restructuring and the market state', in *Health Policy in the Market State*, ed. L. Hancock, Allen & Unwin, Sydney, pp. 48–68.
Hancock, P. and Taylor, M. 2001, *Work, Postmodernism and Organisation: A critical introduction*, Sage, London.
Harcourt, W. 2008, 'Editorial: walking the talk—putting climate justice into action', *Development*, vol. 51, no. 3, special issue on Climate Justice and Development, pp. 307–9.
Hare-Mustin, R. and Marecek, J. 1994, 'Feminism & postmodernism: dilemmas and points of resistance', *Dulwich Centre Newsletter*, no. 4, pp. 13–19.
Harlow, E. 2003, 'New managerialism, social service departments and social work practice today', *Practice*, vol. 15, no. 2, pp. 29–44.
Harris, D.K. 1990, *Sociology of Aging*, 2nd edn, Harper & Row, New York.
Harris, G. 2007, *Seeking Sustainability in an Age of Complexity*, Cambridge University Press, Cambridge.
Harris, J. 2003, *The Social Work Business*, Routledge, London.
Hart, M. 2002, *Seeking Mino-Pimatisiwin: An Aboriginal approach to helping*, Fernwood, Halifax, BC, Canada.
Hart, N. 2007, 'Disciplining through depression: an analysis of contemporary discourse on women and depression', *Women's Studies in Communication*, vol. 30, no. 3, pp. 284–309.
Hartley, R. 1995, *Families and Cultural Diversity in Australia*, Allen & Unwin, Sydney.
Harvey, J. 2000, *Give Sorrow Words: Perspectives on loss and trauma*, Brunner/Mazel, Philadelphia.
Hayes, F. 1992, 'Unionism and community workers: the role of the Australian Social Welfare Union', in *Community Work or Social Change?*, eds R. Thorpe and J. Petruchenia, Hale & Iremonger, Sydney, pp. 180–98.
Haynes, K. and Mickelson, J. 2003, *Affecting Change: Social workers in the political arena*, 5th edn, Pearson Education, Boston.
Healey, L., Boulet, J. and Boulet, J. 2006, 'Volunteering: what's in a name?', *New Community Quarterly*, vol. 4, no. 3, pp. 39–47.
Healy, B. 1993, 'Elements in the development of an Australian radical social work', *Australian Social Work*, vol. 46, no. 1, pp. 3–8.
Healy, K. 1999, 'Power and activist social work', in *Transforming Social Work Practice*, eds B. Pease and J. Fook, Allen & Unwin, Sydney.
——2000, *Social Work Practices: Contemporary perspectives on change*, Sage, London.
——2001, 'Reinventing critical social work: challenges from practice, context and postmodernism', *Critical Social Work*, vol. 2, no. 1, pp. 1–17.
——2005a, *Social Work Theories in Context: Creating frameworks for practice*, Palgrave Macmillan, Basingstoke.
——2005b, 'Under reconstruction: renewing critical social work practices', in *Social Work: A critical turn*, eds S. Hick, J. Fook and R. Pozzuto, Thompson, Toronto, pp. 219–30.
——2005c, 'Modern critical social work: from radical to anti-oppressive', *Social Work Theories in Context: Creating frameworks for practice*, Palgrave Macmillan, Houndmills.
——2005d, 'What is critical social work? Current understandings of critical social work', in *Social Work: A critical turn*, eds S. Hick, J. Fook and R. Pozzuto, Thompson Education, Toronto.

Hearn, J. 1996, 'Is masculinity dead? A critique of the concept of masculinity/masculinities', in *Understanding Masculinities*, ed. M. Mac an Ghaill, Open University Press, Buckingham.

——1998, 'The welfare of men?', in *Men, Gender Divisions and Welfare*, eds J. Popay, J. Hearn and J. Edwards, Routledge, London.

——1999, 'It's time for men to change', in *Working with Men for Change*, ed. J. Wild, UCL Press, London.

——2001, 'Men, social work and men's violence towards women', in *Men and Social Work: Theories and practice*, ed. A. Christie, Palgrave, London.

Hearn, J. and Collinson, D. 1994, 'Theorising unities and differences between men and between masculinities', in *Theorising Masculinities*, eds H. Brod and M. Kaufman, Sage, Thousand Oaks, CA.

Hekman, S. 1999, *The Future of Differences: Truth and method in feminist theory*, Polity Press, Cambridge.

Held, D. 1980, *Introduction to Critical Theory: Horkheimer to Habermas*, Hutchinson, London.

——2004, 'Democratic accountability and political effectiveness from a cosmopolitan perspective', *Government and Opposition*, vol. 39, no. 2, pp. 364–91.

Helfrich, C.A., Fujiura, G.T. and Rutkowski-Smitta, V. 2008, 'Mental health disorders and functioning of women in domestic violence shelters', *Journal of Interpersonal Violence*, vol. 23, no. 4, pp. 437–53.

Hendrick, H. 1997, 'Constructions and reconstructions of British childhood: an interpretative survey, 1800 to the present', in *Constructing and Reconstructing Childhood: Contemporary issues in the sociological study of childhood*, eds. A. James and A. Prout, 2nd edn, Falmer Press, London, pp. 28–56.

Hennig, C. 1975, 'Introduction', in *Working Papers No. 1*, Inside Welfare: Revolutionary Welfare Workers, University of Queensland, Brisbane, pp. 4–7.

Herman, J. 1992, *Trauma and Recovery: From domestic abuse to political terror*, Pandora, London.

Hibbins, R. and Pease, B. 2009, 'Masculinities on the move', in *Migrant Men: Critical studies of masculinities and the migration experience*, eds R. Howson, B. Pease, R. Hibbins and M. Donaldson, Routledge, London.

Hick, S. 2005, 'Reconceptualising critical social work', in *Social Work: A critical turn*, eds S. Hick, J. Fook and R. Pozzuto, Thompson Education, Toronto.

Hick, S., Fook, J. and Pozzuto, R. eds 2005, *Social Work: A critical turn*, Thompson Education, Toronto.

Hick, S. and Pozzuto, R. 2005, 'Introduction: towards "becoming" a critical social worker', in *Social Work: A critical turn*, eds S. Hick, J. Fook and R. Pozzuto, Thompson, Toronto.

Hicks, S. 1996, 'The "last resort"? Lesbian and gay experiences of the social work assessment process in fostering and adoption', *Practice*, vol. 8, no. 2, pp. 15–24.

Higgins, J.R. and Butler, N. 2007, *Indigenous responses to child protection issues*, 'Promising practices in out-of-home care for Aboriginal and Torres Strait Islander carers, children and young people' (booklet 4), Australian Institute of Family Studies, Melbourne.

Higgins, V. and Lockie, S. 2001, 'Getting big and getting out: government policy, self-reliance and farm adjustment', in *Rurality Bites: The social and environmental transformation of rural Australia*, eds S. Lockie and L. Bourke, Pluto Press, Sydney, pp. 178–90.

Hill, B.H. 2003, 'Home: urban and reservation', in *Genocide of the Mind: New Native American writing*, ed. M. Moore, Thunder's Mouth Press/Nation Books, New York, pp. 21–8.

Hiranandani, V. 2005, 'Towards a critical theory of disability in social work', *Critical Social Work*, vol. 6, no. 1, pp. 1–15.

Hiskey, E. 1980, 'Child protection policy in Victoria: part 1', in *Australian Child and Family Welfare*, vol. 5, no. 3, pp. 6–10.

Hitchcock, A. 2001, 'Rising number of dowry deaths in India', World Socialist website, 4 July, <www.wsws.org/articles/2001/jul2001/ind-j04.shtml> [1 August 2008].

Hoatson, L., Dixon, J. and Sloman, D. 1996, 'Community development, citizenship and the contract state', *Community Development Journal*, vol. 31, no. 2, pp. 126–36.

Hobsbawm, E. 2002, *Interesting Times: A twentieth-century life*, Abacus, London.

Hobsbawm, E. with Polito, A. 2000, *On the Edge of the New Century*, The New Press, New York.

Hobson, B., ed. 2002, *Making Men into Fathers*, Cambridge University Press, Cambridge.

Hockey, J. and James, A. 1995, 'Back to our futures: imaging second childhood', in *Images of Aging: Cultural representations of later life*, eds M. Featherstone and A. Wernick, Routledge, London, pp. 135–48.

Hocking, G. 2003, 'Oxfam Great Britain and sustainable livelihoods in the UK', *Community Development Journal*, vol. 38, no. 3, pp. 235–42.

Hollinsworth, D. 1997, 'The work of anti-racism', in *The Resurgence of Racism: Howard, Hanson and the race debate*, Monash Publications in History, No. 24, Monash University, Melbourne.

Hollway, W. 2001, 'The psycho-social subject in "evidence-based practice"', *Journal of Social Work Practice*, vol. 15, no. 1, pp. 9–22.

Holmes, C.A. and Warelow, P.J. 2000, 'Some implications of postmodernism for nursing theory, research and practice', *Canadian Journal of Nursing Research*, vol. 32, no. 2, pp. 89–101.

Holst-Warhaft, G. 2000, *The Cue for Passion: Grief and its political uses*, Harvard University Press, Cambridge.

Hooks, B. 2004, *The Will to Change: Men, masculinity and love,* Washington Square Press, Washington DC.

Hough, G. and Briskman, L. 2003, 'Responding to the socio-political contexts of practice', in *Critical Social Work: An introduction to theories and practices*, eds J. Allan, B. Pease and L. Briskman, Allen & Unwin, Sydney, pp. 202–13.

Houston, S. 1995, 'Transcending the f ssure in risk theory: critical realism and child welfare', *Child and Family Social Work*, vol. 6, pp. 219–28.

——2001, 'Beyond social constructionism: critical realism and social work', *British Journal of Social Work*, vol. 31, pp. 845–61.

——2002, 'Ref ecting on habitus, f eld and capital: towards a culturally sensitive social work', *Journal of Social Work*, vol. 2, pp. 149–67.

Hovdestad, E. 2001, 'Seeking justice: the strategy of the national social action program', *Journal of Social Distress and the Homeless*, vol. 10, no. 1, pp. 105–21.

Howarth, G. 2007, *Death & Dying: A sociological introduction*, Polity Press, Cambridge.

Hugman, R. 2008, 'Invited commentary: social work values: equity or equality? A response to Solas', *Australian Social Work*, vol. 61, no. 2, pp. 141–5.

Human Rights and Equal Opportunity Commission 1997, *Bringing Them Home: Report of the National Inquiry into the Separation of Aboriginal and Islander Children from Their Families*, HREOC, Sydney.

Humphries, B. 2008, *Social Work Research for Social Justice*, Palgrave Macmillan, Basingstoke.

Hurst, M. 1995, 'Counselling women from a feminist perspective', in *Issues Facing Australian Families*, 2nd edn, eds W. Weeks and J. Wilson, Longman, Melbourne, pp. 245–57.

Ife, J. 1995, *Community Development*, Longman, Melbourne.

——1997, *Rethinking Social Work: Towards critical practice*, Longman, Melbourne.

——1999, 'Postmodernism, critical theory and social work', in *Transforming Social Work Practice: Postmodern critical perspectives*, eds B. Pease and J. Fook, Allen & Unwin, Sydney, pp. 211–23.

——2001, *Human Rights and Social Work: Towards rights-based practice*, Cambridge University Press, Cambridge.

——2002, *Community Development: Community-based alternatives in an age of globalisation*, 2nd edn, Pearson Education, Sydney.

——2005a, 'What is critical social work today?', in 'Current Understandings of Critical Social Work', in *Social Work: A critical turn*, eds S. Hicks, J. Fook and R. Pozzuto, Thompson Education, Toronto.

——2005b, 'Human rights and critical social work', in *Social Work: A critical turn*, eds S. Hick, J. Fook and R. Pozzuto, Thompson Education, Toronto.

——2007, 'Cultural relativism and community activism', in *Challenges in Human Rights: A social work perspective*, ed. E. Reichert, Colombia University Press, New York.

——2008a, *Human Rights and Social Work: Towards rights-based practice*, revised edn, Cambridge University Press, Cambridge.

——2008b, 'Ignoring the lessons of community development', Personal communication.

Ife, J. and Tesoreiro, F. 2006, *Community Development: Community based alternatives in an age of globalisation*, 3rd edn, Pearson Education, Sydney.

IFSW (International Federation of Social Work)/IASSW (International Association of Schools of Social Work) 2004, *Ethics in Social Work: Statement of principles*, <www.ifsw.org/en/p38000398.html> [7 October 2008].

Industry Commission 1995, *Charitable Organisations in Australia*, Report no. 45, AGPS, Canberra.

Ingamels, A. 2007, 'Community development and community renewal: tracing the workings of power', *Community Development Journal*, vol. 42, no. 2, pp. 237–50.

Inside Welfare 1975, *Working Papers No. 1*, Inside Welfare, Brisbane.

——1976, *First National Conference Proceedings*, Inside Welfare, Melbourne.

——1979, *An Annotated Bibliography for Marxist Welfare Workers*, Inside Welfare, Sydney.

International Association of Schools of Social Work 2001, *International Definition of Social Work*, <www.iassw.org> [1 July 2008].

International Federation of Social Workers (IFSW) 2005, *International Policy on Women*, <www.ifsw.org/en/f38000075.html> [8 August 2008].

——1996, *International Policy on Human Rights*, <www.ifsw.org> [1 July 2008].

IPP-SHR (International Program of Psycho-Social Health Research) 2008, 'Off the press—drug therapy in psychiatry: the consumers' perspective', *Psycho-Social Update*, vol. 3, no. 2, July, p. 1.

Ishay, M., ed. 1997, *The Human Rights Reader: Major political essays, speeches, and documents from the Bible to the present*, Routledge, New York.

Ivey, A. 2008, 'Complexity and culture', in *New Horizons in Multicultural Counseling*, eds G. Monk, J. Winslade and S. Sinclair, Sage, Thousand Oaks, CA.

Iwaniec, D. 2007, 'Competence in working with families', in *Competence in Social Work Practice: A guidebook for students and professionals*, ed. K. O'Hagan, Jessica Kingsley, London.

Jackson, S. 1999, *Heterosexuality in Question*, Sage, London.

Jackson, S. and Scott, S. 1996, 'Sexual skirmishes and feminist factions', in *Feminism and Sexuality: A reader*, eds S. Jackson and S. Scott, Edinburgh University Press, Edinburgh, pp. 1–34.

Jaggs, D. 1986, *Neglected and Criminal: Foundations of child welfare legislation in Victoria*, Centre for Youth and Community Studies, Phillip Institute of Technology, Melbourne.

Jalland, P. 2006, *Changing Ways of Death in Twentieth-century Australia: War, medicine and the funeral business*, University of New South Wales Press, Sydney.

James, A. and James, A. 2004, *Constructing Childhood: Theory, policy and social practice*, Palgrave Macmillan, London.

James, A. and Prout, A. 1997, '"Re-presenting childhood": time and transition in the study of childhood', in *Constructing and Reconstructing Childhood: Contemporary issues in the sociological study of childhood*, eds A. James and A. Prout, 2nd edn, Falmer Press, London, pp. 230–50.

Jamieson, L. 1998, *Intimacy: Personal relationships in modern societies*, Polity Press, Cambridge.

Jamrozik, A. 2001, *Social Policy in the Post-welfare State: Australians on the threshold of the 21st century*, Pearson Education, Sydney.

Jenkins, A. 1990, *Invitations to Responsibility*, Dulwich Publications, Adelaide.

——1991, 'Intervention with violence and abuse in families: the inadvertent perpetuation of irresponsible behaviour', *ANZJFT*, vol. 12, no. 4, pp. 186–95.

Jenkins, S. 2004, 'Developing a residential programme for children in response to trauma-related behaviours', *Children Australia*, vol. 29, no. 3, pp. 22–9.
Jenks, C. 1996, *Childhood*, Routledge, London.
Jensen, A.M. and Saporiti, A. 1992, *Do Children Count? A statistical compendium*, Eurosocial Report 36/17, European Centre for Social Welfare Policy and Research, Vienna.
Jessop, B. 1993, 'Towards a Schumpetarian workfare state? Preliminary remarks on a post-Fordist political economy', *Studies in Political Economy*, vol. 40, pp. 7–39.
——1994, 'The transition to post-Fordism and the Schumpeterian workfare state', in *Towards a post-Fordist Welfare State?*, eds R. Burrows and B. Loader, Routledge, London, pp. 13–37.
——1999, 'The changing governance of welfare: recent trends in its primary functions, scale, and modes of coordination', *Social Policy and Administration*, vol. 33, pp. 348–59.
——2002a, *The Future of the Capitalist State*, Polity Press, Cambridge.
——2002b, 'Liberalism, neoliberalism and urban governance: a state theoretical perspective', *Antipode*, vol. 3, pp. 452–72.
Jessup, H. and Rogerson, S. 1999, 'Postmodernism and the teaching and practice of interpersonal skills', in *Transforming Social Work Practice*, eds B. Pease and J. Fook, Allen & Unwin, Sydney.
Johansson, T. 2007, 'Intimacy', in *International Encyclopedia of Men and Masculinities*, Routledge, Milton Park.
Johnson, K. 1997, *Deinstitutionalising Women: An ethnographic study of deinstitutionalisation*, Cambridge University Press, Melbourne.
Johnson, K. and Tait, S. 2003, 'Throwing away the key: people with intellectual disabilities and involuntary detention', in *Involuntary Detention and Civil Commitment: International perspectives*, eds I. Freckleton and K. Diesfeld, Bloomsbury, London, pp. 135–58.
Johnson, K., Strong, R., Hillier, L. and Pitts, M. 2002, *Screened Out: Women with disabilities and cervical screening*, The Cancer Council, Melbourne.
Jones, K., Cooper, B. and Ferguson, H. 2008a, 'Concluding ref ections on the nature and future of critical best practice', in *Best Practice in Social Work: Critical perspectives*, eds K. Jones, B. Cooper and H. Ferguson, Palgrave Macmillan, Basingstoke.
——eds 2008b, *Best Practice in Social Work: Critical perspectives*, Palgrave Macmillan, Basingstoke.
Jones, M. and Kriesler, P., eds 1998b, *Globalisation, Human Rights and Civil Society*, Prospect Media, Sydney.
Jouve, E. 1979, 'The ideology of human rights', in *Ecumenical Institute for the Development of Peoples Trilateral Commission, National Security*, Human Rights, Paris, pp. 83–92.
Judge, C. and Van Blummelen F. 2002, *Kew Cottages: The world of Dolly Steiner*, Spectrum, Melbourne.
Kagan, R. and Schlosberg, S. 1989, *Families in Perpetual Crisis*, W.W. Norton, New York.
Kagawa-Singer, M. 1998, 'The cultural context of death rituals and mourning practices', *Oncology Nursing Forum*, vol. 25, pp. 1752–6.
KAMSC (Kimberley Aboriginal Medical Services Council) 2008, 'Protective behaviours community way package', <www.kamsc.org.au/resources.html> [12 September 2008].
Kanner, A.D. and Gomes, M.E. 1995, 'The all-consuming self', in *Ecopsychology: Restoring the earth, healing the mind*, eds T. Roszak, M. Gomes and A. Kanner, Sierra Club Books, San Francisco.
Kaufman, M. 1993, *Cracking the Armour: Power, pain and the lives of men*, Viking, Toronto.
Kay, A. 2006, 'Social capital, the social economy and community development', *Community Development Journal*, vol. 41, no. 2, 160–73.
Kellehear, A., ed. 2000a, *Death and Dying in Australia*, Oxford University Press, Melbourne.
——2000b, 'The Australian way of death: formative historical and social inf uences', in *Death and Dying in Australia*, ed. A. Kellehear, Oxford University Press, Melbourne.
——2005, *Compassionate Cities: Public health and end-of-life care*, Routledge, Milton Park.
——ed. 2001, *Grief and Remembering: 25 Australians tell it like it is*, Rivoli, Melbourne.

Kenny, S. 2006, *Developing Communities for the Future: Community development in Australia*, 3rd edn, Thomas Nelson, Melbourne.

Kermode, S. and Brown, C. 1996, 'The postmodernist hoax and its effects on nursing', *International Journal of Nursing Studies*, vol. 33, no. 4, pp. 375–84.

Kessen, W. 1983, 'The child and other cultural inventions', in *The Child and Other Cultural Inventions*, eds F.S. Kessel and A.W. Siegel, Houston Symposium 4, 1981, Praeger Special Studies, New York, pp. 26–47.

Kilby, P. 1994, 'Human rights and participatory development: stemming the rise of the "new anarchy"', *Development Bulletin*, vol. 32, pp. 20–2.

Kimmel, M. 2000, *The Gendered Society*, Oxford University Press, New York.

Kimmel, M., Hearn, J. and Connell, R., eds 2005, *Handbook of Studies on Men and Masculinities*, Sage, Thousand Oaks, CA.

Kingf sher, C. 1998, 'How providers make policy: an analysis of everyday conversation in a welfare off ce', *Journal of Community and Applied Psychology*, vol. 8, no. 2, pp. 119–36.

Kirk, S.A. 2005, 'Introduction: critical perspectives', in *Mental Disorders in the Social Environment*, ed. S.A. Kirk, Columbia University Press, New York.

Kitzinger, J. 1997, 'Who are you kidding? Children, power and the struggle against sexual abuse', in *Constructing and Reconstructing Childhood: Contemporary issues in the sociological study of childhood*, 2nd edn, eds A. James and A. Prout, Falmer Press, London, pp. 165–89.

Klass, D., Silverman, P. and Nickman, S., eds 1996, *Continuing Bonds: New understandings of grief*, Taylor & Francis, Philadelphia.

Klass, D. and Walter, T. 2001, 'Processes of grieving: how bonds are continued', in *Handbook of Bereavement Research: Consequences, coping, and care*, eds M. Stroebe, R. Hansson, W. Stroebe and H. Schut, American Psychological Association, Washington.

Klosterman, D.M. and Stratton, D.C. 2006, 'Speaking truth to power, Jane Addams's values base for peacemaking', *Affilia, Journal of Women and Social Work*, vol. 21, no. 2, pp. 158–68.

Koenig, M.A., Ahmed, S., Hossain M.B. and Alam Mozumder A.B.M.K. 2003, 'Women's status and domestic violence in rural Bangladesh: individual- and community-level effects', *Demography*, vol. 40, no. 2, pp. 269–88.

Korr, W., Fallon, B. and Brieland, D. 1994, 'UN Convention on the Rights of the Child: implications for social work education', *International Social Work*, vol. 37, no. 4, pp. 333–45.

Korten, D. 1990, *Getting to the 21st Century*, Kumarian, West Hartford.

——1995, *When Corporations Rule the World*, Kumarian, West Hartford.

——2006, *The Great Turning: From empire to earth community*, Berrett-Koehler, San Francisco.

Kovel, J. 2007, *The Enemy of Nature: The end of capitalism or the end of the world?*, Zed Books, London.

Kristjanson, L., Lobb, E., Aoun, S. and Monterosso, L. 2006, A systematic review of the literature on complicated grief, prepared by the WA Centre for Cancer & Palliative Care, Edith Cowan University, Churchlands, Western Australia. <www.health.gov.au/internet/wcms/publishing.nsf/Content/palliative care-pubs-rsch-grief> [7 October 2007].

Kübler-Ross, E. 1970, *On Death and Dying*, Tavistock, London.

Kübler-Ross, E. and Kessler, D. 2005, *On Grief and Grieving: Finding the meaning of grief through the five stages of loss*, Scribner, New York.

Kufeldt, K., Simard, M. and Vachon, J. 2000, *Looking after Children in Canada: Final report*, Submitted to Social Development Partnerships of Human Resources Development, Canada.

Kumsa, M.K. 2007, 'A resettlement story of unsettlement: transformative practices of taking it personally', in *Doing Anti-Oppressive Practice: Building transformative politicized social work*, ed. D. Baines, Fernwood, Halifax, BC, Canada.

Kundnani, A. 2007, *The End of Tolerance: Racism in 21st century Britain*, Pluto Press, London.

Kuper, A. 2004, *Democracy beyond Borders: Justice and representation in global institutions*, Oxford University Press, Oxford.

Ladd, P. 2003, *Understanding Deaf Culture: In search of deafhood*, Random House, London.
Lamb, S. and Coakley, M. 1993, 'Normal childhood sexual play and games—differentiating play from abuse', *Child Abuse and Neglect*, vol. 17, no. 4, pp. 515–26.
Langan, M. 2002, 'The legacy of radical social work', in *Social Work: Themes, issues and critical debates*, 2nd edn, eds R. Adams, L. Dominelli and M. Payne, Palgrave, Houndmills, pp. 209–17.
Langan, M. and Lee, P. 1989, 'Whatever happened to radical social work?', in *Radical Social Work Today*, eds M. Langan and P. Lee, Unwin Hyman, London, pp. 1–18.
Larkins, R. 2007, *Funeral Rights: What the Australian 'death-care' industry doesn't want you to know*, Viking, Melbourne.
Larner, G. 2001, 'The critical practitioner model in therapy', *Australian Psychologist*, vol. 36, no. 1, pp. 36–43.
——2004, 'Family therapy and the politics of evidence', *Journal of Family Therapy*, vol. 26, pp. 17–39.
Larson, A. and Peterson, A. 2001, 'Rethinking responses to "domestic violence" in Australian Indigenous communities', *Journal of Social Welfare and Family Law*, vol. 23, no. 2, pp. 121–34.
Latouche, S. 1993, *In the Wake of Affluent Society*, Zed Books, London.
Lawrence, J. 1965, *Professional Social Work in Australia*, Australian National University, Canberra.
Lawrence, M. 1992, 'Women's psychology and feminist social work practice', in *Women, Oppression and Social Work: Issues in anti-discriminatory practice*, eds M. Langan and L. Day, Routledge, London, pp. 32–48.
Leach, M. 1993, 'Hard yakkin'', *XY: Men, Sex, Politics*, vol 3, no. 3, pp. 14–17.
Lechner, F. and Boli, J., eds 2000, *The Globalization Reader*, Blackwell, Oxford.
Ledwith, M. 2006, *Community Development: A critical approach*, Policy Press, Bristol.
Lee, C. 2008, 'What is Culture', in *New Horizons in Multicultural Counseling*, eds G. Monk, J. Winslade and S. Sinclair, Sage, Thousand Oaks, CA.
Legge, V. and Cant, R. 1995, 'A lonely old age', *Social Alternatives*, vol. 14, no. 2, pp. 44–7.
Leibrich, J. 1998, 'The healer within: a personal view of recovery', in *Folding Back the Shadows*, ed. S.E. Romans, University of Otago Press, Dunedin, New Zealand.
Lennie, I. 1976, 'Inside Welfare', *Arena*, no. 42, pp. 18–22.
Lenore, E. 1994, *Abused Women and Survivor Therapy: A practical guide for the psychotherapist*, American Psychological Association, Washington.
Leonard, P. 1984, *Personality and Ideology: Towards a materialist understanding of the individual*, Macmillan, London.
——1997, *Postmodern Welfare: Reconstructing an emancipatory project*, Sage, London.
——2001, 'The future of critical social work in uncertain conditions', *Critical Social Work*, vol. 2, no. 1, pp. 1–7, <www.criticalsocialwork.com/CSW_2001_1.html> [23 August 2001].
Lev-Wiesel, R., Goldblatt, H., Eisikovits, Z. and Admi, H. 2008, 'Growth in the shadow of war: the case of social workers and nurses working in a shared war reality', *British Journal of Social Work*, Advance Access, 5 March, <http://bjsw.oxfordjournals.org> [15 July 2008].
Lichtenberg, P. 1999, 'Men overview', in *Encyclopedia of Social Work*, 19th edn, National Association of Social Workers, Washington.
Liffman, M. 1978, *Power for the Poor*, Allen & Unwin, Sydney.
Lincoln, Y.S. and Guba, E.G. 2000, 'Paradigmatic controversies, contradictions, and emerging conf uences', in *Handbook of Qualitative Research*, 2nd edn, eds N.K. Denzin and Y.S. Lincoln, Sage, London, pp. 163–88.
Lipsky, M. 1980, *Street Level Bureaucracy: The dilemmas of individuals in the public service*, Sage, Thousand Oaks, CA.
Lisak, D. 1991, 'Sexual aggression, masculinity and fathers', *Signs: Journal of Women, Culture and Society*, vol. 16, no. 2, pp. 239–63.
Lister, R. 1990, *The Exclusive Society: Citizenship and the poor*, Child Poverty Action Group, London.
——2003, *Citizenship: Feminist perspectives*, 2nd edn, Palgrave Macmillan, Houndmills.

Lister, R., Middleton S. and Smith N. 2001, *Young People's Voices: Citizenship education*, Youth Work Press, Leicester.

Little, G. 1999, *The Public Emotions: From mourning to hope*, ABC Books, Sydney.

Llewellyn, S. 1998, 'Boundary work: costing and caring in the social services', in *Accounting, Organisations and Society*, vol. 23, no. 1, pp. 23–47.

Lobb, E., Kristjanson, L., Aoun, S. and Monteresso, L. 2006, 'An overview of complicated grief terminology and diagnostic criteria', *Grief Matters*, vol. 9, no. 2, pp. 28–32.

Lockie, S. and Bourke, L. 2001, *Rurality Bites: The social and environmental transformation of rural Australia*, Pluto Press, Sydney.

Longres, J. and Bailey, R. 1979, 'Men's issues and sexism: a journal review', *Social Work*, January, pp. 26–32.

Lopez, J. and Potter, G. 2005, *After Postmodernism: An introduction to critical realism*, Continuum, New York.

Lowell, R. 2006, *Localising Human Services*, Australian Scholarly Publishing, Melbourne.

Lundy, C. 2004, *Social Work and Social Justice: A structural approach to practice*, Broadview, Ontario.

Lymberry, M. and Butler, S. 2004, 'Introduction', in *Social Work Ideals and Practice Realities*, eds M. Lymberry and S. Butler, Palgrave Macmillan, Basingstoke.

Lynch, T. 2006, 'Understanding psychiatry's resistance to change', *Critical Psychiatry: The limits of madness*, ed. D.B. Double, Palgrave Macmillan, Basingstoke.

Lynn, R. 1998, *'Murri Way!'—Aborigines and Torres Strait Islanders reconstruct social welfare practice*, Centre for Social and Welfare Research, James Cook University, Townsville.

Lyons, M. 1993, 'Data on Australia's third sector: an impossible quest?', in The Centre for Australian Community Organisations and Management (CACOM), *Power, Politics and Performance: Community management in the 1990s*, conference papers, University of Technology, Sydney, pp. 27–36.

——1998, 'The impact of managerialism on social policy', *Public Productivity and Management Review*, vol. 21, no. 4, pp. 419–32.

——2001, *Third Sector: The contribution of nonprofit and cooperative enterprises in Australia*, Allen & Unwin, Sydney.

McBeath, G. and Webb, S. 2005, 'Post-critical social work analytics', in *Social Work: A critical turn*, eds S. Hick, J. Fook and R. Pozzuto, Thompson Education, Toronto.

McBride, J. 1995, *War, Battering and Other Sports*, Humanities Press, Atlantic Highlands, NJ.

McCain, M. and Mustard, J.F. 1999, *Reversing the Real Brain Drain: Early years study final report*, Canadian Institute for Advanced Research, Toronto.

McCoy, B. 2008, *Holding Men*, Aboriginal Studies Press, Canberra.

McDonald, C. 1999, 'Human service professionals in the community service industry', *Australian Social Work*, vol. 52, no. 1, pp. 17–25.

——2003, 'Forward via the past?: Evidence-based practice as a strategy in social work', *The Drawing Board: An Australian Review of Public Affairs*, vol. 3, no. 3, pp. 123–42.

——2006, *Challenging Social Work: The context of practice*, Palgrave Macmillan, Basingstoke.

——2007, 'Wizards of Oz? The radical tradition in Australian social work (and what we can learn from Aotearoa New Zealand', in *International Social Work and the Radical Tradition*, eds M. Lavalette and I. Ferguson, Venture Press, London.

McDonald, C., Harris, J. and Wintersteen, R. 2003, 'Contingent or context? Social work and the state in Australia, Britain and the USA', *British Journal of Social Work*, vol. 33, pp. 191–208.

McDonald, C. and Marston, G. 2005, 'Workfare as welfare: governing unemployment in the advanced liberal state', *Critical Social Policy*, vol. 25, no. 3, pp. 374–401.

MacDonald, L. 1996, 'Dismantling the movement: feminism, postmodernism and political action', *Refractory Girl*, vol. 51, no. 96, pp. 48–51.

McDonald, L. and Collins, A. 2000, *Abuse and Neglect of Older Adults: A discussion paper*, Health Canada, Family Violence Prevention Unit, Ottawa.

McDonald, P. 1994, 'What are the issues?', *Family Matters*, vol. 37, April, pp. 4–5.
Macedo, D. 2000, *Introduction to Pedagogy of the Oppressed*, Continuum, New York.
Macedo, D. and Bartolome, L.I. 1999, *Dancing with Bigotry: Beyond the politics of tolerance*, Palgrave, New York.
Macey, D. 2000, *The Penguin Dictionary of Critical Theory*, Penguin, London.
McFarlane, A. 2008, 'Race, ethnicity, and identity', in *New Horizons in Multicultural Counseling*, eds G. Monk, J. Winslade and S. Sinclair, Sage, Thousand Oaks, CA.
McGurk, H. 1996, 'Child care in a caring society', *Family Matters*, vol. 46, pp. 12–17.
Mack, J. 1995, 'The politics of species arrogance', in *Ecopsychology: Restoring the earth, healing the mind*, eds T. Roszak, M. Gomes and A. Kanner, Sierra Club Books, San Francisco.
Mack, K. 1998, 'Judicial attitudes and women's credibility: barriers to equality in the law', in *Women and the Law*, ed. A. Thacker, Deakin University Press, Geelong.
McKendrick, J. and Thorpe, M. 1998, 'The legacy of colonisation: trauma, loss and psychological distress amongst Aboriginal people', *Grief Matters*, September, pp. 4–8.
McLaughlin, H. 2005, 'Young service users as co-researchers: methodological problems and possibilities,' *Qualitative Social Work*, vol. 4, no. 2, pp. 211–28.
McLellan, G. 1994, 'Feminism, epistemology and postmodernism: ref ections on current ambivalence', *Sites*, vol. 28, pp. 98–124.
McLennan, W. 1999, *Older People, Australia: A social report*, Australian Bureau of Statistics, Canberra.
McMahon, A. 1999, *Taking Care of Men: Sexual politics in the public mind*, Cambridge University Press, Melbourne.
McMaster, K.J. 1997, *Feeling Angry, Playing Fair: Breaking the cycle of abuse*, Reed, Auckland.
——2000, 'Working with male social work students', in *Fieldwork in the Human Services*, eds L. Cooper and L. Briggs, Allen & Unwin, Sydney.
McMaster, K.J. and Swain, P. 1989, *A Private Affair: Stopping men's violence to women*, GP Books, Wellington.
McNeill, T. 2006, 'Evidence-based practice in an age of relativism: towards a model for practice', *Social Work*, vol. 51, no. 2, pp. 147–57.
McNicoll, P. 2004, 'Putting social justice on the agenda: addressing habitual and social barriers', in *Growth and Development through Group Work*, eds C. Carson, A. Fritz, E. Lewis, J. Ramey and D. Sugiuchi, The Haworth Press, New York.
McPhail, B.A., Busch, N.B., Kulkarni, S. and Rice, G. 2007, 'An integrative feminist model: the evolving feminist perspective on intimate partner violence', *Violence Against Women*, vol. 13, no. 8, pp. 817–41.
Mann, P. 1994, *Micro-Politics: Agency in a postfeminist era*, University of Minnesota Press, Minneapolis, MN.
Manning, D. 2007, 'Walk the talk: the journey towards deconstructing the education environment as a model for anti-oppressive social work and community welfare practice', *Practice Reflections*, vol. 1, no. 1. pp. 15–26.
Manning, S. 1998, 'Empowerment in mental health programs: listening to the voices', in *Empowerment in Social Work Practice: A sourcebook*, eds L. Gutierrez, R. Parsons and E. Cox, Brooks/Cole, Pacif c Grove, CA.
Mannino, A. and Deutsch, F. 2007, 'Changing the division of labor: a negotiated process between partners', *Sex Roles*, vol. 56, nos 5–6, pp. 309–24.
Mantysaari, M. 2005, 'Realism as a foundation for social work knowledge', *Qualitative Social Work*, vol. 4, no. 1, pp. 87–98.
Marchant, H. 1985, 'A feminist perspective on the development of the social work profession in New South Wales', *Australian Social Work*, vol. 38, no. 1, pp. 35–43.
Marchant, H. and Wearing, B. 1986a, *Gender Reclaimed: Women in social work*, Hale & Iremonger, Sydney.

——1986b, 'Introduction', in *Gender Reclaimed: Women in social work*, eds H. Marchant and B. Wearing, Hale & Iremonger, Marrickville, pp. 11–13.
Marcuse, P. 1989, 'Dual city: a muddy metaphor for a quartered city', *International Journal of Urban and Regional Research*, vol. 17, pp. 697–708.
Markiewicz, A. 1996, 'The child welfare system in Victoria: changing context and perspectives 1945–1995', *Children Australia*, vol. 21, no. 3, pp. 32–41.
Marris, P. 1996, *The Politics of Uncertainty: Attachment in private and public life*, Routledge, London.
Marsiglio, W. and Pleck, J. 2005, 'Fatherhood and masculinities', in *Handbook on Studies on Men and Masculinities*, eds M. Kimmel, J. Hearn and R. Connell, Sage, Thousand Oaks, CA.
Marston, G. and Watts, R. 2003, 'Tampering with the evidence: a critical appraisal of evidence-based policy making', *The Drawing Board: An Australian Review of Public Affairs*, vol. 3, no. 3, pp. 143–63.
Martin, E. 1990, 'Gender, demand and domain: the social work profession in South Australia 1935–1980', PhD thesis, Department of History, University of Melbourne.
——1992, 'Themes in a history of the social work profession', *International Social Work*, vol. 35, pp. 327–45.
Martin, J. 2003, 'Historical development of critical social work practice', in *Critical Social Work*, eds J. Allan, B. Pease and L. Briskman, Allen & Unwin, Sydney, pp. 17–31.
——2006, 'Migrants and refugees', in *Social Work and Human Services: Best practice*, eds W. Hong Chui and J. Wilson, The Federation Press, Sydney.
Martin, T. and Doka, K. 2000, *Men Don't Cry . . . Women Do: Transcending gender stereotypes of grief*, Brunner/Mazel, Philadelphia.
Mason, J. 2001, 'Social work with families', in *Social Work: Fields of practice*, eds M. Alston and J. McKinnon, Oxford University Press, Melbourne.
——2005, 'Social work with families', in *Social Work: Fields of practice*, eds M. Alston and J. McKinnon, 2nd edn, Oxford University Press, Melbourne, pp. 83–94.
Mathers, C. 2000, 'Men's health in Australia: a statistical prof le', unpublished paper, Australian Institute of Health and Welfare, Canberra.
Matsakis, A. 1998, *Managing Client Anger: What to do when a client is angry with you*, New Harbinger, Oakland.
Maushart, S. 2001, *Wifework: What marriage really means for women*, Text, Melbourne.
Mauss, M. 2002, *The Gift: The form and reason for exchange in archaic societies*, Routledge, London.
Max-Neef, M. et al. 1991, *Human Scale Development*, Apex, New York.
May, R. 2007, 'Working without diagnosis', *The Psychologist*, vol. 20, part 5 (May) www.thepsychologist.org.uk/archive/archive_home.cfm?volumeID=20&editionID=147 [17 February 2009].
Mayo, M. 2005, *Global Citizens: Social movements and the challenge of globalization*, Canadian Scholars Press, Toronto.
Meagher, G. 2000, 'Social sustainability in Australia', *Canberra Bulletin of Public Administration*, no. 96, pp. 63–78.
——2002, *The Politics of Knowledge in Social Service Evaluation*, Uniting Care Burnside, Sydney.
Memmott, P., Stacy, R., Chambers, C. and Keys, C. 2001, *Violence in Indigenous Communities*, Attorney-General's Department, Canberra.
Mendes, P. 2001, 'Public attacks on social work in Australia: the two *Bulletin* Affairs', *Australian Social Work*, vol. 54, no. 3, pp. 55–62.
——2005, 'The history of social work in Australia: a critical literature review', *Australian Social Work*, vol. 58, no. 2, pp. 121–31.
——2007, 'Social workers and social activism in Victoria, Australia', *Journal of Progressive Human Services*, vol. 18, no. 1, April, pp. 25–44.
——2008, 'Integrating social work and community development practice in Victoria, Australia', *Asia Pacific Journal of Social Work and Development*, vol. 18, no. 1, pp. 14–25.

Mental Health Council of Australia 2005, *Not for Service: Experiences of injustice and despair in mental health care in Australia*, Mental Health Council of Australia, Canberra.

Mercia, K. and Julien, I. 1988, 'Race, sexual politics and black masculinity: a dossier', in *Male Order: Unwrapping masculinity*, eds R. Chapman and J. Rutherford, Lawrence & Wishart, London.

Merry, S.E. 2006, *Human Rights and Gender Violence: Translating international law into local justice*, University of Chicago Press, Chicago.

Middleman, R. and Goldberg, G. 1974, *Social Service Delivery: A structural approach to social work practice*, Columbia University Press, New York.

Middleton, S., Ashworth, K. and Walker, R. 1994, *Family Fortunes: Pressures on parents and children in the 1990s*, Child Poverty Action Group, London.

Mies, M. and Shiva, V. 1993, *Ecofeminism*, Zed Books, London.

Millear, A. with Johnson, K. 2000, '39 months under the *Disability Discrimination Act*', in *Women with Intellectual Disabilities: Finding a place in the world*, eds R. Traustadottir and K. Johnson, Jessica Kingsley, London, pp. 239–52.

Millei, Z. and Lee, L. 2007, '"Smarten up the parents": whose agendas are we serving? Governing parents and children through the Smart Population Foundation Initiative in Australia', *Contemporary Issues in Early Childhood*, vol. 8, no. 3, pp. 208–21, online only, <www.wwwords.co.uk/ciec/content/maincontents.asp> [3 March 2008].

Miller, E. and Omarzu, J. 1998, 'New directions in loss research', in *Perspectives on Loss: A sourcebook*, ed. J. Harvey, Brunner/Mazel, Philadelphia.

Miller, K., Kulkarni, M. and Kushner, H. 2006, 'Beyond trauma-focused psychiatric epidemiology: bridging research and practice with war-affected populations', *American Journal of Orthopsychiatry*, vol. 76, issue 4, pp. 409–22.

Miller, S. 1996, 'Class, power and social construction: issues of theory and application in thirty years of rural studies', *Sociologia Ruralis*, vol. 36, no. 1, pp. 93–116.

Milner, J. 2001, *Women and Social Work: Narrative approaches*, Palgrave, New York.

Mitchell, G. 1999, 'Evidence-based practice: critique and alternative view', *Nursing Science Quarterly*, vol. 12, no. 1, pp. 30–5.

Mmatli, T. 2008, 'Political activism as a social work strategy in Africa', *International Social Work*, vol. 51, no. 3, pp. 297–310.

Mooney Cotter, A.M. 2004, *Gender Injustice: A comparative analysis of women in employment*, Ashgate, Aldershot.

Moore, N. 1996, '"Me operation": Abortion and class in Australian women's novels, 1920s–1950', *Hecate*, vol. xxii, no. 1, pp. 27–46.

Moreau, M. 1977, 'A structural approach to social work', unpublished paper, School of Social Work, Carleton University, Ottawa.

——1979, 'A structural approach to social work practice', *Canadian Journal of Social Work Education*, vol. 5, no. 1, pp. 78–94.

——1990, 'Empowerment through advocacy and consciousness raising: implications of a structural approach to social work', *Journal of Sociology and Social Welfare*, vol. 17, no. 2, pp. 78–94.

Moreau, M., Frosst, S., Frayne, G., Hlywa, M., Leonard, L. and Rowell, M. 1993, *Empowerment II: Snapshots of the structural approach in action*, Carleton University Press, Ottawa.

Moreau, M. in collaboration with Leonard, L. 1989, *Empowerment through a Structural Approach to Social Work: A report from practice*, École de service sociale, Université de Montreal and Carleton University School of Social Work and Health and Welfare Canada, Montreal and Ottawa.

Moreton-Robinson, A. 2000, *Talkin' Up to the White Woman: Indigenous women and feminism*, University of Queensland Press, Brisbane.

Morgan, D. 2005, 'Class and masculinity', in *Handbook on Studies on Men and Masculinities*, eds M. Kimmel, J. Hearn and R. Connell, Sage, Thousand Oaks, CA.

Morgan, J. 2000, 'Boxes and remembering in the time of AIDS', *Dulwich Centre Journal*, no. 4, Morgan, J. and The Bambanani Women's Group 2003, *Long Life . . . Positive HIV Stories*, ABC Press, Cape Town.

Morley, C. 2003, 'Towards critical social work practice in mental health: a review', *Journal of Progressive Human Services*, vol. 14, no. 1, pp. 61–84.

——2004, 'Critical ref ection in social work: A response to globalisation?', *International Journal of Social Welfare*, vol. 13, no. 2, pp. 297–303.

——2005, 'Collaborative social work practice in opposing paradigms: issues to emerge from a sexual assault and mental health project', *Women Against Violence: An Australian Feminist Journal*, no. 16, pp. 4–14.

——2007, 'Engaging practitioners in critical ref ection: issues and dilemmas', *Journal of Reflective Practice*, vol. 8, no. 1, pp. 16–74.

Morley, C. and Macfarlane, S., 2008, 'The continued importance of a feminist analysis: making gendered inequalities visible through a critique of Howard government policy on domestic violence', *Just Policy: A Journal of Australian Social Policy*, no. 47. pp. 31–8.

Morrow, L., Verins, I. and Willis, E. 2002, 'Introduction', in *Mental Health and Work: Issues and perspectives*, eds L. Morrow, I. Verins and E. Willis, Commonwealth of Australia, Auseinet: The Australian Network for Promotion, Prevention and Early Intervention for Mental Health, Adelaide.

Moss, M. and Moss, S. 2003, 'Doubly disenfranchised grief in old age', *Grief Matters*, vol. 6, no. 1, pp. 4–6.

Mossakowski, K. 2003, 'Coping with perceived discrimination: does ethnic identity protect mental health?', *Journal of Health and Social Behavior*, vol. 44, no. 3, pp. 318–31.

Mowbray, M. 2000, 'Community development and local government: an Australian response to globalization and economic fundamentalism', *Community Development Journal*, vol. 35, no. 3, pp. 215–23.

——2005, 'Community capacity building or state opportunism?', *Community Development Journal*, vol. 40, no. 3, pp. 255–64.

Muetzelfeldt, M. 1992, 'Economic rationalism in its social context', in *Society, State and Politics in Australia*, ed. M. Muetzelfeldt, Pluto Press, Leichhardt.

Mullaly, B. 1993, *Structural Social Work: Ideology, theory and practice*, McClelland & Stewart, Toronto.

——1997, *Structural Social Work: Ideology, theory and practice*, 2nd edn, Oxford University Press, Toronto.

——2002, *Challenging Oppression: A critical social work approach*, Oxford University Press, Ontario.

——2007, *The New Structural Social Work*, 3rd edn, Oxford University Press, Don Mills.

Mullender, A. and Ward, D. 1991, *Self-Directed Groupwork: Users take action for empowerment*, Whiting & Birch, London.

Muller, U. 2007, 'Men's relations with women', in *International Encyclopedia of Men and Masculinities*, eds M. Flood, J. Gardiner, B. Pease and K. Pringle, Routledge, Milton Park.

Mullings, L. and Schulz, A. 2006, 'Intersectionality and health: an introduction', in *Gender, Race, Class & Health: Intersectional approaches*, eds L. Mullings and A. Schulz, Jossey-Bass, San Francisco.

Mulroney, J. and Chan, C. 2005, 'Men as victims of domestic violence', *Australian Domestic and Family Violence Clearinghouse*, Sydney, <www.austdvclearinghouse.unsw.edu.au/topics/topics_pdf_f les/Men_as_Victims.pdf> [2 August 2008].

Mulvey, A., Terenzio, M., Hill, J., Bond, M.A., Huygens, I., Hamerton, H.R. and Cahill, S. 2000, 'Stories of relative privilege: power and social change in feminist community psychology', *American Journal of Community Psychology*, vol. 28, no. 6, pp. 883–911.

Munro, E. 1998, *Understanding Social Work: An empirical approach*, Athlone Press, London.

——2001, 'Empowering looked after children', *Child and Family Social Work*, vol. 6, no. 2, pp. 129–37.
Murphy, C. ed. 2003, *Egalitarian Politics in the Age of Globalization*, Palgrave Macmillan, Houndmills.
Myerhoff, B. and Ruby, J. 1992, 'A crack in the mirror: ref exive perspectives in anthropology', in *Remembered Lives: The work of ritual, storytelling and growing older*, eds B. Myerhoff with D. Metzger, J. Ruby and V. Tufte, University of Michigan Press, Ann Arbor, pp. 307–40.
Nancarrow, N. 2006, 'In search of justice for domestic and family violence', *Theoretical Criminology*, vol. 10, no. 1, pp. 87–106.
Narrandera 2002, 'The Narrandera Koori community gathering', Dulwich Centre, <www.dulwichcentre.com.au/Narrandera.htm> [4 October 2008].
National Children's Bureau, UK 2007, <www.ncb.org.uk/Page.asp?originx2572po_27291116328194w8n1361462404> [26 February 2008].
Nay, R. 1993, 'Benevolent oppression: lived experiences of nursing home life', PhD thesis, School of Sociology, University of New South Wales.
Ndione, E.S. 1992, *Le Don et le Recours*, Enda Eds, Dakar.
——ed. 1994, *Réinventer le Présent*, Enda Graf Sahel, Dakar.
Neill, R. 2002, *White Out: How politics is killing black Australia*, Allen & Unwin, Sydney.
Neimeyer, R. 2000, *Lessons of Loss: A guide to coping*, PsychoEducational Resources, Keystone Heights.
——ed. 2001, *Meaning Reconstruction & the Experience of Loss*, American Psychological Association, Washington, DC.
——R. ed. 2006, 'Making meaning in the midst of loss', *Grief Matters*, vol. 9, no. 3, pp. 62–5.
Nelson, R. 2007, 'Taking a journey toward greater cultural understanding', unpublished paper, Robynne Nelson Consulting, Melbourne.
New, C. 1996, 'Man bad, woman good? Essentialisms and ecofeminisms', *New Left Review*, no. 216, pp. 79–94.
Nichols, J. 1973, 'The silent majority', *Australian Social Work*, vol. 26, no. 4, pp. 35–43.
——1977, 'Social work education and women's lib: a dead issue?', *Contemporary Social Work Education*, vol. 1, no. 2, pp. 52–4.
Nicholson, L. and Seidman, S., eds 1995, *Social Postmodernism: Beyond identity politics*, Cambridge University Press, Cambridge, MA.
Nicolson, R.I. and Fawcett, A.J. 2007, 'Procedural learning diff culties: reuniting the developmental disorders', *Trends in Neurosciences*, vol. 30, no. 4, pp. 135–42.
Niskanen, W.A. 1971, *Bureaucracy and Representative Government*, Aldine, Chicago.
Noble, C. and Briskman, L. 2000, 'AASW Code of Ethics: the impact of progressive theory on moral and ethical assumptions', *Advances in Social Work and Welfare Education*, vol. 3, no. 1, pp. 89–103.
Nyland, J. 1993, 'Little f ngers of the State: aggressive instrumentalism in the Australian Welfare State', in *Power, Politics and Performance*, Conference Papers, Book 2 CACOM, University of Technology, Sydney, pp. 100–17.
O'Brien, M. and Penna, S. 1998, 'Oppositional postmodern theory and welfare analysis: anti-oppressive practice in a postmodern frame', in *Postmodernity and the Fragmentation of Welfare*, ed. J. Carter, Routledge, New York.
O'Connor, I., Smyth, P. and Warburton, J., eds 2000, *Contemporary Perspectives on Social Work and the Human Services: Challenges and change*, Layman, Melbourne.
O'Connor, I., Wilson, J. and Setterlund, D. 2003, *Social Work and Welfare Practice*, 4th edn, Pearson Education, Sydney.
O'Connor, J.S., Orloff, A.S. and Shaver, S. 1999, *States Markets and Families*, Cambridge University Press, Cambridge, MA.

O'Hagan, K. 1997, 'The problem of engaging men in child protection work', *British Journal of Social Work*, vol. 27, pp. 25–42.

O'Hagan, M. 2004, 'Recovery in New Zealand: lessons for Australia?', *Australian e-Journal for the Advancement of Mental Health*, vol. 3, no. 1, pp. 1–30.

——2008, 'Creating the future for recovery-based services', *New Paradigm*, Psychiatric Disability Support Services of Victoria (VICSERV), Winter, pp. 15–19.

O'Shea, L. 2005, 'Contemporary Gestalt: the application of key principles to grief work', *Grief Matters*, vol. 8, no. 2, pp. 35–7.

Oakley, A. 1981, *Subject Women*, Fontana, Oxford.

——2000, *Experiments in Knowing: Gender and method in the social sciences*, Polity Press, Cambridge.

Off ce of Seniors Interests 1997, *Breaking the Ice: A guide to marketing to maturity*, Off ce of Seniors Interests, Perth.

Oliver, M. 1996, *Understanding Disability: From theory to practice*, Macmillan, London.

——2004, 'The social model in action: if I had a hammer', in *Implementing the Social Model of Disability: Theory and research*, eds C. Barnes and G. Mercer, Disability Press, Leeds.

Olson, M. 1965, *The Logic of Collective Action*, Harvard University Press, Cambridge, MA.

Orme, J., Dominelli, L. and Mullender, A. 2000, 'Working with violent men from a feminist social work perspective', *International Social Work*, vol. 43, no. 1, pp. 89–105.

Osborne, D. and Gaebler, T. 1992, *Reinventing Government: How the entrepreneurial spirit is transforming the public sector—from schoolhouse to statehouse, city hall to the Pentagon*, Addison Wesley, Reading, MA.

Osmond, J. and O'Connor, I. 2006, 'Use of theory and research in social work practice: implications for knowledge-based practice', *Australian Social Work*, vol. 59, no. 1, pp. 5–19.

Padgett, D. 1998, *Qualitative Methods in Social Work Research*, Sage, Thousand Oaks, CA.

Papilloud, C. 2004, 'Three conditions of human relations: Marcel Mauss and Georg Simmel', *Philosophy and Social Criticism*, vol. 30, no. 4, pp. 431–44.

Pardeck, J.T. and Murphy, J.W. 1993, 'Postmodernism and clinical practice: a critical analysis of the disease model', *Psychological Reports*, vol. 72, no. 3, part 2, pp. 1187–94.

Parker, J. 2001, 'Social movements and science: the question of plural knowledge systems', in *After Postmodernism: An introduction to critical realism*, eds J. Lopez and G. Potter, Athlone Press, New York.

Parker, R., Ward, H., Jackson, S., Aldgate, J. and Wedge, P. 1991, *Looking After Children: Assessing outcomes in child care*, HMSO, London.

Parker, S., Fook, J. and Pease, B. 2005, 'Empowerment: the modern social work concept par excellence', in *Transforming Social Work Practice: Postmodern critical perspectives*, eds B. Pease and J. Fook, Routledge, London, pp. 150–9.

Parkes, C. 1996, *Bereavement: Studies of grief in adult life*, 3rd edn, Penguin, Harmondsworth.

Parsons, I. 1994, *Oliver Twist has Asked for More: The politics and practice of getting justice for people with disabilities*, Villamanta, Geelong.

Parton, N. 1991, *Governing the Family: Child care, child protection and the state*, Macmillan, London.

——2003, 'Rethinking professional practice: the contributions of social constructionism and the feminist "ethics of care"', *British Journal of Social Work*, vol. 33, no. 1, pp. 1–16.

Parton, N. and O'Byrne, P. 2000a, *Constructive Social Work: Towards a new practice*, Macmillan, Houndmills.

——2000b, 'What do we mean by constructive social work'?, *Critical Social Work*, vol. 1, no. 2, pp. 1–22, <www.criticalsocialwork.com/CSW_2000_2.html> [23 August 2001].

Pawson, R. 2002, 'Evidenced-based policy: the promise of a realist synthesis', *Evaluation*, vol. 8, no. 3, pp. 340–58.

Payne, M. 1997, *Modern Social Work Theory*, 2nd edn, Macmillan, Basingstoke.

——2005, *Modern Social Work Theory*, 3rd edn, Palgrave Macmillan, Basingstoke.

Pearce, F. and Woodiwiss, T. 2001, 'Reading Foucault as a realist', in *After Postmodernism: An introduction to critical realism*, eds J. Lopez and G. Potter, Athlone Press, New York.

Pease, B. 1996, 'Naming violence as a gender issue: victimisation, blame and responsibility', *Women Against Violence*, no. 1, pp. 33–9.

——1997, *Men and Sexual Politics*, Dulwich, Adelaide.

——2000, *Recreating Men: Postmodern masculinity politics*, Sage, London.

——2001, 'Theoretical issues and political dilemmas in working with men', in *Working with Men in the Human Services*, eds B. Pease and P. Camilleri, Allen & Unwin, Sydney.

——2002a, 'Rethinking empowerment: a postmodern reappraisal for emancipatory practice', *British Journal of Social Work*, vol. 32, pp. 135–47.

——2002b, *Men and Gender Relations*, Tertiary Press, Melbourne.

——2003a, 'Critical ref ections on profeminist practice in men's groups', in *Gender and Social Groupwork*, eds M. Cohen and A. Mullender, Routledge, London.

——2003b, 'Men and masculinities: profeminist approaches to changing men', in *Critical Social Work: An introduction to theories and practices*, eds J. Allan, B. Pease and L. Briskman, Allen & Unwin, Sydney.

——2004, 'Decentring white men: critical ref ections on masculinity and white studies', in *Whitening Race: Essays in cultural and social criticism*, ed. A. Moreton-Robinson, Aboriginal Studies Press, Canberra.

——2004–05, 'Rethinking profeminist men's behaviour change programs', *Women Against Violence: An Australian Feminist Journal*, no. 16, pp. 32–40.

——2006a, 'Encouraging critical ref ections on privilege in social work and the human services', *Practice Reflexions*, vol. 1, no. 1, pp. 15–26.

——2006b, 'Gendering men: implications for gender equality', in *Men and Gender Equality: Towards progressive policies*, eds J. Varanka, A. Narhinen and R. Siukola, Ministry of Social Affairs and Health, Helsinki.

——2008, *Engaging Men in Violence Prevention: Exploring the tensions, dilemmas and possibilities*, Australian Domestic and Family Violence Clearinghouse, Issues Paper 17, August.

——2009, 'Racialised masculinities and the health of immigrant and refugee men', in *Men's Health: Body, identity and context*, eds A. Broom and P. Tovey, John Wiley & Sons, Chichester.

Pease, B., Allan, J. and Briskman, L. 2003, 'Introducing critical social work', *Critical Social Work: An introduction to theories and practices*, eds J. Allan, B. Pease and L. Briskman, Allen & Unwin, Sydney.

Pease, B. and Camilleri, P. 2001, *Working with Men in the Human Services*, Allen & Unwin, Sydney.

Pease, B. and Fook, J. 1999a, 'Postmodern critical theory and emancipatory social work practice', in *Transforming Social Work Practice*, eds B. Pease and J. Fook, Allen & Unwin, Sydney, pp. 1–22.

——eds. 1999b, *Transforming Social Work Practice: Postmodern critical perspectives*, Allen & Unwin, Sydney.

Peck, J. 2001 *Workfare States*, The Guilford Press, New York.

Peck, J., Leitner, H. and Sheppard, E.S. 2007, *Contesting Neoliberalism: Urban frontiers*, The Guilford Press, New York.

Peile, C. and McCouat, M. 1997, 'The rise of relativism: the future of theory and knowledge development in social work', *British Journal of Social Work*, vol. 27, pp. 343–60.

Pemberton, A. and Locke, R. 1971, 'Towards a radical critique of social work and welfare ideology', *Australian Journal of Social Issues*, vol. 6, no. 2, pp. 95–107.

Perlesz, A. 1999, 'Complex responses to trauma: challenges in bearing witness', *Australian and New Zealand Journal of Family Therapy*, vol. 20, no. 1, pp. 11–19.

Perry, B. 1997, 'Incubated in terror: neurodevelopmental factors in the cycle of violence', in *Children, Youth and Violence: Searching for solutions*, ed. J. Osofsky, The Guilford Press, New York.

——2002, *Brain Structure and Function 1*, W.W. Norton, New York.

——2005, 'The real crisis of Katrina', *The National Association to Protect Children*, <www.childtrauma.org> [4 October 2008].

Petr, C. and Walter, U. 2005, 'Best practices inquiry: a multidimensional, value-critical framework', *Journal of Social Work Education*, vol. 41, no. 2, pp. 251–67.

Pettman, J. 1992, *Living in the Margins*, Allen & Unwin, Sydney.

Pheterson, G. 1986, 'Alliances between women: overcoming internalised oppression and internalised domination', *Signs: Journal of Women, Culture and Society*, vol. 12, no. 1, pp. 146–60.

Phillips, R. 2006, 'Undoing an activist response: feminism and the Australian government's domestic violence policy', *Critical Social Policy*, vol. 26, no. 1, pp. 192–219.

Pine, D.W. 1996, 'Post-modernist analysis a valuable tool for feminists', *Refractory Girl*, vol. 51, no. 96, pp. 4–7.

Plath, D. 2006, 'Evidence-based practice: current issues and future directions', *Australian Social Work*, vol. 59, no. 1, pp. 56–72.

Plummer, K. 2003, *Intimate Citizenship, Private Decisions and Public Dialogues*, University of Washington Press, Washington.

——2005, 'Male sexualities', in *Handbook of Studies on Men and Masculinities*, eds M. Kimmel, J. Hearn and R. Connell, Sage, Thousand Oaks, CA.

Polanyi, M. 1958, *Personal Knowledge: Towards a post critical philosophy*, Routledge, London.

Pollock, L. 1983, *Forgotten Children: Parent–child relations from 1500 to 1800*, Cambridge University Press, Cambridge, MA.

——1987, *A Lasting Relationship: Parents and children over three centuries*, Fourth Estate, London.

Porter, S. 1998, *Social Theory and Nursing Practice*, Macmillan, Basingstoke.

Porter, T. 1995, *Trust in Numbers: The pursuit of objectivity in science and public life*, Princeton University Press, Princeton, NJ.

Potter, G. and Lopez, J. 2001, 'After postmodernism: the millennium', in *After Postmodernism: An introduction to critical realism*, eds J. Lopez and G. Potter, Athlone Press, New York.

Potter, J. 1996, *Representing Reality*, Sage, London.

Powell, F. 2001, *The Politics of Social Work*, Sage, London.

Powell, J.L. 2006, *Social Theory and Aging*, Rowman & Littlef eld, Lanham, MD.

Power, M. 1999, *The Audit Society: Rituals of verification*, Oxford University Press, Oxford.

Poynting, S., Tabar, P. and Noble, G. 2009, 'Looking for respect: Lebanese immigrant young men in Australia', in *Migrant Men: Critical studies of masculinities and the migration experience*, eds R. Howson, B. Pease, R. Hibbins and M. Donaldson, Routledge, London.

Pozzuto, R. 2000, 'Notes on a possible critical social work', *Critical Social Work*, vol. 1, no. 1, pp. 1–5, <www.criticalsocialwork.com/CSW_2000_1.html> [23 August 2001].

Pozzuto, R., Brent Angell, G. and Dezendorf, P. 2005, 'Therapeutic critique: traditional versus critical perspectives', in *Social Work: A critical turn*, eds S. Hick, J. Fook and R. Pozzuto, Thompson Education, Toronto.

Preston-Shoot, M. 2007, *Effective Groupwork*, 2nd edn, Palgrave Macmillan, Houndmills.

Prieto, A. ed. with de Ungria, R. 2006, *Fallen Cradle: Parents on the loss of a child*, Anvil, Manila.

Prigerson, H., Vanderwerker, L. and Maciejewski, P. 2008, 'A case for inclusion of prolonged grief disorder in DSM-IV', *Grief Matters*, vol. 11, no. 1, pp. 23–32.

Pringle, K. 1995, *Men, Masculinities and Welfare*, UCL Press, London.

——1997, 'Men challenging gender oppression on social work programmes in higher education: a framework for action', *Social Work Education*, vol. 16, no. 4, pp. 55–69.

——1998a, 'Current profeminist debates regarding men and social welfare: some national and transnational perspectives', *British Journal of Social Work*, vol. 28, pp. 623–33.

——1998b, 'Men and child care: policy and practice', *Men, Gender Divisions and Welfare*, eds J. Popay, J. Hearn and J. Edwards, Routledge, London.

——2001, 'Men in social work: the double edge', in *Men and Social Work: Theories and practice*, ed. A. Christie, Palgrave, London.

Pryjmachuk, S. 1998, 'Sexuoerotic development in children and young people', in *Children and Sexuality: Perspectives in health care*, ed. T. Harrison, Baillière Tindall, London, pp. 42–66.

Purvis, T. and Hunt, A. 1993, 'Discourse, ideology, discourse, ideology, discourse, ideology . . .', *British Journal of Sociology*, vol. 44, no. 3, pp. 473–99.

Pyke, K. 1996, 'Class-based masculinities: the interdependence of gender, class and interpersonal power', *Gender and Society*, vol. 10, no. 5, pp. 527–49.

Pyles, L. 2005, 'Understanding the engaged Buddhist movement: implications for social development practice', *Critical Social Work*, vol. 6, no. 1, <http://bjsw.oxfordjournals.org/cgi/context/abstract/bcn032v1> [19 January 2009].

Quinn, M. 2003, 'Immigrants and refugees: towards anti-racist and culturally aff rming practices', in *Critical Social Work: An introduction to theories and practices*, eds J. Allan, B. Pease and L. Briskman, Allen & Unwin, Sydney, pp. 75–91.

Rabin, C. 1996, *Equal Partners—Good Friends*, Routledge, New York.

Ramia, G. and Carney, T. 2001, 'Contractualism, managerialism and welfare: the Australian experiment with marketised employment services', in *Policy and Politics*, vol. 29, no. 1, pp. 59–83.

Ramon, S., Campbell, J., Lindsay, J., McCrystal, P. and Baidoun, N. 2006, 'The impact of political conf ict on social work: experiences from Northern Ireland, Israel and Palestine', *British Journal of Social Work*, vol. 36, no. 3, pp. 435–50.

Rando, T. 1993, *Treatment of Complicated Mourning*, Research Press, Illinois.

Ranson, G. 2007, 'Fatherhood and paid work', in *International Encyclopedia of Men and Masculinities*, eds M. Flood, J. Gardiner, B. Pease and K. Pringle, Routledge, Milton Park.

Raphael, B. 2000, 'Grief and loss in Australian society', in *Death and Dying in Australia*, ed. A. Kellehear, Oxford University Press, Melbourne.

Rea, N. and Messner, J. 2008, 'Constructing Aboriginal NRM livelihoods: Anmatyerr employment in water management', *Rangeland Journal*, no. 30, pp. 85–93.

Read, J. 2007, 'Why promoting biological ideology increases prejudice against people labelled "schizophrenic"', *Australian Psychologist*, vol. 42, no. 2, pp. 118–28.

Rees, S. 1991, *Achieving Power: Practice and policy in social welfare*, Allen & Unwin, Sydney.

Rees, S. and Pease B. 2007, 'Domestic violence in refugee families in Australia: rethinking settlement policy and practice', *Journal of Immigrant & Refugee Studies*, vol. 5, no. 2, pp. 1–19.

Rees, S. and Wright, S., eds 2000, *Human Rights and Corporate Responsibility: A dialogue*, Pluto Press, Sydney.

Reichert, E. 1998, 'Women's rights are human rights: platform for action', *International Social Work*, vol. 41, no. 3, pp. 371–84.

——2003, *Social Work and Human Rights: A foundation for policy and practice*, Columbia University Press, New York.

——2006, *Understanding Human Rights: An exercise book*, Sage, Thousand Oaks, CA.

——ed. 2007, *Challenges in Human Rights: A social work perspective*, Columbia University Press, New York.

Rein, M. 1970, *Social Policy: Issues of choice and change*, Random House, New York.

Reisch, M. and Andrews, J. 2001, *The Road Not Taken: A history of radical social work in the United States*, Brunner Routledge, Philadelphia.

Renouf, N. and Bland, R. 2005, 'Navigating stormy waters: challenges and opportunities for social work in mental health', *Australian Social Work*, vol. 58, no. 4, pp. 419–30.

Resurgence 2008, *Indigenous Intelligence: Diverse solutions for the 21st century*, no. 250, September.

Reynolds, J. 2002, 'Disenfranchised grief and the politics of helping: social policy and its clinical implications', in *Disenfranchised Grief: New directions, challenges, and strategies for practice*, ed. K. Doka, Research Press, Champaign, IL.

Richardson, S. and Bacon, H., eds 1991, *Child Sexual Abuse: Whose problem? Reflections from Cleveland*, Venture Press, Birmingham.

Richmond, M. 1917, *Social Diagnosis*, Russell Sage Foundation, New York.

Ridge, T. 2002, *Childhood Poverty and Social Exclusion: From a child's perspective*, Policy Press, Bristol.

Rioux, M. and Zubrow, E. 2001, 'Social disability in the public good', in *The Market or the Public Domain: Global governance and the asymmetry of power*, ed. D. Drache, Routledge, London, pp. 148–71.

Robinson, E. 2007, 'Long term outcomes of losing a child through adoption: the impact of disenfranchised grief', *Grief Matters*, vol. 10, no. 1, pp. 8–11.

Robinson, P. 2008, *The Changing World of Gay Men*, Palgrave, London.

Robinson, V. 2007, 'Heterosexuality', in *International Encyclopedia of Men and Masculinities*, eds M. Flood, J. Gardiner, B. Pease and K. Pringle, Routledge, Milton Park.

Rogers, A. and Pilgrim, D. 2003, *Mental Health and Inequality*, Palgrave Macmillan, Basingstoke.

Rolfe, S. 2004, *Rethinking Attachment for Early Childhood Practice*, Allen & Unwin, Sydney.

Rose, N. 1979, 'The psychological complex: mental measurement and social administration', *Ideology and Consciousness*, vol. 5, pp. 5–68.

——1990, 'The gaze of the psychologist', in *Governing the Soul: The shaping of the private self*, Routledge, London.

Rose, S. 2000, 'Heterosexism and the study of women's romantic and friend relationships', *Journal of Social Issues*, vol. 56, no. 2, pp. 315–28.

Rosenblatt, P. 2008, 'Recovery following bereavement: metaphor, phenomenology and culture', *Death Studies*, vol. 32, no. 1, pp. 6–16.

Rossetti, S.J. 1996, *A Tragic Grace: The Catholic Church and child sexual abuse*, Interfaith Sexual Trauma Institute, Liturgical Press, Collegeville.

Rossiter, A. 2005, 'Discourse analysis in critical social work: from apology to question', *Critical Social Work*, vol. 6, no. 1, <www.criticalsocialwork.com/units/socialwork/critical.nsf/8c20dad9f1c4be3a85256d6e006d1089/f55933acd8333f4385256fd700606f86?OpenDocument> [5 November 2007].

Rowan, J. 1997, *The Horned God: Feminism as wounding and healing*, Routledge, London.

Russell, G. and Hwang, C. 2004, 'The impact of workplace practice on father involvement', in *The Role of the Father in Child Development*, ed. M. Lamb, John Wiley, New York.

Russell, M. 1995, *Confronting Abusive Beliefs: Group treatment for abusive men*, Sage, Thousand Oaks, CA.

Ryan, A. 2000, *A Silent Love: Personal stories of coming to terms with miscarriage*, Penguin Books, Ringwood.

Ryan, W. 1976, *Blaming the Victim*, 2nd edn, Vintage Books, New York.

Sachs, W., ed. 1993, *The Development Dictionary: A guide to knowledge as power*, Zed Books, London.

——1995, 'Global ecology and the shadow of "development"', in *Deep Ecology for the 21st Century*, ed. G. Sessions, Shambala, Boston, pp. 428–44.

Sadler, P. 2006, *Elder Abuse: A holistic response. Background paper*, Aged & Community Services Australia, Sydney.

Said, E. 1993, *Culture and Imperialism*, Vintage, London.

Saleebey, D. 1997, *The Strength Perspective in Social Work Practice*, Longman, New York.

——ed. 2006, *The Strength Perspective in Social Work Practice*, 4th edn, Pearson/Allyn & Bacon, Boston.

Sanders, W. 2004, 'Indigenous centres in the policy margins: the CDEP scheme over 30 years', *Centre for Aboriginal Economic Policy Research*, Australian National University, Canberra.

Sanderson, I. 2002, 'Evaluation, policy learning and evidence-based policy making', *Public Administration*, vol. 80, no. 1, pp. 1–22.

Sands, R.G. 1996, 'The elusiveness of identity in social work practice with women: a postmodern feminist perspective', *Clinical Social Work Journal*, vol. 24, no. 2, pp. 167–86.

Sands, R. and Nuccio, K. 1992, 'Postmodern feminist theory and social work', *Social Work*, vol. 37, no. 6, pp. 489–94.
Sassen, S. 1991, *The Global City*, Princeton University Press, Princeton, NJ.
Sattel, J. 1989, 'The inexpressive male: tragedy or sexual politics', in *Men's Lives*, eds M. Kimmel and M. Messner, Macmillan, New York.
Sattem, L., Savells, J. and Murray, E. 1984, 'Sex role stereotypes and commitment to rape', *Sex Roles*, vol. 11, nos 9/10, pp. 849–60.
Saunders, P. 1994, *Welfare and Inequality: National and international perspectives on the Australian welfare state*, Cambridge University Press, Melbourne.
Sax, S. 1993, *Ageing and Public Policy in Australia*, Allen & Unwin, Sydney.
Schacht, S. and Atkinson, P. 1992, 'Heterosexual instrumentalism: past and future directions', *Feminism and Psychology*, vol. 2, no. 3, pp. 37–53.
Schatz, M., Tracy, J. and Tracy, S. 2006, 'Overcoming social oppression: using dialogue and theatre to reveal oppression and foster healing', *Critical Social Work*, vol. 7, no. 2, <www.criticalsocialwork.com/units/socialwork/critical.nsf/982f0e5f06b5c9a285256d6e006cff78/f655e425a85322ae85257277002cb1d0?OpenDocument> [5 November 2007].
Scheyett, A. 2006, 'Silence and surveillance: mental illness, evidence-based practice and a Foucauldian lens', *Journal of Progressive Human Services*, vol. 17, no. 1, pp. 71–92.
Schneider, R. and Lester, L. 2001, *Social Work Advocacy*, Brooks/Cole, Stamford.
Schön, D. 1983, *The Reflective Practitioner*, Temple Smith, London.
Scott, D. and Swain, S. 2002, *Confronting Cruelty: Historical perspectives on child protection in Australia*, Melbourne University Press, Melbourne.
Scott, D., Walker, L. and Gilmore, K. 1995, 'Counselling support for adults who have been sexually assaulted', *Breaking the Silence: A guide to supporting adult victim/survivors of sexual assault*, 2nd edn, CASA House, Royal Women's Hospital, Melbourne, pp. 53–71.
Scourf eld, J. 2003, *Gender and Child Protection*, Palgrave Macmillan, London.
Scutt, J. 1998, 'Character, credit, context: women's lives, judicial reality', in *Balancing the Scales: Rape Law Reform and Australian Culture*, ed. P. Easteal, Federation Press, Sydney, pp. 159–73.
Searing, H. 2003, 'The continuing relevance of casework ideas to long-term child protection work', *Child and Family Social Work*, vol. 8, pp. 311–20.
Segal, L. 1990, *Slow Motion: Changing masculinities, changing men*, Virago, London.
——1995, 'Feminism and the family', in *Gender, Power and Relationships*, eds C. Burke and B. Speed, Routledge, London, pp. 248–66.
——1999, *Why Feminism?*, Polity Press, Cambridge.
Seidman, S. 1994, *Contested Knowledge: Social theory in a postmodern era*, Blackwell, Oxford.
Sev'er, A. and Yurdakul, G. 2001, 'Culture of honor, culture of change: a feminist analysis of honor killings in rural Turkey', in *Violence Against Women*, vol. 7, no. 9, pp. 964–98.
Shakespeare, T. 2006, *Disability Rights and Wrongs*, Routledge, London.
Shapiro, E. 1994, *Grief As a Family Process: A developmental approach to clinical practice*, The Guilford Press, New York.
——1996, 'Family bereavement and cultural diversity: a social developmental model', *Family Process*, vol. 35, no. 4, pp. 313–32.
Sharma, S. and Rees, S. 2007, 'Consideration of the determinants of women's mental health in remote Australian mining towns', *Australian Journal of Rural Health*, no. 15, pp. 1–7.
Shaw, M. 2008, 'Community development and the politics of community', *Community Development Journal*, vol. 43, no. 1, pp. 24–36.
Shearing, H. 2005, 'Barefoot social worker: the voice of radical social work in Britain', <www.radical.org.uk/barefoot> [5 February 2008].
Sheldon, B. 2000, 'Cognitive-behavioural models in social care: a look at the evidence', in *Social Work*

Models, Methods and Theories: A framework for practice, eds P. Stepney and D. Ford, Russell House, Lyme Regis.
Shepard, P. 1995, 'Nature and madness', in *Ecopsychology: Restoring the earth, healing the mind*, eds T. Roszak, M. Gomes and A. Kanner, Sierra Club Books, San Francisco.
Sheppard, M. 1998, 'Practice validity, ref exivity and knowledge for social work', *British Journal of Social Work*, vol. 28, pp. 763–81.
Shortall, S. 2005, 'Social or economic goals, civic inclusion or exclusion? An analysis of rural development theory and practice', *Sociologia Ruralis*, vol. 44, no. 1, pp. 10–23.
Shortall, S. and Shucksmith, M. 2001, 'Rural development in practice: issues arising in Scotland and Northern Ireland', *Community Development Journal*, vol. 36, no. 2, pp. 122–33.
Sigurjonsdottir, H.B. and Traustadottir, R. 2000, 'Motherhood, family and community life', in *Women with Intellectual Disabilities: Finding a place in the world*, Jessica Kingsley, London, pp. 253–70.
Silverman, P. 1986, *Widow-to-Widow*, Springer, New York.
Silverman, P. and Klass, D. 1996, 'Introduction: what's the problem?', in *Continuing Bonds: New understandings of grief*, eds D. Klass, P. Silverman and S. Nickman, Taylor & Francis, Philadelphia.
Simpkin, M. 1979, *Trapped Within Welfare*, Macmillan, London.
Sin, R. 2007, 'Community action research: lessons from the Chinese communities', in *Doing Anti-Oppressive Practice: Building transformative politicized social work*, ed. D. Baines, Fernwood, Halifax, BC, Canada.
Sinclair, R. and Albert, J. 2008, 'Social work and the anti-oppressive stance: does the emperor really have new clothes?', *Critical Social Work*, vol. 9, no. 1, <www.criticalsocialwork.com/units/socialwork/critical.nsf/982f0e5f06b5c9a285256d6e006cff78/833a864e85f358668525744c0076eeb5?OpenDocument> [12 August 2008].
Skenridge, P. and Lennie, I. 1978, 'Social work: the wolf in sheep's clothing', *Arena*, no. 51, pp. 47–92.
Small, N. 2001, 'Theories of grief: A critical review', in *Grief, Mourning and Death Ritual*, eds J. Hockey, J. Katz and N. Small, Open University Press, Buckingham.
Smith, C. 2001, 'Trust and conf dence: possibilities for social work in "high modernity"', *British Journal of Social Work*, vol. 31, no. 2, pp. 287–305.
Smith, D. 2004, 'Introduction: some versions of evidence-based practice', in *Social Work and Evidence-Based Practice*, ed. D. Smith, Jessica Kingsley, London.
Smith, J. 2007, 'Beyond masculine stereotypes: moving men's health promotion forward in Australia', *Health Promotion Journal of Australia*, vol. 18, no. 1, pp. 20–5.
Smith, K. 2007, 'Social work, restructuring and everyday resistance: "Best practices" gone underground', in *Doing Anti-Oppressive Practice: Building transformative politicized social work*, ed. D. Baines, Fernwood, Halifax, BC, Canada.
Smith, L. 2008, 'Climate change "will lead to warfare over food and water"', *The Times*, 24 January, <www.timesonline.co.uk/tol/news/environment/article3241362.ece> [2 August 2008].
Smith, R. and van den Anker, C. eds 2005, *The Essentials of Human Rights*, Hodder Arnold, London.
SNAICC 2008, *Secretariat National Aboriginal and Islander Child Care*, <www.snaicc.asn.au>.
Solas, J. 2000, 'Can a radical social worker believe in human rights?', *Australian Social Work*, vol. 53, no. 1, 65–70.
——2008, 'Social work and social justice: what are we f ghting for?', *Australian Social Work*, vol. 61, no. 2, pp. 124–36.
Sorensen, H. and Black, B. 2001, 'Advocacy and ageing', *Australasian Journal on Ageing*, vol. 20, no. 3, pp. 27–34.
Soros, G. 1998, *The Crisis of Global Capitalism: Open society endangered*, Little, Brown, London.
——2008, *The New Paradigm for Financial Markets: The credit crash of 2008 and what it means*, Public Affairs, New York.

South Eastern Centre Against Sexual Assault (SECASA) 2004a, *Practical Help for Men*, <www.secasa.com.au/infosheet/infosheet_2004.pdf> [5 August 2008].

——2004b, *Sexual Assault and Oral Health*, <www.secasa.com.au/infosheet/dental_survivors.pdf> [5 August 2008].

Spratt, T. 2005, 'Radical drama with children: working with children using critical social work methods', in *Social Work: A critical turn*, eds S. Hick, J. Fook and R. Pozzuto, Thompson Education, Toronto.

Stafford Smith, M. 2008, 'The "desert syndrome"—causally linked factors that characterize outback Australia', *Rangeland Journal*, no. 30, pp. 3–14.

Stainton, T. 2007, 'Case management in a rights-based environment: structure, context and roles', in *Planning Support for People with Intellectual Disabilities: Issues for case managers and other professionals*, eds C. Bigby, C. Fyffe and L. Ozanne, Jessica Kingsley, London, pp. 90–107.

Stanley, J. and Goddard, C. 2002, *In the Firing Line: Violence and power in child protection work*, Wiley, Chichester.

Staples, L. 2004, 'Social action groups', in *Handbook of Social Work with Groups*, eds C. Garvin, L. Gutierrez and M. Galinsky, The Guilford Press, New York.

——1989, 'Masculinity and race: the dual dilemma of black men', in *Men's Lives*, eds M. Kimmel and M. Messner, Macmillan, New York.

Stenner, P. and Taylor, D. 2008, 'Psychosocial welfare: ref ections on an emerging f eld', *Critical Social Policy*, vol. 28, no. 4, pp. 415–37, <http://csp.sagepub.com/cgi/content/refs/28/4/415> [8 November 2008].

Stepney, P. 2006, 'Mission impossible? Critical practice in social work', *British Journal of Social Work*, vol. 36, pp. 1289–307.

Stern, N. 2006, *The Economics of Climate Change*, Cambridge University Press, Cambridge.

Stickley, T. 2006, 'Should service user involvement be consigned to history? A critical realist perspective', *Journal of Psychiatric and Mental Health Nursing*, no. 13, pp. 570–7.

Stiglitz, J. 2006, *Making Globalization Work*, Penguin. London.

Streeck-Fischer, A. and van der Kolk, B. 2000, 'Down will come baby, cradle and all: diagnostic and therapeutic implications of chronic trauma on child development', *Australian and New Zealand Journal of Psychiatry*, no. 346, pp. 903–18.

Strega, S. 2005, 'The view from poststructural margins: epistemology and methodology reconsidered', in *Research as Resistance: Critical, Indigenous and anti-oppressive approaches*, eds L. Brown and S. Strega, Canadian Scholars' Press, Toronto.

Stroebe, M. and Schut, H. 2001, 'Models of coping with bereavement: a review', in *Handbook of Bereavement Research: Consequences, coping, and care*, eds M. Stroebe, R. Hansson, W. Stroebe and H. Schut, American Psychological Association, Washington, DC.

——2008, 'The dual process model of coping with bereavement: overview and update', *Grief Matters*, vol. 11, no. 1, pp. 4–10.

Stroebe, M., Schut, H. and Stroebe, W. 1998, 'Trauma and grief: a comparative analysis' in *Perspectives on Loss: A sourcebook*, ed. J. Harvey, Brunner/Mazel, Philadelphia.

Stromquist, N. 2000, 'The challenges to emancipation in higher education', *World Studies in Education*, vol. 1, no. 1, pp. 61–77.

Stuart, D. 1993, 'No real harm done: sexual assault and the criminal justice system', in *Without Consent: Confronting adult sexual violence*, ed. P. Easteal, Proceedings of a conference held 27–29 October 1992, pp. 95–105.

Sue, D.W. 2003, *Overcoming Our Racism: The journey to liberation*, Jossey-Bass, San Francisco.

Sullivan, N., Mesbur, E., Lang, N., Goodman, D. and Mitchell, L, eds. 2003, *Social Work with Groups: Social justice through personal, community and social change*, The Haworth Press, New York.

Swain, S. 2000, 'Confronting cruelty: writing a history of the detection and treatment of child abuse', *Victorian Historical Journal*, vol. 71, no. 1, pp. 6–18.

Swensen, G. 1995, 'Female genital mutilation and human rights', *Australian Social Work*, vol. 48, no. 2, pp. 27–33.

Tabb, W. 2002, *Unequal Partners: A primer on globalization*, The New Press, New York.

Taffel, R. 2001, 'The wall of silence', *Psychotherapy Networker*, vol. 25, no. 3, pp. 52–64.

Taylor, C. and White, S. 2000, *Practising Reflectivity in Health and Welfare: Making knowledge*, Open University Press, Buckingham.

Taylor, J. 1990, *Giving Women Voice*, Brotherhood of St Laurence, Melbourne.

Taylor, J., Brown, D. and Bell, M. 2006, 'Population dynamics and demographic accounting in arid and savanna Australia: methods, issues and outcomes', Report 16, *Desert Knowledge CRC*, Alice Springs.

Taylor, S. 1996, 'Court-licensed abuse and the construction of the "incest" victim', in *Balancing the Scales: National Conference of Sexual Assault*, Proceedings of a conference held in June 1996, WA Sexual Assault Referral Centre, Perth.

Taylor-Gooby, P. 1993, *Postmodernism and Social Policy: A great leap backwards*, Social Policy Research Centre Discussion Paper No. 45, University of New South Wales, Sydney.

Taylor-Ide, D. and Taylor, C.E. 2002, *Just and Lasting Change: When communities own their futures*, Johns Hopkins University Press, Baltimore, MD.

Tew, J. 2002, *Social Theory, Power and Practice*, Palgrave Macmillan, Houndmills.

——2005, 'Power relations, social order and mental distress', in *Social Perspectives in Mental Health: Developing social models to understand and work with mental distress*, ed. J. Tew, Jessica Kingsley, London.

Think Safe 2008, <www.juniorcitizen.org.uk/kids/strangerdanger/> [16 June 2008].

Thomas, C. 2007, *Sociologies of Disability and Illness: Contested ideas in disability studies and medical sociology*, Palgrave Macmillan, London.

Thomas, P. and Bracken, P. 2004, 'Critical psychiatry in practice', *Advances in Psychiatric Treatment*, vol. 10, pp. 361–70.

Thompson, N. 1995, 'Men and anti-sexism', *British Journal of Social Work*, vol. 25, pp. 459–75.

——1998, *Promoting Equality: Challenging discrimination and oppression in the human services*, Macmillan, Houndmills.

——2000, *Theory and Practice in Human Services*, Open University Press, Buckingham.

——2003, *Promoting Equality: Challenging discrimination and oppression*, 2nd edn, Palgrave Macmillan, New York.

——2006, *Anti-discriminatory practice*, 4th edn, Palgrave Macmillan, New York.

Thorne-Finch, R. 1992, *Ending the Silence: The origins and treatment of male violence against women*, University of Toronto Press, Toronto.

Thorpe, R. and Irwin, J., eds 1996, *Women and Violence: Working for change*, Hale & Iremonger, Sydney.

Thorpe, R. and Petruchenia, J. 1990, 'Introduction', in *Social Change & Social Welfare Practice*, eds R. Thorpe and J. Petruchenia, Hale & Iremonger, Sydney, pp. 11–17.

Thorson, J.A. 2000, *Aging in a Changing Society*, 2nd edn, Brunner/Mazel, Philadelphia.

Throssell, H. 1975, 'Social work overview', in *Social Work: Radical Essays*, University of Queensland Press, Brisbane, pp. 3–25.

——1976, 'A critical appraisal of social work', in *The Professions in Australia: A critical appraisal*, eds P. Boreham, A. Pemberton and P. Wilson, University of Queensland Press, Brisbane, pp. 179–19.

Thyer, B.A. 1989, *Behavioral Family Therapy*, Charles Thomas, Springf eld, IL.

Tierney, L. 1963, *Children Who Need Help: A study of child welfare policy and administration in Victoria*, Melbourne University Press, Melbourne.

Tilbury, C. 2006, 'Accountability via performance measurement: the case of child protection services', *Australian Journal of Public Administration*, vol. 65, no. 3, pp. 48–61.

Timimi, S. 2005, 'Institutionalised racism lies at the heart of the conceptual systems we use in psychiatry', *Mental Health Today*, April, p. 21.

Tolman, R., Mowry, D., Jones, L. and Brekke, J. 1986, 'Developing a profeminist commitment among men in social work', *Feminist Visions for Social Work*, eds. N. Van Den Bergh and L. Cooper, National Association of Social Workers, New York.

Tomlinson, J. 1975, 'Client power: helping clients gain their welfare rights', in *Social Work: Radical essays*, ed. H. Throssell, University of Queensland Press, Brisbane, pp. 115–24.

——1977, *Is Band-Aid Social Work Enough?*, Wobbly Press, Darwin.

Tonts, M. 2005, 'Government policy and rural sustainability', in *Sustainability and Change in Rural Australia*, eds C. Cocklin and J. Dibden, University of New South Wales Press, Sydney, pp. 194–211.

Towney, L. 2005, 'The power of healing in the yarn: working with Aboriginal men', *International Journal of Narrative Therapy and Community Work*, no. 1, pp. 39–43.

Trainor, T. 1996, *Radicalism, Feminism and Fanaticism: Social work in the nineties*, Avebury, Aldershot.

Trinder, L. 2000, 'A critical appraisal of evidence-based practice', in *Evidence-Based Practice: A critical appraisal*, eds L. Trinder and S. Reynolds, Blackwell, Oxford.

Trotter, C. 2006, *Working with Involuntary Clients: A guide to practice*, Allen & Unwin, Sydney.

Tucci, J, Mitchell J. and Goddard, C. 2006, 'Out of sight out of mind: community attitudes about child abuse and child protection in Australia', Australian Childhood Foundation, <www.childhood.org.au/downloads/2006/mind.pdf> [15 September 2008].

——2008, 'Children's experiences of childhood in contemporary Australia', Australian Childhood Foundation, <www.childhood.org.au/downloads/2006/mind.pdf> [15 September 2008].

Turner, A. 1994, 'Genetic and hormonal inf uences on male violence', in *Male Violence*, ed. J. Archer, Routledge, London.

Turner, M. and Beresford, P. 2005, *User Controlled Research: Its meanings and potential—final report*, Shaping Our Lives and the Centre for Citizen Participation, Brunel University, <www.shapingourlives.org.uk> [9 July 2008].

United Nations 1948, *Universal Declaration of Human Rights*, <www.un.org> [1 July 2008].

United Nations 2006, *The Convention on the Rights of Persons with Disabilities*, United Nations, New York.

United Nations 2007, *The Convention on the Elimination of All Forms of Discrimination against Women (CEDAW)*, Division for the Advancement of Women, Department of Economic and Social Affairs, <www.un.org/womenwatch/daw/cedaw/text/econvention.htm#intro> [20 October 2007].

United Nations Center for Human Rights 1992, *Teaching and Learning about Human Rights: A manual for schools of social work and the social work profession*, United Nations, New York.

United Nations Development Fund for Women (UNIFEM) n.d. 'Facts and f gures on violence against women', *Working for Women's Empowerment and Gender Equality*, <www.unifem.org/gender_issues/violence_against_women/facts_f gures.php> [4 July 2008].

United Nations Educational, Scientif c and Cultural Organization (UNESCO) 2002, *Abuse of Older Persons: Recognizing and responding to abuse of older persons in a global context*, Commission for Social Development acting as the preparatory committee for the Second World Assembly on Aging, New York.

——2004, *Trafficking Statistics Project*, <www.unescobkk.org/f leadmin/user_upload/culture/Traff cking/project/Graph_Worldwide_Sept_2004.pdf> [1 August 2008].

United Nations High Commissioner for Human Rights 1997–2003, <www.unhchr.ch/html/menu3/b/k2crc.htm> [3 March 2008].

VACCA 2008, *Victorian Aboriginal Child Care Agency*, <www.vacca.org/01_program/lakidjeka_acsass.html> [13 September 2008].

Valsler, J. 1996, 'Elder abuse', in *Care of the Older Person: A handbook for care assistants*, eds C. McMahon and R. Isaacs, Blackwell, Cambridge, pp. 93–117.

Van Den Bergh, N. and Cooper, L.B, eds 1986, *Feminist Visions for Social Work*, National Association of Social Workers, Silver Spring, pp. 101–27.

Vasta, E. and Castles, S. 1996, *The Teeth are Smiling: The persistence of racism in multicultural Australia*, Allen & Unwin, Sydney.

Verhelst, T. 1990, *No Life Without Roots*, Zed Books, London.

Victorian Health Promotion Foundation 2005, *A Plan for Action 2005–2007: Promoting mental health and wellbeing*, Mental Health and Wellbeing Unit, Victorian Health Promotion Foundation, Melbourne, <www.vichealth.vic.gov.au> [9 September 2008].

Vincent, J.A. 1999, *Politics, Power and Old Age*, Open University Press, Buckingham.

Vinson, T. 2004, 'Community adversity and resilience', Jesuit Social Services, <www.jss.org.au> [13 September 2008].

Voydanoff, P. and Donnelly, B.W. 1990, *Adolescent Sexuality and Pregnancy*, Sage, Newbury Park, CA.

Wacquant, L. 1999, 'How penal common sense comes to Europeans: notes on the transatlantic diffusion of the neoliberal *doxa*', *European Societies*, vol. 1, pp. 319–52.

Waddell, M. 1989, 'Living in two worlds: psychodynamic theory and social work practice', *Free Associations*, vol. 15, pp. 11–35.

Wadsworth, Y. 2007, 'Is it safe to talk about systems again yet? Self organising processes for complex living systems and the dynamics of human inquiry', *Systemic Practice and Action Research*, Vol. 21, no. 2, pp. 153–70.

Walby, S. 1992, 'Post-post-modernism? Theorising social complexity', in *Destabilising Theory: Contemporary feminist debates*, eds M. Barrett and A. Phillips, Stanford University Press, Stanford, CN.

Waldegrave, C. 1990, 'Just therapy', *Dulwich Centre Newsletter*, no. 1, Adelaide, pp. 5–47.

Waldman, A. 2001, 'Behind the burka: women subtly fought Taliban', *New York Times*, <www.dpo.uab.edu/~svan/behindburka.html> [1 August 2008].

Walle, A. 2004, 'Native people and the DSMIV-TR: expanding diagnostic criteria to ref ect minority trauma', *Journal of Ethnicity in Substance Abuse*, vol. 3, no. 3, pp. 49–65.

Wallerstein, I. 1995, 'The insurmountable contradictions of liberalism: human rights and the rights of peoples in the geoculture of the modern world-system', *South Atlantic Quarterly*, vol. 94, no. 4, pp. 1161–78.

Walmsley, J. 2005, 'Institutionalization: a historical perspective', in *Deinstitutionalization and People with Intellectual Disabilities: In and out of institutions*, eds R. Traustadottir and K. Johnson, Jessica Kingsley, London, pp. 50–65.

Walter, T. 1996, 'A new model of grief: bereavement and biography', *Mortality*, vol. 1, no. 1, pp. 7–25.

——1999, *On Bereavement: The culture of grief*, Open University Press, Buckingham.

——2006, 'What is complicated grief? A social constructionist perspective', *Omega: Journal of Death and Dying*, vol. 52, pp. 71–9.

Ward, J. 2000, 'Queer sexism: rethinking gay men and masculinity', *Gay Masculinities*, ed. P. Nardi, Sage, Thousand Oaks, CA.

Waring, M. 1999, *Counting for Nothing: What men value and what women are worth*, 2nd edn, University of Toronto Press, Toronto.

Warr, D.J. 2005, 'Social networks in a "discredited" neighbourhood', *Journal of Sociology*, vol. 41, no. 3, pp. 285–308.

Watermeyer, B. and Swartz, L. 2008, 'Conceptualising the psycho-emotional aspects of disability and impairment: the distortion of personal and psychic boundaries', *Disability and Society*, vol. 23, no. 6, pp. 599–610.

Wattam, C. and Parton, N. 1999, 'Introduction: impediments to implementing a child-centred approach', in *Child Sexual Abuse: Responding to the experiences of children*, eds. N. Parton and C. Wattam, John Wiley & Sons, Chichester, pp. 1–18.

Watts, R. 1979, 'Two Bo-Peeps amongst the Sheep: a comment on wolf in sheep's clothing', *Arena*, no. 52, pp. 91–102.

Webb, D. 1981, 'Themes and continuities in radical and traditional social work', *British Journal of Social Work*, vol. 11, no. 2, pp. 143–58.
Webb, S. 2001, 'Considerations on the validity of evidence based practice in social work', *British Journal of Social Work*, vol. 31, no. 1, pp. 57–79.
——2006, *Social Work in a Risk Society: Social and political perspectives*, Palgrave Macmillan, Basingstoke.
Weber, L. 2006, 'Reconstructing the landscape of health disparities research: promoting dialogue and collaboration between feminist intersectional and biomedical paradigms', *Gender, Race, Class & Health: Intersectional approaches*, eds L. Mullings, and A. Schulz, Jossey-Bass, San Fransisco.
Weedon, C. 1987, *Feminist Practice and Poststructuralist Theory*, 2nd edn, Blackwell, Oxford.
Weeks, W. 2000, 'Ref ections on social work and human service theory and practice with families and communities', in *Issues Facing Australian Families*, 3rd edn, eds W. Weeks and M. Quinn, Pearson Education, Sydney, pp. 119–36.
——2003, 'Women: developing feminist practice in women's services', *Critical Social Work: An introduction to theories and practices*, eds J. Allan, B. Pease and L. Briskman, Allen & Unwin, Sydney, pp. 107–23.
Weeks, W., Hoatson, L. and Dixon, J. 2003, *Community Practices in Australia*, Pearson Education, Sydney.
Weinberg, M. 2008, 'Structural social work: a moral compass for ethics in practice', *Critical Social Work*, vol. 9, no. 1, <www.criticalsocialwork.com/units/socialwork/critical.nsf/982f0e5f06b5c9a285256d6e006cff78/3fc6041e5a0302358525744d0006b1a7?OpenDocument> [12 August 2008].
Weingourt, R., Maruyama, T., Sawada, I. and Hoshino, J. 2001, 'Domestic violence and women's mental health in Japan', *International Nursing Review*, vol. 48, no. 2, pp. 102–8.
Weiss, L. 1998, *The Myth of the Powerless State*, Polity Press, Cambridge.
West, R. 2000, 'Discovering a sister', in *Women with Intellectual Disabilities: Finding a place in the world*, eds R. Traustadottir and K. Johnson, Jessica Kingsley, London, pp. 34–52.
Westen, D. and Bradley, R. 2005, 'Empirically supported complexity: rethinking evidence-based practice in psychotherapy', *Current Directions in Psychological Science*, vol. 14, no. 5, pp. 266–71.
Westhorp, G. and Sebastian, A. 1997, *Advocacy Training Program: Introduction to advocacy—a learning package*, Disability Action, Mile End.
Whipple, V. 2007, 'Working with lesbian widows', *Grief Matters*, vol. 10, no. 1, pp. 4–7.
White, D. and Woollett, A. 1992, *Families: A context for development*, Falmer Press, London.
White, M. 1988, 'Saying hullo again: the incorporation of the lost relationship in the resolution of grief', *Dulwich Centre Newsletter*, Spring, pp. 7–11.
——1992, 'Deconstruction and therapy', in *Experience, Contradictions, Narratives and Imagination*, eds D. Epston and M. White, Dulwich Centre Publications, Adelaide.
——1993, 'Deconstruction and therapy', in *Therapeutic Conversations*, eds S. Gilligan and R. Price, W.W. Norton, New York.
——2000, *Reflections on Narrative Practice: Essays and interviews*, Dulwich Centre Publications, Adelaide.
White, M. and Epston, D. 1990, *Narrative Means to Therapeutic Ends*, W.W. Norton, New York.
Whitehead, S. 1992, 'The social origins of normalization', in *Normalisation: A reader for the nineties*, eds H. Brown and H. Smith, Tavistock/Routledge, London, pp. 47–59.
Wilensky, H.L. and Lebeaux, C.N. 1965, *Industrial Society and Social Welfare*, The Free Press, New York.
Willett, G. 2000, *Living Out Loud: A history of gay and lesbian activism in Australia*, Allen & Unwin, Sydney.
Williams, J. 2005, 'Women's mental health: taking inequality into account', in *Social Perspectives in Mental Health: Developing social models to understand and work with mental distress*, ed. J. Tew, Jessica Kingsley, London.
Williamson, O. 1985, *Economic Institutions of Capitalism*, The Free Press, New York.

Willow, C., Marchant, R., Kirby, P. and Neale, B. 2004, *Young Children's Citizenship: Ideas into practice*, <www.jrf.org.uk/bookshop> [22 February 2004].
Wilson, R. 1997, *The Stolen Generations Report*, Human Rights and Equal Opportunity Commission, Sydney.
Wilson, V. 2006, 'Critical realism as emancipatory action: the case for realistic evaluation in practice development', *Nursing Philosophy*, vol. 7, pp. 45–57.
Wingard, B. 2001a, 'Finding our own ways to grieve, to remember and to heal', in *Telling Our Stories in Ways that Make Us Stronger*, eds B. Wingard and J. Lester, Dulwich Centre, Adelaide.
—2001b, 'Grief: remember, ref ect, reveal', in *Telling Our Stories in Ways that Make Us Stronger*, eds B. Wingard and J. Lester, Dulwich Centre, Adelaide.
Wingard, B. and Lester, J., eds 2001, *Telling Our Stories in Ways that Make Us Stronger*, Dulwich Centre, Adelaide.
Wise, S. 1995, 'Feminist ethics in practice', in *Ethical Issues in Social Work*, eds R. Hugman and D. Smith, Routledge, London, pp. 85–101.
——2001, 'A framework for responding to vulnerable children and their families', *Family Matters*, no. 59, pp. 16–21.
——2002, 'An evaluation of a trial of "Looking After Children" in the state of Victoria', *Children and Society*, no. 16, pp. 1–15.
——2003, 'Using "Looking After Children" to create an Australian out of home care database', *Children Australia*, vol. 28, no. 2, pp. 38–44.
Wiseman, J. 1978, 'Power handout at the Family Centre?', *Arena*, no. 51, pp. 155–62.
Withorn, A. 1984, *Serving the People: Social services and social change*, Columbia University Press, New York.
Witkin, S. 1996, 'If empirical practice is the answer, then what is the question?', *Social Work Research*, vol. 20, no. 2, pp. 69–75.
Wolch, J. 1989, *The Shadow State*, Foundation Press, New York.
Wong, Y. 2004, 'Knowing through discomfort: a mindfulness-based critical social work pedagogy', *Critical Social Work*, vol. 5, no. 1, <www.criticalsocialwork.com/units/socialwork/critical.nsf/8c20dad9f1c4be3a85256d6e006d1089/dd7c350ba0866ae785256ec20063c090?OpenDocument> [5 November 2007].
Wood, G. Goldberg and Middleman, R. 1989, *Social Service Delivery: The structural approach to direct practice in social work*, rev. edn, Columbia University Press, New York.
Wood, J.T. 2001, 'The normalization of violence in heterosexual romantic relationships: women's narrative of love and violence', *Journal of Social and Personal Relationships*, vol. 18, no. 2, pp. 239–54.
Woodroofe, K. 1968, *From Charity to Social Work*, Routledge & Kegan Paul, London.
Worden, W. 1991, *Grief Counselling and Grief Therapy*, 2nd edn, Springer, New York.
World Health Organization 2008a, <www.who.int/social_determinants/en/> [August 2008].
——2008b, *Female Genital Mutilation, Key Facts*, <www.who.int/mediacentre/factsheets/fs241/en/> [1 August 2008].
Wright, A. 2004, *Religion, Education and Postmodernity*, Routlege Falmer, London.
Wronka, J. 1992, *Human Rights and Social Policy in the 21st Century: A history of the idea of human rights and comparison of the United Nations Universal Declaration of Human Rights with United States federal and state constitutions*, University Press of America, Lanham, MD.
Yanay, U. and Benjamin, S. 2005, 'The role of social workers in disasters: the Jerusalem experience', *International Social Work*, vol. 48, no. 3, pp. 263–76.
Yeatman, A. 1994, *Postmodern Revisionings of the Political*, Routledge, London.
——1998a, 'Introduction', in *Activism and the Policy Process*, ed. A. Yeatman, Allen & Unwin, Sydney.
——1998b, 'Interpreting contemporary contractualism', in *Governing Australia: Studies in the contemporary rationalities of government*, eds M. Dean and B. Hindess, Cambridge University Press, Melbourne.

——2000, 'Social policy and the global economy', in *Contemporary Perspectives on Social Work and the Human Services: Challenges and change*, eds I. O'Connor, P. Smyth and J. Warburton, Pearson Education, Sydney, pp. 60–72.

Yeatman, A. and Penglase, J. 2004, 'Looking After Children: a case of individualised services delivery', *Australian Journal of Social Issues*, no. 393, pp. 233–47.

Yip, K. 2006a, 'Self-ref ection in ref ective practice: a note of caution', *British Journal of Social Work*, vol. 36, pp. 777–88.

——2006b, 'Developing social work students' ref ectivity in cultural indigenisation of mental health practice', *Reflective Practice*, vol. 7, no. 3, pp. 393–408.

Young, I.M. 1997, *Intersecting Voices, Dilemmas of Gender, Political Philosophy, and Policy*, Princeton University Press, Princeton, NJ.

Young, M. and Guenther, J. 2008, 'The shape of Aboriginal learning and work opportunities in desert regions', *Rangeland Journal*, no. 30, pp. 177–86.

Young, S. 2004, 'Social work theory and practice: the invisibility of whiteness', in *Whitening Race*, ed. A. Moreton-Robinson, Aboriginal Studies Press, Canberra.

Yurchesyn, K., Keith, A. and Renner, E. 1992, 'Contrasting perspectives on the nature of sexual assault provided by a service for sexual assault victims and the law courts', *Canadian Journal of Behavioural Science*, vol. 24, no. 1, pp. 71–85.

Zifcak, S. 2001, 'Contractualism, democracy and ethics', *Australian Journal of Public Administration*, vol. 60, no. 2, pp. 86–98.

index

For Product Safety Concerns and Information please contact our EU representative GPSR@taylorandfrancis.com Taylor & Francis Verlag GmbH, Kaufingerstraße 24, 80331 München, Germany

Batch number: 10732716

Printed by Printforce, the Netherlands